Psychiatry and Biological Factors

Psychiatry and Biological Factors

Edited by

Edouard Kurstak

Faculty of Medicine
University of Montreal
Montreal, Quebec, Canada

Plenum Medical Book Company • New York and London

Library of Congress Cataloging-in-Publication Data

Psychiatry and biological factors / edited by Edouard Kurstak.
p. cm.
Includes bibliographical references and index.
ISBN-13: 978-1-4684-5813-8 e-ISBN-13: 978-1-4684-5811-4
DOI: 10.1007/978-1-4684-5811-4
1. Mental illness--Etiology. 2. Mental illness--Physiological aspects. 3. Mental illness--Immunological aspects. 4. Virus diseases--Psychological aspects. 5. Virus diseases--Animal models. 6. Nervous system--Diseases--Animal models. I. Kurstak, Edouard.
[DNLM: 1. Adjuvants, Immunologic. 2. Fatigue Syndrome, Chronic. 3. Mental Disorders--immunology. 4. Schizophrenia--etiology. 5. Schizophrenia--immunology. 6. Virus Diseases--complications. 7. Viruses--pathogenicity. WM 203 P9732]
RC455.4.B5P74 1991
616.89'071--dc20
DNLM/DLC
for Library of Congress 91-3750
CIP

ISBN-13: 978-1-4684-5813-8

Softcover reprint of the hardcover 1st edition 1991
233 Spring Street, New York, N.Y. 10013

Plenum Medical Book Company is an imprint of Plenum Publishing Corporation

Contributors

Jay D. Amsterdam
Depression Research Unit
Department of Psychiatry
University of Pennsylvania School of Medicine
Philadelphia, Pennsylvania 19104
and
The Wistar Institute
Philadelphia, Pennsylvania 19104

Björn Appelberg
Department of Psychiatry
University of Helsinki
SF-00180 Helsinki, Finland

P. Babál
Department of Pathology
Medical Faculty
Bratislava, Czechoslovakia

Melvyn J. Ball
Departments of Pathology, Clinical Neurological Sciences, and Psychiatry
University of Western Ontario
London, Ontario N6A 5C1, Canada

Christopher E. Barr
Department of Psychology
University of Southern California
Los Angeles, California 90089-1111

Daniel Becker
Department of Psychiatry
Chaim Sheba Medical Center
Tel-Aviv University
Sackler School of Medicine
Tel-Hashomer 52621, Israel

D. Ben-Nathan
Department of Virology
Israel Institute for Biological Research
Ness-Ziona, Israel

Ann E. Bowler
Twin Studies Unit
NIMH Neurosciences Center
St. Elizabeths Hospital
Washington, D.C. 20032

Susanna Brambilla
Institute of Clinical Psychiatry
University of Milan
20122 Milan, Italy

Robert W. Buchanan
Maryland Psychiatric Research Center
Department of Psychiatry
University of Maryland School of Medicine
Baltimore, Maryland 21228

Kari Cantell
National Public Health Institute
Helsinki, Finland

Domenico Caputo
Multiple Sclerosis University Center "Don C. Gnocchi"
20148 Milan, Italy

William T. Carpenter, Jr.
Maryland Psychiatric Research Center
Department of Psychiatry
University of Maryland School of Medicine
Baltimore, Maryland 21228

Donald R. Carrigan
Department of Pathology
Medical College of Wisconsin
Milwaukee, Wisconsin 53226

Carlo Lorenzo Cazzullo
Institute of Clinical Psychiatry
University of Milan
20122 Milan, Italy

Mark A. Coggiano
Neuropsychiatry Branch
Intramural Research Program
National Institute of Mental Health
Washington, D.C. 20032

Timothy J. Crow
Division of Psychiatry
Clinical Research Centre
Northwick Park Hospital
Harrow, Middlesex, HA1 3UJ
United Kingdom

Anne M. Deatly
Department of Microbiology
Mount Sinai School of Medicine
New York, New York 10029

Anita Feenstra
Neuropsychiatry Branch
Intramural Research Program
National Institute of Mental Health
Washington, D.C. 20032
Present address:
Zentrum für Molekulare Biologie Heidelberg
D-6900 Heidelberg, Federal Republic of Germany

Pasquale Ferrante
Multiple Sclerosis University Center "Don C. Gnocchi"
20148 Milan, Italy

G. Feuerstein
Department of Neurology
USUHS
Bethesda, Maryland 20814

Bernhard Fleckenstein
Institute of Clinical Virology
University of Erlangen–Nuremberg
Erlangen, Federal Republic of Germany

Susy Floru
Department of Psychiatry
Chaim Sheba Medical Center
Tel-Aviv University
Sackler School of Medicine
Tel-Hashomer 52621, Israel

M. M. Garayev
Biotechnology Laboratory of the Ivanovsky Virology Institute
USSR Academy of Medical Sciences
123098 Moscow, USSR

Kavita Goel
Department of Psychiatry
University of Michigan Medical Center
Ann Arbor, Michigan 48109

Joann Goodson
Department of Psychiatry
University of Michigan Medical Center
Ann Arbor, Michigan 48109

Tamar Gotlieb-Stematsky
The Central Virology Laboratory
Chaim Sheba Medical Center
Tel-Aviv University
Sackler School of Medicine
Tel-Hashomer 52621, Israel

John F. Greden
Department of Psychiatry, the Alcohol Research Center, and Midwest AIDS Biobehavioral Research Center,
University of Michigan
Ann Arbor, Michigan 48109

Ashley T. Haase
Department of Microbiology
University of Minnesota
Minneapolis, Minnesota 55455

Edgar P. Heimer
Hoffman–LaRoche, Inc.
Nutley, New Jersey 07110

P. M. Hoffman
Veterans Administration Medical Center
Baltimore, Maryland 21218

J. Daniel House
Department of Psychiatry
University of Michigan Medical Center
Ann Arbor, Michigan 48109
and
Northern Illinois University
DeKalb, Illinois 60115

N. G. Ignatova
N. F. Gamaleya Institute of Epidemiology and Microbiology of the USSR Academy of Medical Sciences
123098 Moscow, USSR

A. Ivanushkin
All Union Mental Health Research Center of the USSR Academy of Medical Sciences
113152 Moscow, USSR

I. U. Karas
Immunobiology Laboratory of the Mental Health Research Institute
Tomsk Scientific Center of the USSR Academy of Medical Sciences
634014 Tomsk-14, USSR

Heikki Katila
Department of Psychiatry
University of Helsinki
SF-00180 Helsinki, Finland

Darrell G. Kirch
Neuropsychiatry Branch
Intramural Research Program
National Institute of Mental Health
Washington, D.C. 20032

G. Kolyaskina
All Union Mental Health Research Center of the USSR Academy of Medical Sciences
113152 Moscow, USSR

J. Krajčík
Regional Psychiatry Hospital
Pezinok, Czechoslovakia

Eli Kritschmann
Department of Psychiatry
Chaim Sheba Medical Center
Tel-Aviv University
Sackler School of Medicine
Tel-Hashomer 52621, Israel

Ziad A. Kronfol
Department of Psychiatry
University of Michigan Medical Center
Ann Arbor, Michigan 48109

M. Kúdelová
Institute of Virology
Slovak Academy of Sciences
Bratislava, Czechoslovakia

G. V. Logvinovich
Clinics of the Mental Health Research Institute
Tomsk Scientific Center of the USSR Academy of Medical Sciences
634014 Tomsk-14, USSR

S. Lustig
Department of Virology
Israel Institute for Biological Research
Ness-Ziona, Israel

Greg Maislin
Depression Research Unit
Department of Psychiatry
University of Pennsylvania School of Medicine
Philadelphia, Pennsylvania 19104

Roberta Mancuso
Multiple Sclerosis University Center "Don C. Gnocchi"
20148 Milan, Italy

J. L. Martin
Veterans Administration Medical Center
Baltimore, Maryland 21218

D. Martišová
Regional Psychiatry Hospital
Pezinok, Czechoslovakia

Cinzia Masserini
Institute of Clinical Psychiatry
University of Milan
20122 Milan, Italy

Sarnoff A. Mednick
Department of Psychology
University of Southern California
Los Angeles, California 90089-1111

T. Micheeva
All Union Mental Health Research Center of the USSR Academy of Medical Sciences
113152 Moscow, USSR

Hans W. Moises
Department of Genetics
Stanford University School of Medicine
Stanford, California 94305
Present address:
Department of Psychiatry
Kiel University Hospital
D-2300 Kiel 1, Federal Republic of Germany

P. Morozov
All Union Mental Health Research Center of the USSR Academy of Medical Sciences
113152 Moscow, USSR

V. Mucha
Institute of Virology
Slovak Academy of Sciences
Bratislava, Czechoslovakia

M. Murányiová
Mental Research Laboratory
Institute of Medical Bionics
Bratislava, Czechoslovakia

N. N. Naidyonova
Immunobiology Laboratory of the Mental Health Research Institute
Tomsk Scientific Center of the USSR Academy of Medical Sciences
634014 Tomsk-14, USSR

Madhavan P. N. Nair
Departments of Psychiatry, Pediatrics, and Epidemiology
University of Michigan Medical Center
Ann Arbor, Michigan 48109

N. B. Nefedova
N. F. Gamaleya Institute of Epidemiology and Microbiology of the USSR Academy of Medical Sciences
123098 Moscow, USSR

T. I. Nevidimova
Immunobiology Laboratory of the Mental Health Research Institute
Tomsk Scientific Center of the USSR Academy of Medical Sciences
634014 Tomsk-14, USSR

Heikki Nikkilä
Department of Psychiatry
University of Helsinki
SF-00180 Helsinki, Finland

W. P. Paré
Veterans Administration Medical Center
Perry Point, Maryland 21902

J. Pogády
Mental Research Laboratory
Institute of Medical Bionics
Bratislava, Czechoslovakia
and
Regional Psychiatry Hospital
Pezinok, Czechoslovakia

Raveendran Pottathil
Hoffman–LaRoche, Inc.
Nutley, New Jersey 07110

J. Rajčáni
Institute of Virology
Slovak Academy of Sciences
Bratislava, Czechoslovakia
and
Regional Psychiatry Hospital
Pezinok, Czechoslovakia

Suraiya Rasheed
Laboratory of Viral Oncology and AIDS Research
University of Southern California
Los Angeles, California 90032-3626

Robert Rawlings
Division of Biometry and Epidemiology
National Institute on Alcohol Abuse and Alcoholism
Rockville, Maryland 20857

Gavin P. Reynolds
Department of Pathology
University of Nottingham Medical School
Nottingham, United Kingdom

Ranan Rimón
Department of Psychiatry
University of Helsinki
SF-00180 Helsinki, Finland

D. S. Robbins
Veterans Administration Medical Center
Baltimore, Maryland 21218

Rüdiger Rüger
Institute of Clinical Virology
University of Erlangen–Nuremberg
Erlangen, Federal Republic of Germany
Present address:
Boehringer Mannheim
Department of Genetics
Penzberg, Federal Republic of Germany

A. A. Rzhaninova
D. I. Ivanovsky Institute of Virology of the USSR Academy of Medical Sciences
123098 Moscow, USSR

Emilio Sacchetti
Institute of Clinical Psychiatry
University of Milan
20122 Milan, Italy

Stanley A. Schwartz
Departments of Pediatrics and Epidemiology
University of Michigan Medical Center
Ann Arbor, Michigan 48109

T. Sekirina
All Union Mental Health Research Center of the USSR Academy of Medical Sciences
113152 Moscow, USSR

V. Y. Semke
Clinics of the Mental Health Research Institute
Tomsk Scientific Center of the USSR Academy of Medical Sciences
634014 Tomsk-14, USSR

M. Shchurin
All Union Mental Health Research Center of the USSR Academy of Medical Sciences
113152 Moscow, USSR

A. M. Shevchenko
The Chair of Childhood Neuropathology of the Bielorussian State Institute for Advanced Medical Training
220714 Minsk, USSR

Yaffa Shlomo-David
The Central Virology Laboratory
Chaim Sheba Medical Center
Tel-Aviv University
Sackler School of Medicine
Tel-Hashomer 52621, Israel

Y. Y. Tentsov
D. I. Ivanovsky Institute of Virology of the USSR Academy of Medical Sciences
123098 Moscow, USSR

E. Fuller Torrey
Twin Studies Unit
NIMH Neurosciences Center
St. Elizabeths Hospital
Washington, D.C. 20032

M. Tsutsulkovskaya
All Union Mental Health Research Center of the USSR Academy of Medical Sciences
113152 Moscow, USSR

Carlo Ezio Vaccari
Multiple Sclerosis University Center "Don C. Gnocchi"
20148 Milan, Italy

O. A. Vasiljeva
Immunobiology Laboratory of the Mental Health Research Institute
Tomsk Scientific Center of the USSR Academy of Medical Sciences
634014 Tomsk-14, USSR

T. P. Vetlugina
Immunobiology Laboratory of the Mental Health Research Institute
Tomsk Scientific Center of the USSR Academy of Medical Sciences
634014 Tomsk-14, USSR

Antonio Vita
Institute of Clinical Psychiatry
University of Milan
20122 Milan, Italy

T. Voronkova
All Union Mental Health Research Center of the USSR Academy of Medical Sciences
113152 Moscow, USSR

Royce W. Waltrip II
Maryland Psychiatric Research Center
Department of Psychiatry
University of Maryland School of Medicine
Baltimore, Maryland 21228

Simon Wessely
Department of Psychological Medicine
Institute of Psychiatry
Camberwell, London SE5 8AF
United Kingdom

Richard Jed Wyatt
Neuropsychiatry Branch
Intramural Research Program
National Institute of Mental Health
Washington, D.C. 20032

A. I. Zhankov
Immunobiology Laboratory of the Mental Health Research Institute
Tomsk Scientific Center of the USSR Academy of Medical Sciences
634014 Tomsk-14, USSR

V. A. Zuev
N. F. Gamaleya Institute of Epidemiology and Microbiology of the USSR Academy of Medical Sciences
123098 Moscow, USSR

Preface

The main purpose of the volume *Psychiatry and Biological Factors* is to provide a comprehensive, state-of-the-art overview of the current research linked essentially to virus infections, immunity functions, and mental diseases.

In recent years substantial advances have been registered in the physiopathology of mental and neurological disorders. As a result, partial control of certain psychoses, anxiety syndromes, epilepsy, and Parkinson's disease is now possible. However, despite progress in biomedical research, numerous mental and neurological disorders afflict up to 15% of all individuals and little is known about the causes, prevention, and treatment of these diseases.

Several epidemiological investigations demonstrated a high prevalence of functional psychoses and organic mental disorders, and recent data show that biological components appear as a major etiologic factor. In this respect it could be stressed that viral and immunologic hypotheses should be investigated seriously and systematically in relation to the mechanisms of several mental and neurological diseases.

Neuropsychiatric consequences of AIDS related to human immunodeficiency virus infection are now well documented. A variety of behavioral symptoms and psychiatric syndromes with paranoid features are frequent concomitants of AIDS. Other retroviruses are associated with neurological disorders and behavioral symptoms, like HTLV-1, the etiologic factor of tropical spastic paraparesis. It is known that chronic Epstein-Barr virus infection and the resulting infectious mononucleosis are associated with cerebral dysfunction and depression and that after measles or recurrent herpes simplex virus infections, a residual mental disorder occurs. Human cytomegalovirus (CMV) antigen replication was found in the brain of schizophrenic patients. The latent viral infections within CNS could be found in a substantial part of the human population. Periodic reactivation of such infections could lead to CNS dysfunction and behavioral alterations. Also, prenatal viral infection, e.g., by the influenza virus, is postulated to be an etiologic agent of adult schizophrenia. The schizophrenia viral etiology hypothesis is still attractive, and numerous investigators continue to formulate conceptual virus-associated immunopathological theories of schizophrenia.

There are exciting research data on unconventional pathogenic viruses or amyloid agents in the transmissible dementias and other disorders found in the brains of patients with kuru and Creutzfeldt-Jakob disease.

Immune abnormalities and dysfunctions among patients with psychiatric problems were noted by several investigators. In 20% of chronic psychiatric patients hospitalized, antinuclear antibodies were found at a high level and antibodies to brain tissue in sera from schizophrenic patients were reported, as was the evidence of lymphocyte abnormality. Other dysfunctions like decreased macrophage functioning and decreased natural killer cell activity were also noted.

The action of immunomodulators, like interferon, in schizophrenic patients and the linkage of depression to altered immune function are interesting observations. Reported effects of interferon and other immunomodulators when used as a therapeutic modality indicated some relief of symptoms in schizophrenic patients. However, interferon possesses a wide range of biological activities, including neurotoxin function. Focal induction of interferon during viral infections, especially in cases of encephalitis, could lead to its interaction within the CNS and to neurologic disorders. The high production of interferon in the brains of patients infected with the rabies virus was suggested to be responsible for severe psychotic disorders observed shortly before death. In fact, the neurotoxicity of interferon, which production level is also high in AIDS patients, schizophrenic patients, and viral encephalitis cases, opens new avenues for research on the role of immunomodulators in the etiology of mental diseases.

For these reasons I organized two international conferences on these subjects. The volume *Psychiatry and Biological Factors* is one of the results of the recent meeting held in Montreal, Canada, which was well attended by psychiatrists, virologists, immunologists, neurologists, and geneticists.

This volume is divided into five major parts: I—Mental Pathology and Virogene Theory; II—Virological and Immunological Study of Schizophrenia; III—Immunomodulators and Psychiatric Disorders; IV—Viral Fatigue Syndrome and Antivirals; and V—Animal Models in Virus Neuropathology.

In the 26 well-documented chapters the recognized experts in their fields present the latest fundamental and clinical research data, overviews, and hypotheses related to psychiatry and to the role of biological factors in the etiology of mental diseases. One of the great advantages of this volume is its multidisciplinary approach towards biological psychiatry.

I wish to express my sincere thanks to each contributor for a thoughtful treatment of his subject and for providing unpublished data. Special thanks go to Dr. Peter V. Morozov, Program Director at All Union Mental Health Research

Center, Moscow, USSR, and to Dr. Norman Sartorius, Director of the Division of Mental Health of the World Health Organization, Geneva, Switzerland, who co-chaired with me the Montreal Conference, as well as to the Mérieux Foundation, the Department of Health and Welfare, and the Medical Research Council of Canada. Its President, Dr. Pierre Bois, from the beginning encouraged investigators in biological psychiatry, and his support and encouragement are highly appreciated.

My thanks and gratitude are also addressed to the staff of Plenum Publishing Corporation for their part in the production of *Psychiatry and Biological Factors*.

Edouard Kurstak

Montreal, Canada

Contents

Introduction

Edouard Kurstak

Numerous mental and neurological disorders in recent years have been linked to biologic factors, and in this respect extensive research has been directed toward viral infections and immune dysfunction.

Psychiatric patients reveal disturbances in the highest integrative functions of the neurons of the brain caused by bacterial or viral infections in the body of the neuron, its axon, dendrites, or associated cells. A viral hypothesis for schizophrenia and other mental diseases, initially suggested, has now been reinforced by recent findings of the neuropathologic effects of persistent and defective viruses. The viral hypothesis of mental disorders should essentially be in accordance with the following basic principles for pathology and epidemiology of viral diseases in general: (1) the virus involved may cause several different forms of clinical disease varying from inapparent or abortive immunizing infection to various localized or systemic, acute, chronic, or slow, benign, severe, or fatal disease, (2) one type of clinical infection—encephalitis, meningitis, pneumonia or upper respiratory, or gastrointestinal diseases—may be caused by viruses of different taxa as well as different chemical structure or virion size or shape, (3) schizophrenia or other mental disorders show markedly variable symptoms and clinical causes. Should a virus be involved in the pathogenesis, according to Libikova (1983) the following postulates would seem logical:

1. The putative virus involved interacts with other markers—human leukocyte antigens (HLA), endocrine and enzymatic factors, and neuropathologic anomalies.

Edouard Kurstak • *Department of Microbiology and Immunology, Faculty of Medicine, University of Montreal, Montreal, Quebec, Canada H3C 3J7.*

2. Each of these factors may itself be altered before or as a consequence of viral infection.
3. Various biologically and epidemiologically suitable viruses rather than one virus have a hypothetical chance of being involved in schizophrenia or other mental disorder.
4. That more than one agent may persist in any individual cannot be excluded. Furthermore, another problem in psychovirology could emerge if unconventional scrapie-like agents were considered to be the cause not only of kuru or Creutzfeld-Jakob disease but also of the discrete infections of humans.

It is known that retroviruses can be associated with pathologic processes in a host species which frequently involve the nervous system. Veterinary clinicians for decades linked the ovine visna/maedi encephalitis to a retrovirus (Sigurdsson, 1954) and medical clinicians isolated retroviruses (HTLV-1) from patients with neurologic diseases, namely tropical spastic paraparesis or myelopathy (Gessain *et al.*, 1985; Osame *et al.*, 1987; Kayembe *et al.*, 1990). The observations that these diseases are associated with retroviruses, that the source of infection is breast milk, semen, or blood transfusion, and that the virus genome is integrated into the host genome (Bhagavati *et al.*, 1988) are one of the most significant advances in neurologic sciences in the last five years.

Recent epidemiologic data are regarded as supportive of the viral etiology of schizophrenia but results obtained have been rather inconsistent and do not seem to implicate any particular virus with a significant role in this disease. However, Crow (1987) suggested that a retrovirus that exists within the CNS in the form of viral DNA integrated into the cellular genome near the cerebral dominance gene or pseudoautosomal region of the sex chromosome is responsible for schizophrenia.

Typhus and typhoid fever, influenza and malaria, cholera and tuberculosis, meningitis and epidemic encephalitis—all capable of provoking a schizophrenialike syndrome—have been implicated in the causation of mental disorders but despite numerous attempts no clear-cut etiologic relationship is obvious.

From a theoretical point of view, the pathogenesis of mental illness resulting from a viral infection may involve one or more of several possible routes (Lipowski, 1985): (1) the virus may cause local or widespread brain damage or dysfunction and hence elicit one of the organic or mental syndromes such as delirium or dementia, (2) a viral infection may precipitate a reactive psychiatric disorder as a response to a change in mental functioning, somatic perception, or body image, (3) a psychiatric illness, depression for example, resulting from economic and social consequences of having the viral disease, (4) a dreadful viral disease, lethal as well as socially stigmatized such as AIDS, may induce a fear of contracting it (Jenike and Pato, 1986).

Patients with AIDS show a broad range of neuropathologic dysfunctions.

Early clinical neurologic manifestations in human immunodeficiency virus (HIV)-infected individuals include psychomotor dysfunctions, forgetfulness, poor concentration, and hallucination (De la Monte *et al.*, 1987). Some of these symptoms precede the diagnosis of AIDS and may include subacute encephalitis, aseptic meningitis, and peripheral neuropathies. Although several cell types have been shown to serve as reservoirs for dissemination of HIV throughout the body, the predominant cell type in the HIV-infected brain is one of macrophage/monocyte lineage (Koenig *et al.*, 1986) and entry of HIV from cerebrospinal fluid (CSF) to neuronal cells that bear CD4-like receptors may also be facilitated by receptor-mediated endocytosis of HIV particles in complex to antibodies, nonspecific phagocytosis of the virus, or entry via a non-CD4 or Fc-like receptor (Homsy *et al.*, 1989). Intrathecal HIV antibodies may bind to hormone receptors and inhibit production of specific hormones necessary for normal brain functions.

Recurrent herpesvirus reactivation events may play a role in the degeneration of specific areas of the CNS and may cause a dementia state like Alzheimer's disease. In support of the hypothesis that herpes simplex virus may be associated with Alzheimer's disease, herpesvirus DNA was detected by hybridization analysis in the CNS of normal patients and two patients with chronic psychiatric disorders and neuropathologic changes characteristic of Alzheimer's disease dementia (Sequiera *et al.*, 1979).

The occurrence of psychosis following epidemics of influenza was reportedly noted as early as 1846 (Rorie, 1901) and the possibility that the influenza virus might be acquired early in life and cause schizophrenia-like disease many years later was suggested in the 1980s (Watson *et al.*, 1984; Torrey *et al.*, 1988; Mednick *et al.*, 1988). A conclusion from one of these studies was that there was a "specific relationship" between winter schizophrenic births and prevalence of both pneumonia and influenza. Despite the general failure to link perinatal influenza infections to schizophrenic births, a viral cause for the observed schizophrenic birth seasonality continues to be a reasonable as well as an attractive hypothesis.

In recent years, several studies have examined the relationship between viruses and schizophrenia using isolation techniques, antibody investigations, and molecular biology approaches for the research of viral nucleic acids in the brain or other biological materials from patients (Crow, 1983) and partly discordant results suggested antibody response anomalies to viruses, particularly herpes simplex virus. Evaluation on the basis of the presence or lack of ventricular dilatation and/or cortical atrophy in schizophrenic patients in comparison to a group of healthy controls has been of recent interest. Another approach involves investigation of lymphocyte subsets in drug-free schizophrenic patients (Villemain *et al.*, 1989).

There is now substantial evidence indicating that the CNS and immune system are closely interrelated, and several immune abnormalities such as lymphocytopenia, reduction in circulating T cell numbers, impairment in mitogen-induced lymphocyte proliferation, and decrease in natural killer (NK) cell activity in patients with psychiatric disorders have been identified. Abnormalities in immune regulation in schizophrenia, such as an increase in the number of B lymphocytes, a decrease in NK cell activity, and an increase in the level of specific immunoglobulins and/or specific antibrain antibodies, have also been reported. Cytotoxic immune systems constitute an important part of the host defense mechanisms and provide protection against a variety of pathogens including virus-infected cells, and in addition to NK and cytotoxic T lymphocytes, a new cytotoxic immune system—lymphokine-activated killer (LAK) cytotoxicity—is now known. An impairment in LAK cell activity in psychiatric patients, if confirmed, would provide another example of immune dysregulation in psychiatric illness.

Contradictory findings on a wide spectrum of antibodies to neurotropic viruses paved the way for the search for a nonspecific indicator of viral infection such as interferon (IFN). Raised levels of IFN were demonstrated in some schizophrenic patients (Preble and Torrey, 1985) but not in others (Ahokas *et al.*, 1987).

"Chronic fatigue syndrome" (CFS) has been used in reference to various illnesses such as "myalgic encephalomyelitis" or "Royal Free Disease" in Britain and Australia and "chronic Epstein-Barr virus (EBV) infection" or "chronic mononucleosis" in the United States. The current hypothesis is that a viral illness is a cause of chronic fatigue and reportedly the majority of CFS patients exhibit recognizable psychiatric disorder (Denman, 1990). The viruses that are claimed to be responsible for fatigue are common, with exposure to EBV being nearly universal, but conclusive evidence of a direct link between viruses and chronic fatigue remains elusive. Perhaps the availability of reliable epidemiological data would broaden our understanding of CFS.

Biological factors such as viruses or viral components, immune dysfunctions, immunomodulators, and genetic alterations related to mental disorders are currently being actively investigated in several laboratories worldwide. Since the failure to explain mental disorders on the basis of chemical factors, the importance of biological factors has risen immensely and provides hope for a better understanding of the mechanisms of mental pathologies and, hence, their treatment, prevention, and control. The contents of this volume on Psychiatry and Biological Factors provide an insight into the research efforts presently directed toward achieving this goal.

REFERENCES

Ahokas, A., Ramon, R., Koskiniemi, M., Vaheri, A., Julkunen, I., and Saona, S., 1987, Viral antibodies and interferon in acute psychiatric disorders, *J. Clin. Psychiatry* **48:**194–196.

Bhagavati, S., Ehrlich, G., and Kula R. W., 1988, Detection of human T-cell lymphoma leukemia virus type 1 DNA and antigen in spinal fluid and blood of patients with chronic progressive myelopathy, *N. Engl. J. Med.* **318:**1141–1144.

Crow, T. J., 1983, Is schizophrenia an infectious disease? *Lancet* **1**:173–175.

Crow, T. J., 1987, Genes and viruses in schizophrenia: The retrovirus transposon hypothesis, in: *Viruses, Immunity and Mental Disorders* (E. Kurstak, Z. J. Lipowski, and P. V. Morozov, eds.), Plenum Medical, New York, pp. 125–134.

De la Monte, S. M., Ho, D. D., Scharley, R. T., Hirsch, M. S., and Richardson, E. P., 1987, Subacute encephalomyelitis of AIDS and its reaction to HTLV-III infection, *Neurology* **37**:562–569.

Denman, A. M., 1990, The chronic fatigue syndrome: A return to common sense, *Postgrad. Med. J.* **66**:499–501.

Gessain, A., Barin, F., and Vernant, J. C., 1985, Antibodies to human T-lymphotropic virus type 1 in patients with tropical spastic paraparesis, *Lancet* **2**:407–409.

Homsy, J., Meyer, M., Tatino, M., Clarkson, S. J., and Levi, A., 1989, The Fc and not CD4 receptor mediates antibody enhancement of HIV infection in human cells, *Science* **244**:1357–1360.

Jenike, M. A., and Pato, C., 1986, Disabling fear of AIDS responsive to imipramine, *Psychosomatics* **27**:143–144.

Kayembe, K., Goubau, P., Desmyter, J., Vlietinck, R., and Carton, H., 1990, A cluster of HTLV-1 associated tropical spastic paraparesis in Equateur (Zaire) ethnic and familial distribution, *J. Neurol. and Neurosurg. Psychiatry* **53**:4–10.

Koenig, S., Genselsmon, H. E., and Ovenstein, J. M., 1986, Detection of AIDS virus in macrophages in brain tissue from AIDS patients with encephalopathy, *Science* **207**:1089–1093.

Libikova, H., 1983, Schizophrenia and viruses: Principles and ecologic studies, *Adv. Biol. Psychiatry* **12**:20–51.

Lipowski, Z. J., 1985, *Psychosomatic Medicine and Liaison Psychiatry: Selected Papers*, Plenum Press, New York.

Mednick, S. A., Machon, R. A., and Huttunen, M. O., 1988, Adult schizophrenia following prenatal exposure to an influenza epidemic, *Arch. Gen. Psychiatry* **45**:189–192.

Osame, M., Matsumoto, M., and Usuku, K., 1987, Chronic progressive myelopathy with elevated antibodies to human T lymphotropic virus type 1 and adult T-cell leukemia-like cells, *Ann. Neurol.* **21**:117–120.

Preble, O. T., and Torrey, E. F., 1985, Serum interferon in patient with psychosis, *Am. J. Psychiatry* **142**:184–186.

Rorie, G. A., 1901, Post-influenzal insanity in the Cumberland and Westmoreland asylum, with statistics of sixty-eight cases, *J. Ment. Sci.* **47**:317–326.

Sequiera, L. W., Jennings, L. C., Carasco, L. H., Lord, M., Curry, A., and Sutto, R. N. P., 1979, Detection of herpes simplex virus genome in brain tissue, *Lancet* **2**:608–612.

Sigurdsson, B., 1954, Chronic encephalitis of sheep, with general remarks on infections which develop slowly and some of their special characteristics, *Bri. Vet. J.* **110**:341–352.

Torrey, E. F., Rawlings, R., and Waldman, I. N., 1988, Schizophrenic births and viral diseases in two states, *Schiz. Res.* **1**:73–77.

Villemain, F., Chatenaud, L., Galinowski, A., Homo-Delarche, F., Ginestet, D., Loo, H., Zarifian, E., and Bach, J. F., 1989, Aberrant T-cell mediated immunity in untreated schizophrenic patients. Deficient interleukin-2 production, *Am. J. Psychiatry* **146**:609–615.

Watson, C. G., Kulcala, T., and Tilleskjor, C., 1984, Schizophrenic birth seasonality in relation to the incidence of infectious diseases and temperature extremes, *Arch. Gen. Psychiatry* **41**:85–90.

Part **I**

Mental Pathology and Virogene Theory

Chapter 1

The Virogene Hypothesis of Psychosis

Current Status

Timothy J. Crow

BACKGROUND

The viral hypothesis of psychosis has its origin in the concept that there are major environmental determinants of the onset of psychosis, and in observations that schizophrenic psychoses sometimes occur in relation to infective illness. Thus, on the basis of the psychoses seen in association with the influenza epidemic of 1918, both Menninger (1928) and Goodall (1932) proposed that schizophrenia might be due to a virus. If, as seems probable, these postinfluenzal psychoses were a direct manifestation of infection with the influenza virus, this would demonstrate that schizophrenia-like illnesses can be caused by a viral encephalitis. The major question at issue is whether schizophrenia as it commonly occurs could be due to an as yet unidentified agent, perhaps interacting with a genetic predisposition.

Epidemiological observations are relevant. If there are significant geographical and temporal variations in incidence, this would favor an environmental influence and be consistent with spread within populations. Torrey (1980) in particular has argued that variations in incidence across the world are greater than is often thought, although the findings of the recent WHO catchment area studies

Timothy J. Crow • *Division of Psychiatry, Clinical Research Centre, Northwick Park Hospital, Harrow, Middlesex, HA1 3UJ, United Kingdom.*

(Sartorius *et al.*, 1986) suggest that such variations are not large. Hare (1983) has defended the view that there was a significant rise in incidence in the course of the 19th century. Both Hare and Torrey consider an infective etiology.

A peculiarity of schizophrenia that requires explanation is age of onset. This is uncommon before puberty but then rises rapidly—to a peak in the third decade of life—with a mean age of onset around 25 years for males and 28 years for females. It is tempting to suppose that an environmental factor has something to do with this pattern but the regularities of incidence, including the sex difference, pose some problems for a viral or other environmental theory.

Some laboratory findings have also appeared to support a viral theory. We observed that CSF from patients with psychotic illness and some other forms of neuropsychiatric disease (e.g., Huntington's chorea) induced a cytopathic effect when inoculated into human embryonic fibroblast cultures (Tyrrell *et al.*, 1979). The characteristics of this effect—e.g., abolition by filters of pore size less than 50 nm, sensitivity to lipid solvents, and resistance to DNA synthesis inhibition—initially suggested that the cytopathic effect might be due to a small RNA virus. However, passage was not demonstrated and subsequent work appears to rule out that a replicating virus is involved. Thus, the effect, although replicable, is not abolished by either nucleic acid or protein synthesis inhibition, and is not associated with the synthesis of new proteins or the presence of viruslike particles (Taylor *et al.*, 1987). The nature of the effect remains unclear—it could be that a toxin is associated with a fragment of degenerating tissue—but it now seems unlikely that a virus, or other etiologically significant agent, is responsible.

In two further series of experiments, cytopathic CSF from patients with schizophrenia and other neuropsychiatric disease was injected into the brains of marmosets. In the first series, significant differences in activity between animals injected with cytopathic and control CSF developed several months after the injection although no histopathological differences between the brains of the two groups were observed (Baker *et al.*, 1983). These behavioral changes were not found when the study was repeated (Baker *et al.*, 1989). It was concluded that in these, as in the earlier studies of the cytopathic effect, no firm evidence for the presence of a virus or other transmissible agent had been obtained.

IS THERE A NON-GENETIC FACTOR?

Another approach to the viral hypothesis is to ask whether the epidemiological evidence is consistent with horizontal transmission. Is there any reason to think that the disease is passed from affected to nonaffected (but perhaps genetically predisposed) individuals?

An analysis of data from family studies (Crow, 1983) suggested that some findings (e.g., that pairs of siblings were more likely than would otherwise be expected to be of the same sex) not readily accounted for on a genetic basis might be explained in terms of physical proximity, i.e., horizontal transmission. This hypothesis was later subjected to scrutiny in the existing literature with respect to the question of whether, when illness occurs in pairs of siblings, it occurs at the same age or at the same time (Crow and Done, 1986). Although on first analysis it appeared that onset in the younger sibling is systematically at a younger age—i.e., that the illnesses occur at the same time rather than at the same age—more critical appraisal indicates that this is an artifact that arises from underascertainment of later onsets in younger siblings. When this bias is taken into account, it is clear that onset occurs at the same age and not at the same time. This finding is damaging for any theory (e.g., the "contagion" hypothesis) that invokes an environmental agent with an impact in postnatal life.

If onset of illness is genetically programmed, this suggests that the disease is determined by genetic factors to a greater extent than is often thought. Two further considerations support this conclusion. First, adoption away from a family that includes members with the disease does not reduce risk (Karlsson, 1970). Second, the relative constancy of incidence across countries with widely differing social, geographical, and industrial environments, as demonstrated in the recent WHO studies (Sartorius *et al.*, 1986), suggests that rates of illness are relatively independent of any obvious environmental variable. It may be that the origins of psychosis are to be sought in the human genome rather than in the environment. If this is true, it seems that the only viable form of the viral hypothesis is that the disease is due to a "virogene," i.e., a sequence (e.g., a retrovirus or other type of mobile element) that forms part of the human genome (Crow, 1984, 1988b).

CLUES TO THE NATURE AND LOCATION OF THE PSYCHOSIS GENE

A degree of enlargement of the lateral ventricle was first demonstrated by computerized tomography (CT) by Johnstone *et al.* (1976), but earlier suggested by air encephalography (e.g., by Haug, 1962). The finding is now generally accepted in schizophrenia, particularly in studies that have included patients with chronic and deteriorating forms of illness. The meaning of these changes, in particular at what stage of the disease they occur, i.e., whether they precede the onset of illness or progress during its course, has been unclear. One suggestion has been that they are a result of physical treatments; this is ruled out by observations that they are as marked in patients without such treatments as in those who have had substantial amounts (Johnstone *et al.*, 1976; Weinberger *et al.*, 1979) even when the groups are carefully matched for other relevant variables (Owens *et al.*, 1985).

In a recent CT study (Johnstone *et al.*, 1989), three structural changes were detected (see Table 1).

Lateral and third ventricular enlargement have been noted in a number of

Table 1. Schizophrenic (n = 127) versus Nonschizophrenic Psychiatric Patients (n = 45)

VBR	Increased by 10%	$p < 0.05$
Third ventricular area	Increased by 16%	$p < 0.05$
Brain area	Decreased by 3%	$p < 0.01$

studies. In this investigation we found that various indices of ventricular enlargement were intercorrelated—there was no clear indication that there were independently varying components. A reduction in brain area has not previously been emphasized. Although the magnitude of the change was relatively small, it was significant at the 1% level. While ventricular enlargement might well be regarded as a consequence of degeneration, a reduction in brain area (unless the loss of brain substance was very large) is less likely. Such reduction is more readily explained as a failure of development. In support of this view we found that while in the schizophrenic patient group as a whole there were few significant relationships between structural change and psychological impairments, such correlations were present in the subgroup with age of onset below the mean (25 years for males and 28 years for females), and when present the correlations were with brain area rather than ventricular size. The findings suggest that relationships between brain structure and cognitive function are established early in the course of the illness: they are compatible with the notion that the disease is an anomaly of development rather than a degenerative process caused by an exogenous pathogen.

In these chronic patients we found that when other relevant variables (e.g., age and duration of illness) were controlled, age of onset predicted a number of aspects of outcome. Thus, patients who were first admitted to hospital at an age below the mode for the group as a whole were more likely than those who were first admitted at a later age to show negative symptoms, intellectual impairment (e.g., age disorientation), and behavioral deterioration. On this basis it might be expected that age of onset would be a determinant of the structural changes. Surprisingly we found that the three measures (lateral and third ventricular area and brain area) that distinguished patients with schizophrenia from other subjects did not separate patients with early from those with late age of onset. However, a further structural index—the difference between the widths of the two sides of the brain in the posterior segments—did distinguish these groups. Patients with early onset had significant ($p < 0.01$) reductions in the relative width of the left hemisphere in measures taken in the occipital and temporal regions (Crow *et al.*, 1989c). It seemed that early onset had arrested the development of the normal asymmetries in the posterior part of the brain.

The nature of the brain changes and their location are further elucidated by two recent postmortem studies. The first study (Brown *et al.*, 1986) compared patients with schizophrenia with those with affective disorder who had died in the same institution. Brains were excluded from both groups if there was identifiable microscopic pathology (e.g., Alzheimer-type change or vascular disease). Brain structures were assessed on a photograph of a coronal brain section at the level of the interventricular foramina. The main findings were that when age, sex, and year of birth were controlled, (1) brain weight was reduced (by 5 to 6%) in the patients with schizophrenia, (2) lateral ventricular area was modestly (by 15%) but not significantly increased, (3) temporal horn area was significantly ($p < 0.01$) increased, the relative increase being over 80%, and (4) the width of the parahippocampal gyrus was reduced ($p < 0.01$). Reduction of parahippocampal gyrus width was reported in another recent postmortem study (Bogerts *et al.*, 1985). Of particular interest in our study (Brown *et al.*, 1986) was a diagnosis by side interaction, the differences between the groups being significantly ($p < 0.02$) greater on the left side.

The second postmortem study (Crow *et al.*, 1988, 1989a) further emphasizes the relevance of asymmetry. Brains of patients with schizophrenia were compared with age-matched controls. The components of the lateral ventricle were assessed on X-ray images following infusion of radiopaque medium into the ventricular spaces after formalin fixation. The posterior and particularly the temporal horn of the lateral ventricle was increased in patients with schizophrenia, in the latter case by a factor of 80% relative to the control group. In cases of Alzheimer-type dementia studied at the same time, ventricular enlargement was more generalized affecting the anterior horns and body as well as the temporal and posterior horns of the ventricle. The changes in schizophrenia therefore are most marked in the temporal lobe. Of particular interest was the finding that the change in schizophrenia was selective to the left side of the brain (ANOVA $p < 0.001$), while in the Alzheimer cases there was no such lateralization. Selectivity for the left side was present in both males and females and was unaffected by inclusion or exclusion of brains in which histopathological changes could be detected.

The question raised by these findings is whether laterality of change relates to the disease process or to the normal asymmetries in the human brain, i.e., do they indicate that the disease process itself is lateralized or do they reflect an interaction between a bilateral process and normal anatomical and chemical asymmetries? The findings of the second postmortem study (Crow *et al.*, 1989a) answer this question. Temporal horn enlargement is present in Alzheimer-type dementia but it is not lateralized; when present in schizophrenia it is selective to the left hemisphere. The findings rather strongly support the view that the disease process in schizophrenia is in some way associated with the mechanisms that determine the asymmetries in the human brain.

That there are such asymmetries has been known since the work of Dax (1865) and Broca (1861) on aphasia in the last century. In recent years the anatomical basis has been much clarified by the work of Geschwind and colleagues. They found that in most people, particularly right-handers, the lateral sulcus extends back further on the left than on the right side of the brain (Geschwind and Levitsky, 1968). This is because there are structures in the left temporal lobe, for example including the planum temporale, that forms part of the superior temporal gyrus, that are larger on the left than on the right. These encompass those areas of association cortex, including Wernicke's area, that are responsible for speech and communication.

There must be a gene or genes that determine these developments, and these genes are among those that particularly distinguish man from other primates. The cerebral dominance gene or right shift factor is known from the studies of Annett (1985), McManus (1985), and others on handedness. It is transmitted as an autosomal dominant, although its location is unknown. Thirty thousand genes are said to be expressed in the brain. Of these the cerebral dominance gene seems the best candidate for the psychosis gene that we now have.

A PSEUDOAUTOSOMAL LOCUS FOR THE PSYCHOSIS GENE?

The concept that there is a continuum of psychosis that extends from unipolar and bipolar affective illness through schizoaffective psychosis to schizophrenia without and then with a defect state (Crow, 1986) is consistent with the findings of some recent family studies (e.g., Angst *et al.*, 1983; Angst and Scharfetter, 1989, 1990; Gershon *et al.*, 1982, 1988). Such a concept implies that there is a single locus at which genetic variation occurs, and that this variation accounts for the different forms of psychosis. This concept is challenged by the observation that affective disorders at least are transmitted in a manner that sometimes appears sex-linked and sometimes autosomal (Leader, 1987). Such heterogeneity appears contrary to the continuum hypothesis: the only possible resolution of the contradiction being that the locus is pseudoautosomal (Crow, 1987, 1988a).

The pseudoautosomal region is that region of the short arms of the X and Y chromosomes within which recombination occurs in male meiosis (Burgoyne, 1986). Within this region there is strict homology of genes on the two sex chromosomes although outside it there is divergence. Because a single obligatory crossover occurs within the region in male meiosis, there is a high rate of recombination relative to other parts of the genome. Another peculiarity is that the region is not subject to inactivation in the female.

A pseudoautosomal locus for psychosis could account for the tendency [first noted by Mott (1911), and later by Penrose (1942) and Rosenthal (1962)] for pairs of relatives to be more often than would be expected of the same sex. With a pseudoautosomal locus, same sex concordance arises because when the gene is transmitted from a father it is passed either on the X chromosome to daughters or on the Y chromosome to sons. Because there is a gradient of sex linkage within the region (a single obligatory crossover occurs in each male meiosis) the size of the effect gives an indication of the location of the gene—the effect being maximal with a gene at the centromeric limit and absent with a gene at the telomere.

The prediction that concordance by sex is related to paternal inheritance has been tested in a series of 120 pairs of siblings with schizophrenia collected with the help of the National Alliance for the Mentally Ill in the United States and at a District General Hospital in North West London (Crow *et al.*, 1989b). When parental derivation was determined by a "hierarchical" system (i.e., one according to which schizophrenia in the parent or parental relative takes precedence over psychosis NOS (not otherwise specified) and this takes precedence over a diagnosis of affective disorder), an excess of same sex pairs was observed in the paternally but not in the maternally derived sibships (Table 2). A similar excess was seen when parental derivation was determined by two other methods—classification by presence of any psychiatric illness on one but not the other side, and classification by the nearest relative to be affected by such illness.

The excess of same sex cases in paternally derived pairs is also seen when concordance is assessed pairwise (i.e., including information from sibships with more than two affected members) rather than sibshipwise. Further evidence for a pseudoautosomal locus is available from a molecular study with a telomeric probe (Collinge *et al.*, 1989a, 1991).

A locus for psychosis within the pseudoautosomal region provides an explanation for the more than twofold excess of cases of sex chromosome aneuploidy (XXY, XXX, and possibly XYY) seen in populations of patients with psychosis (Forssman, 1970; DeLisi *et al.*, 1988; Crow, 1988a). Indeed it can be argued that the finding of this excess is in itself evidence for a pseudoautosomal location of the psychosis gene. If the gene were located elsewhere on the X chromosome, according to the rule that whatever the number of X chromosomes an individual may possess all but one are inactivated, no excess of cases would be expected in the XXX and XXY syndromes. However, the pseudoautosomal region is not subject to

Table 2. Concordance by Sex in Sibships with Schizophrenia Classified by a "Hierarchical" System of Assessing Family History[a]

	Paternal	Maternal	Both	Neither	Totals
Same sex	17	12	11	23	63
Mixed sex	7	23	6	21	57
	0.008*				

[a]From Crow *et al.* (1989b).
*Fisher's exact *p* (two-tailed).

inactivation. Therefore, one must consider either the possibility that the genetic mechanism underlying psychosis in sex chromosomal anomalies is unrelated to schizophrenia in general, or the possibility of a pseudoautosomal locus.

LOCATION OF THE CEREBRAL DOMINANCE GENE

If psychosis is a disorder of the cerebral dominance gene, and the psychosis locus is in the pseudoautosomal region, it follows that the cerebral dominance gene should be located within the pseudoautosomal region. There is evidence that this is the case (Crow, 1989) from the studies of the neuropsychology of Turner's and Klinefelter's syndromes that have been conducted by Netley and Rovet (1982, 1987) (see Table 3).

Turner's syndrome cases lack an X chromosome and Klinefelter's have an extra X. Netley and Rovet found that on IQ tests they have reciprocal deficits—in Turner's there is a performance deficit (Netley and Rovet, 1982), and in Klinefelter's a verbal deficit (Netley and Rovet, 1987). The obvious interpretation is that in Turner's there is a right hemisphere deficit and in Klinefelter's a left hemisphere deficit. Thus, some factor which is located on the X chromosome is responsible for the relative development of the two hemispheres. However, because in normal females one X chromosome is inactivated, the abnormalities in Turner's syndrome are attributable to those parts of the X that are not inactivated. These include particularly the pseudoautosomal region. Therefore, this suggests that the cerebral dominance gene is in the same part of the genome as the putative psychosis locus.

NATURE OF THE VIROGENE

According to the virogene hypothesis, the psychosis gene is an element with a degree of potential autonomy. That is to say, it is a genomic component with the capacity to replicate in defiance of normal regulatory controls and thus to disrupt cellular function. Animal models of disease caused by such mechanisms are

Table 3. Neuropsychological Performance of Individuals with Turner's (XO) and Klinefelter's (XXY)[a]

	Chromosomes	*n*	Verbal IQ	Performance IQ
Turner's syndrome	XO	35	100	88
Klinefelter's syndrome	XXY	24	83	100

[a]Note: in a collated sample of XXX girls, a verbal–performance discrepancy similar to, but of lesser magnitude than, that in XXY males was seen (adapted from Netley and Rovet, 1982, 1987).

available; for example, mammary tumors and leukemia in the mouse can both be caused by endogenous retroviruses that are inherited in a Mendelian manner (Teich, 1982). A type of motor neuron disease also is described that is caused by an interaction between an endogenous retrovirus and lactate dehydrogenase virus (Murphy *et al.*, 1983). Besides demonstrating that disease can be caused by viral sequences that are part of the host genome, these animal models have two features that are of relevance to the psychoses: (1) the viruses are expressed in a tissue-specific manner, and (2) the diseases that they cause are manifest at a particular point in the life span of the host. In two further respects, however, these diseases do not mirror the psychoses: (1) transmission conforms closely to a Mendelian dominant pattern, whereas in the psychoses the mode of transmission is uncertain, and (2) only certain mouse strains are affected, while psychotic illness is widely distributed in the human species.

A number of mobile elements have been described in the human genome; these include retroviral sequences, short- and long-interspersed nuclear elements (SINEs and LINEs), and transposons apparently specific to man (Paulson *et al.*, 1985). A feature of the virogene hypothesis is that by postulating an interaction between an endogenous viral sequence and a growth factor (or proto-oncogene) it provides a possible explanation for selectivity to the left hemisphere. Proto-oncogene/transposon interactions are described for some mobile elements (e.g., Katzir *et al.*, 1985). Of particular interest are the sequences which give rise to intracisternal A-type particles (Kuff *et al.*, 1983). These have homologies with retroviruses and are sometimes expressed, e.g., in the embryo, as intracellular viruslike particles; they may play a role in development. Such an element might have both a normal regulatory role and a capacity for uncontrolled replication.

There is already a case that one form of neuropsychiatric disease is caused by a virogene. The Gerstmann–Straussler syndrome is a dementing illness that is inherited as an autosomal dominant. The disease can be transmitted to the marmoset by intracerebral inoculation of brain material (Baker *et al.*, 1985); it appears to be an inherited form of Creutzfeldt-Jakob disease. On the basis of the findings in these families, we have argued that the agent arises not from the environment but from the human genome (Baker *et al.*, 1985). In recent studies we have shown that affected family members have mutations [in some families an insertion (Owen *et al.*, 1989, 1990; Collinge *et al.*, 1989b) and in other families a single base change (Hsiao *et al.*, 1989)] in the prion gene, the single-copy gene on chromosome 20 that codes for a normal membrane protein and also for the amyloid material that accumulates in the brains of affected individuals in this and other transmissible encephalopathies. This protein is closely associated with infectivity and is probably a component of the transmissible agent. These mutations thus render pathogenic and transmissible a structure which originates in the host genome. Thus, we have a disease that is caused by an agent that at least in part is coded by the human genome, and variations in host gene sequence are related to the form of the disease that it can induce.

CONCLUSIONS

That schizophrenia might be caused by a virus was first suggested by the phenomenology of the psychoses associated with the influenza epidemic of 1918. However, a number of observations stand against the view that there are major environmental contributions to the etiology of schizophrenia: (1) the disease occurs across the world in populations exposed to widely differing industrial, geographical, and social environments; (2)adoption away from a family that includes schizophrenic members does not reduce risk of disease; and (3) onset of illness when it occurs in pairs of siblings is at the same age and not at the same time. Thus, it appears that the cause of the disease must be sought in the human genome.

Two clues to the nature and location of the psychosis gene are available: (1) recent neuroradiological and postmortem studies support the view that the disease is in some way related to the determinants of cerebral asymmetry, and (2) concordance by sex for psychosis within sibships is associated with paternal transmission. This finding is consistent with a locus within the pseudoautosomal region, and there are other grounds for supposing that the cerebral dominance gene, the genetic determinant of asymmetry in the human brain, is located within this region.

According to the "virogene" hypothesis, episodes of psychosis are due to the autonomous expression of a retroviral or other potentially mobile sequence, a normal component of the human genome, that is closely related to and may form part of the cerebral dominance gene or right shift factor responsible for the asymmetric development of the human brain. The symbiotic relationship between growth factor and virogene is assumed to have developed early in man's evolution from other primates. The gene complex (i.e., virogene plus right shift factor) includes a component that is subject to significant variation between individuals. This component is responsible for variations in expression including those that lead to psychosis. According to this concept, the psychosis virogene is no more than a labile and potentially deleterious variant of the cerebral dominance gene which itself is variable between individuals.

REFERENCES

Angst, J., and Scharfetter, C., 1989, Familial aspects of bipolar schizoaffective disorder, in: *Affective Disorders, World Psychiatric Association Symposium, Athens, 1985*, Abstract S104.

Angst, J., and Scharfetter, C., 1990, *Schizoaffective Psychosen. Ein Nosologischer Aergernis*, in *Affective Psychoses* (R. J. Witkowski, ed.), Schattauer Verlag, Stuttgart.

Angst, J., Scharfetter, C., and Stassen, H. H., 1983, Classification of schizo-affective patients by multidimensional scaling and cluster analysis, *Psychiatr. Clin.* **16**:254–264.

Annett, M., 1985, *Left, Right, Hand and Brain: The Right Shift Theory*, Erlbaum, London.

Baker, H. F., Ridley, R. M., Crow, T. J., Bloxham, C., Parry, R. P., and Tyrrell, D. A. J., 1983, An investigation of the effects of intracerebral injection in the marmoset of cytopathic csf from patients with schizophrenia and neurological disease, *Psychol. Med.* **13**:449–511.

Baker, H. F., Ridley, R. M., and Crow, T. J., 1985, Experimental transmission of an autosomal dominant spongiform encephalopathy: Does the infectious agent originate in the human genome? *Br. Med. J.* **291**:299–302.

Baker, H. F., Ridley, R. M., Crow, T. J., and Tyrrell, D. A. J., 1989, A re-investigation of the behavioural effects of intracerebral injection in marmosets of cytopathic csf from patients with schizophrenia or neurological disease, *Psychol. Med.* **19**:325–329.

Bogerts, B., Meertz, E., and Schonfeldt-Bausch, R., 1985, Basal ganglia and limbic system pathology in schizophrenia, *Arch. Gen. Psychiatry* **42**:784–791.

Broca, P., 1861, Perte de la parole. Ramollisement chronique et déstruction partielle du lobe antérieur gauche du cerveau, *Bull. Soc. Anthropol.* **2**:219–235.

Brown, R., Colter, N., Corsellis, J. A. N., Crow, T. J., Frith, C. D., Jagoe, R., Johnstone, E. C., and Marsh, L., 1986, Post-mortem evidence of structural brain changes in schizophrenia, *Arch. Gen. Psychiatry* **43**:36–42.

Burgoyne, P. S., 1986, Mammalian X and Y crossover, *Nature* **319**:258–259.

Collinge, J., Boccio, A., DeLisi, L. E., Johnstone, E. C., Lofthouse, R., Owen, F., Poulter, M., Risby, D., Shah, T., and Crow, T. J., 1989a, Evidence for a pseudoautosomal locus for schizophrenia: A sibling pair analysis, *Cytogenetics and Cell Genetics* **51**:978.

Collinge, J. S., Harding, A. E., Owen, F., Poulter, M., Lofthouse, R., Boughey, A. M., Shah, T., and Crow, T. J., 1989b, Diagnosis of Gerstmann-Straussler syndrome in familial dementia with prion protein gene analysis, *Lancet* **2**:15–17.

Collinge, J., DeLisi, L. E., Boccio, A., Johnstone, E. C. Lowe, A., Larkin, C., Leach, M. Lofthouse, R., Owen, F., Poulter, M., Shah, T., Walsh, C. and Crow, T. J., 1991, Evidence for a pseudo-antosomal locus for schizophenia using the method of affected sibling pairs, *Br. J. Psychiatry* **158** (in press).

Crow, T. J., 1983, Is schizophrenia an infectious disease? *Lancet* **1**:173–175.

Crow, T. J., 1984, A re-evaluation of the viral hypothesis: Is psychosis the result of retroviral integration at a site close to the cerebral dominance gene? *Br. J. Psychiatry* **145**:243–253.

Crow, T. J., 1986, The continuum of psychosis and its implication for the structure of the gene, *Br. J. Psychiatry* **149**:419–429.

Crow, T. J., 1987, Pseudoautosomal locus for psychosis? *Lancet* **2**:1532.

Crow, T. J., 1988a, Sex chromosomes and psychosis: The case for a pseudoautosomal locus, *Br. J. Psychiatry* **153**:675–683.

Crow, T. J., 1988b, The viral theory of schizophrenia, *Br. J. Psychiatry* **153**:564–566.

Crow, T. J., 1989, Pseudoautosomal locus for the cerebral dominance gene, *Lancet* **2**:339–340.

Crow, T. J., and Done, D. J., 1986, Age of onset of schizophrenia in siblings: A test of the contagion hypothesis, *Psychiatry Res.* **18**:107–117.

Crow, T. J., Colter, N., Brown, R., Bruton, C. J., and Johnstone, E. C., 1988, Lateralised asymmetry of temporal horn enlargement in schizophrenia, *Schizophrenia Res.* **1**:155.

Crow, T. J., Ball, J., Bloom, S. R., Brown, R., Bruton, C. J., Colter, N., Frith, C. D., Johnstone, E. C., Owens, D. G. C., and Roberts, G. W., 1989a, Schizophrenia as an anomaly of development of cerebral asymmetry, *Arch. Gen. Psychiatry* **46**:1145–1150.

Crow, T. J., DeLisi, L. E., and Johnstone, E. C., 1989b, Concordance by sex in sibling pairs with schizophrenia is paternally inherited: Evidence for a pseudoautosomal locus, *Br. J. Psychiatry* **154**:92–97.

Crow, T. J., Colter, N., Frith, C. D., Johnstone, E. C., and Owens, D. G. C., 1989c, Developmental arrest of cerebral asymmetries in early onset schizophrenia, *Psychiatry Res.* **29**:247–253.

Dax, M., 1865, Lesions de la moitié gauche de l'éncephale coincident avec l'oublie des signes de la pensée. Lu a congres meridionel tenu a Montpellier en 1836, *Gaz. Hebd. Med. Chir.* **11**:259–260.

DeLisi, L. E., Reiss, A. L., White, B. J., and Gershon, E. S., 1988, Cytogenetic studies of males with schizophrenia: Screening for the fragile X chromosome and other chromosomal abnormalities, *Schizophrenia Res.* **1**:277–281.

Forssman, H., 1970, The mental implications of sex chromosome aberrations, *Br. J. Psychiatry* **117**:353–363.

Gershon, E. S., Hamovit, J., Guroff, J. J., Dibble, E., Leckmann, J. F., Sceery, W., Targum, S. D., Nurnberger, J. I., Goldin, L. R., and Bunney, W. E., 1982, A family study of schizo-affective, bipolar I, bipolar II, unipolar and normal control patients, *Arch. Gen. Psychiatry* **39**:1157–1167.

Gershon, E. S., DeLisi, L. E., Hamovit, J., Nurnberger, J. I., Maxwell, M. E., Schreiber, J., Dauphinais, D., Dingman, C. W., and Guroff, J. J., 1988, A controlled family study of chronic psychoses: Schizophrenia and schizo-affective disorder, *Arch. Gen. Psychiatry* **45**:328–336.

Geschwind, N., and Levitsky, W., 1968, Left-right asymmetry in temporal speech region, *Science* **161**:186–187.

Goodall, E., 1932, The exciting cause of certain states, at present classified under schizophrenia by psychiatrists, may be infection, *J. Ment. Sci.* **78**:746–755.

Hare, E. H., 1983, Was insanity on the increase? *Br. J. Psychiatry* **142**:439–455.

Haug, J. O., 1962, Pneumoencephalographic studies in mental disease, *Acta Psychiatr. Scand.* **38**(Suppl):165.

Hsiao, K., Baker, H. F., Crow, T. J., Poulter, M., Owen, F., Terwilliger, J. D., Westaway, D., Ott, J., and Prusiner, S. B., 1989, Linkage of a prion protein mis-sense variant to Gerstmann-Straussler syndrome, *Nature* **338**:342–345.

Johnstone, E. C., Crow, T. J., Frith, C. D., Husband, J., and Kreel, L., 1976, Cerebral ventricular size and cognitive impairment in chronic schizophrenia, *Lancet* **2**:924–926.

Johnstone, E. C., Owens, D. G. C., Bydder, G. M., Colter, N., Crow, T. J., and Frith, C. D., 1989, The spectrum of structural brain changes in schizophrenia: Age of onset as a predictor of cognitive and clinical impairments and their cerebral correlates, *Psychol. Med.* **19**:91–103.

Karlsson, J. L., 1970, The rate of schizophrenia in foster-reared close relatives of schizophrenic index cases, *Biol. Psychiatry* **2**:285–290.

Katzir, N., Rechavi, G., Cohen, J. B., Unger, T., Simoni, F., Segul, S., Cohen, D., and Givol, D., 1985, "Retroposon" insertion into the cellular oncogene c-myc in canine transmissible venereal tumour, *Proc. Nat. Acad. Sci. USA* **82**:1054–1058.

Kuff, E. L., Feenstra, A., Lueders, K., Smith, L., Hawley, R., Hozumi, N., and Shulman, M., 1983, Intracisternal A-particle genes as movable elements in the mouse genome, *Proc. Nat. Acad. Sci. USA* **80**:1992–1996.

Leader, 1987, A continuum of psychosis? *Lancet* **2**:889–890.

McManus, I. C., 1985, Handedness, language dominance and aphasia: A genetic model, *Psychol. Med. Suppl.* **8**:1–40.

Menninger, K. A., 1928, The schizophrenia syndrome as the product of infectious disease, *Arch. Neurol. Psychiatry* **20**:464–481.

Mott, F. W., 1911, Hereditary aspects of nervous and mental disease, *Br. Med. J.* **2**:1013–1020.

Murphy, W. H., Nawrocki, J. F., and Pease, L. R., 1983, Age-dependent paralytic viral infection in C58 mice: Possible implications for human neurologic disease, *Prog. Brain Res.* **59**:291–303.

Netley, C. T., 1986, Summary overview of behavioural development in individuals with neonatally identified X and Y aneuploidy, *Birth Defects* **22**:293–306.

Netley, C. T., and Rovet, J., 1982, Atypical hemispheric lateralization in Turner syndrome subjects, *Cortex* **18**:377–384.

Netley, C. T., and Rovet, J., 1987, Relations between a dermatoglyphic measure, hemispheric specialization, and intellectual abilities in 47,XXY males, *Brain & Cognition* **6**:153–160.

Owen, F., Poulter, M., Lofthouse, R., Collinge, J., Crow, T. J., Risby, R., Baker, H. F., Ridley, R. M., Hsiao, K., and Prusiner, S. B., 1989, Insertion in prion protein gene in familial Creutzfeldt-Jakob disease, *Lancet* **1**:51–52.

Owen, F., Poulter, M., Shah, T., Collinge, J., Lofthouse, R., Baker, H., Ridley, R., McVey, J., and Crow, T. J., 1990, An in-frame insertion in the prior protein gene in familial Creutzfeldt-Jakob disease, *Mol. Brain Res.* **7**:273–276.

Owens, D. G. C., Johnstone, E. C., Crow, T. J., Frith, C. D., Jagoe, J. R., and Kreel, L., 1985, Cerebral ventricular enlargement in schizophrenia: Relationship to the disease process and its clinical correlates, *Psychol. Med.* **15**:27–41.

Paulson, K. E., Doka, N., Schmid, G. W., Misra, R., Schindler, C. W., Rush, M. G., Kadyk, L., and Leinwand, L., 1985, A transposon-like element in human DNA, *Nature* **316**:359–361.

Penrose, L. S., 1942, Auxiliary genes for determining sex as contributory causes of mental illness, *J. Ment. Sci.* **88**:308–316.

Rosenthal, D., 1962, Familial concordance by sex with respect to schizophrenia, *Psychol. Bull.* **59**: 401–421.

Sartorius, N., Jablensky, A., Korten, A., Ernberg, G., Anker, M., Cooper, J. E., and Day, R., 1986, Early manifestations and first contact incidence of schizophrenia in different cultures, *Psychol. Med.* **16**:909–928.

Taylor, G. R., Carter, G. I., and Crow, T. J., 1987, Cytotoxic csf from neurological and neuropsychiatric patients, in *Viruses, Immunity and Mental Disorders* (E. Kurstak, Z. J. Lipowski, and P. V. Morozov, eds.), Plenum Press, New York, pp. 161–171.

Teich, N., 1982, Endogenous viruses, in: *RNA Tumour Viruses*, 2nd ed. (R. Weiss, N. Teich, H. Varmus, and J. Coffin, eds.), Cold Spring Harbor Laboratory, Cold Spring Harbor, N.Y., pp. 1109–1203.

Torrey, E. F., 1980, *Schizophrenia and Civilization*, Aronson, New York.

Tyrrell, D. A. J., Crow, T. J., Parry, R. P., Johnstone, E. C., and Ferrier, I. N., 1979, Possible virus in schizophrenia and some neurological disorders, *Lancet* **1**:839–841.

Weinberger, D. R., Torrey, E. F., Neophytides, A. N., and Wyatt, R. H., 1979, Lateral cerebral ventricular enlargement in chronic schizophrenia, *Arch. Gen. Psychiatry* **36**:735–739.

Chapter **2**

A Virus-Associated Immunopathological Theory of Schizophrenia

Royce W. Waltrip II, Donald R. Carrigan,
Robert W. Buchanan, and William T. Carpenter, Jr.

INTRODUCTION

Schizophrenia is a clinical syndrome which is increasingly considered to be a neurological disease with behavioral symptoms that primarily manifest as dysfunction of frontal and limbic brain areas. Hypotheses of the etiology or etiologies of schizophrenia have tended to be limited to intrinsic central nervous system (CNS) processes, such as neurotransmitter dysregulation or neuroanatomical models. These models have a correspondingly limited predictive validity. An alternate and potentially more useful perspective of the disease would be one that takes into account its pleomorphic nature. Schizophrenia has a broad spectrum of associated findings suggesting involvement of developmental processes and a pathophysiology that may be systemic in nature. Viral hypotheses have been one way that the issue of pleomorphism has been addressed.

Menninger (Menninger, 1926, 1928) and others (McCowan and Cook, 1928; Sands, 1928; Hendrick, 1928) associated cases of schizophrenia with influenza,

Royce W. Waltrip II, Robert W. Buchanan, and William T. Carpenter, Jr. • *Maryland Psychiatric Research Center, Department of Psychiatry, University of Maryland School of Medicine, Baltimore, Maryland 21228.* Donald R. Carrigan • *Department of Pathology, Medical College of Wisconsin, Milwaukee, Wisconsin 53226.*

following the pandemic in the early part of this century. Recent epidemiological data are regarded as supportive of a viral etiology by some authors (Torrey *et al.*, 1988; Stevens, 1988), although this interpretation is not shared by others (Murray and Reveley, 1983). Numerous investigators have searched for evidence of active viral replication within the CNS of schizophrenic patients (Libikova *et al.*, 1979; Rimón *et al.*, 1978; Shrikhande *et al.*, 1985; Albrecht *et al.*, 1980) and for serological evidence of viral involvement in the disease (King *et al.*, 1985, 1985a, b; Ahokas *et al.*, 1987; Libikova *et al.*, 1979; Gotlieb-Stematsky *et al.*, 1987; Kaufmann *et al.*, 1983; Robert-Guroff *et al.*, 1985). In general, the results obtained have been inconsistent and do not implicate any particular viral pathogen as playing an important role in schizophrenia.

The lack of direct evidence for viral involvement has led Crow (1984, 1986) to formulate more elaborate hypotheses regarding the type of virus that might be present and to propose that the viral agent may be acting by altering neuronal systems in such a way as to produce changes consistent with those predicted by the dopamine hypothesis of schizophrenia (Snyder, 1973). Specifically, he suggests that the viral agent involved is a retrovirus that exists within the CNS in the form of viral DNA integrated into the cellular genome near the cerebral dominance gene (Crow, 1987b) or pseudoautosomal region of the sex chromosomes (Crow, 1987a). Integration near the cerebral dominance gene is proposed to explain the association between concordance in monozygotic twins of schizophrenia and right-handedness (Boklage 1977, cited in Crow, 1987b) and the observation that right-handed individuals with schizophrenia have a milder form of the disease than do those who are left-handed (Luchins *et al.*, 1979, cited in Crow, 1987b). Integration near the pseudoautosomal region of the sex chromosomes is proposed to explain X-linkage.

The need for such complex and elaborate postulates to relate viruses to schizophrenia and the failure of numerous studies to identify a specific viral cause of schizophrenia may result from the implicit assumption that if a virus is involved in the pathogenesis of schizophrenia, then it must be a single, particular virus. Stated another way, the lack of clear evidence for a particular virus being the cause of schizophrenia suggests one of two things: (1) that there is no virus involved or (2) that the virus is very elusive, such as Crow's integrated viral DNA or the prion agent associated with kuru and Creutzfeldt-Jakob disease (Gajdusek, 1985), and cannot be readily transmitted to other primates or cultured using standard techniques (Baker *et al.*, 1983). However, a third possibility exists and forms the conceptual basis for the hypothesis presented here. Specifically, it is possible that no particular virus causes schizophrenia, but that any one of several viruses that commonly infect the normal CNS can interact with host defense mechanisms in genetically susceptible individuals in such a way as to cause the disease. A number of different viral agents could trigger a common sequence of physiological events that result in the CNS dysfunction underlying schizophrenia (Waltrip *et al.*, 1990).

The present discussion will cover broad areas of clinical and basic science and attempt to integrate them with respect to the proposed theory. To establish a common framework for discussion, brief overviews of latent viral infections of the human CNS and the biology of interferon will be presented as well as a perspective on schizophrenic symptomatology. Then the proposed theory will be considered in some detail with emphasis being placed on how various aspects of schizophrenia can be explained by it. Finally, a program of research with questions that can be addressed will be discussed.

LATENT VIRAL INFECTIONS OF THE HUMAN CNS

Recent studies in a number of laboratories have shown that CNS tissues from normal individuals, in addition to those with known neurological disease, contain genetic materials of a variety of viral agents. Haase *et al.* (1984) using the method of *in situ* hybridization detected measles virus RNA in the brains of 13 of 25 multiple sclerosis patients and in 5 of 18 neurologically normal control patients. This apparent neurotropism of measles virus is consistent with the electroencephalographic (EEG) changes and the cerebrospinal fluid (CSF) pleocytosis that occur during acute rubeola (Reinicke *et al.*, 1974; Hanninen *et al.*, 1980) and suggests that invasion of the CNS by the virus occurs in a substantial proportion of normal individuals. That this neuroinvasion is not always harmless is indicated by the occurrence of fatal subacute measles encephalitis in immunocompromised individuals and of subacute sclerosing panencephalitis (SSPE), a fatal disease of children and young adults, in a small proportion of measles-infected individuals (Johnson and Carrigan, 1981).

The immunological mechanisms responsible for maintaining measles virus in a latent state within the CNS are unknown. However, the failure of patients with the acquired immunodeficiency syndrome (AIDS) or other severely immunocompromised adults to develop measles virus-associated CNS disease (Elder and Sever, 1988) suggests that a very low level of residual immunity is adequate to maintain the infection in a suppressed state. Viral reactivation is prevented, or contained, by local defensive responses within the CNS, such as interferon (IFN) or other cytokine production by microglia or other CNS cells (Giulian *et al.*, 1986; Larsson *et al.*, 1978). The production of IFN in the brains of patients with SSPE and several other viral infections of the CNS has recently been directly demonstrated by immunohistochemical procedures (Traugott and Lebon, 1988).

Work by Brahic *et al.* (1985), also using the *in situ* hybridization procedure, found genetic material related to poliovirus in the brains of one patient with amyotrophic lateral sclerosis and one normal control. The normal neurotropism of poliovirus, and indeed of picornaviruses as a family, has been well documented. Examples of acute encephalitides include classical poliomyelitis caused by poliovirus (Melnick, 1985) and the meningoencephalitis caused by echovirus in neonates and immunocompromised patients (Reiss-Levy *et al.*, 1986; Prentice *et al.*, 1985). Examples of chronic neurological diseases caused by picornaviruses are

Theiler's virus encephalomyelitis in mice (Rodriguez *et al.*, 1983) and chronic echovirus meningoencephalitis in patients with agammaglobulinemia (McKinney *et al.*, 1987). Immunological mechanisms involved in these chronic infections and in the persistence of picornavirus genomes in normal CNS tissues are not understood. However, as with measles virus above, the absence of CNS disease caused by reactivation of picornaviruses in severely immunosuppressed patients suggests that either low levels of immunological reactivity are sufficient to maintain the suppressed state, local defensive responses, such as IFN, are responsible for the suppression, or the viral genome is incapable of reactivating at all.

Perhaps the best studied and understood instance of latent viral infection of the CNS is that of herpes simplex virus (HSV) infection of the spinal ganglia (Roizman and Sears, 1987). It has now been demonstrated by both Southern blot (Fraser *et al.*, 1981) and *in situ* hybridization (Sequiera *et al.*, 1979) techniques that HSV can latently infect the brain as well as spinal ganglion neurons. Specifically, Fraser *et al.* (1981) detected HSV DNA sequences in brain from four of five patients with multiple sclerosis and three of five normal individuals with no neurological disease. In a similar study, Sequiera *et al.* (1979) found HSV DNA sequences in the brains of three of four elderly patients with chronic psychiatric illnesses associated with significant neuropathological changes. Two other patients with histories of acute psychotic episodes but with no significant histopathological abnormalities were negative for HSV.

Recent findings in one of our own laboratories have added human cytomegalovirus (HCMV) to the list of viruses that frequently establish latent infections in the human CNS (Toorkey and Carrigan, 1989). Briefly, immunohistochemical procedures were used to detect expression of one of the immediate early (IE) antigens of HCMV in brain tissue from several normal individuals who were seropositive for HCMV and who died of trauma or acute myocardial infarction. It has been suggested that such antigens serve as markers for cells latently infected with other members of the herpesvirus family, such as HSV and varicella-zoster virus (VZV) (Vafai *et al.*, 1988). Initially, HCMV IE antigen was detected in one of seven normal brains examined (Toorkey and Carrigan, 1989). However, by examining additional sections of brain tissue from the IE antigen-negative cases, this proportion has been raised to three of the seven cases examined. The mechanism by which this latent infection, as with the other infections outlined above, is maintained is not understood. However, it is likely that the latent HCMV in the brain is subject to periodic reactivation as has been described for latent HCMV infections in the periphery (Winston *et al.*, 1985). Interestingly, numerous studies have described increased HCMV antibody levels in patients with schizophrenia compared to normal individuals (Torrey *et al.*, 1982; Albrecht *et al.*, 1980b), and there is one report of HCMV antigens being expressed in the brain of a schizophrenic patient (Stevens *et al.*, 1984). However, several other studies have failed to confirm these results (Shrikhande *et al.*, 1985; Taylor *et al.*, 1985).

In summary, sufficient evidence exists to conclude that a substantial percentage of the human population carries within their CNS tissues one or more latent viral infections. In the majority of people, these viruses cause no overt disease or symptoms. However, through periodic reactivations they may induce severe, and even life-threatening, infections in immunocompromised individuals, such as HCMV encephalitis in patients with AIDS (Masdeu *et al.*, 1988), or in otherwise normal people, such as sporadic HSV encephalitis (Johnson, 1982). By analogy to the periodic reactivations of HSV and HCMV that are known to occur in peripheral organs (Baringer, 1975; Jordan, 1983), it is likely that subclinical reactivations of latent viruses within the CNS occur with some regularity in most infected people. In certain, predisposed individuals these reactivational events may set into motion immunopathological responses that lead to specific and focal CNS dysfunctions. As alluded to above, it is likely that alpha IFN (aIFN) may play an important role in this process.

THE BIOLOGY OF aIFN

The term interferon refers to a class of polypeptides that have in common the ability to induce an antiviral state in cells characterized by a general resistance toward infection by a wide variety of viruses. Three major types of interferon are known and have been designated alpha (aIFN), beta (bIFN), and gamma (gIFN). The three differ from one another antigenically and with respect to many of their biological properties. In this discussion, only aIFN will be considered. aIFN actually is a family of closely related proteins that share amino acid sequence homologies and many biological properties, although there is accumulating evidence that different aIFN subtypes may vary in their specific physiological functions (Creasey *et al.*, 1988). For the purposes of this discussion no distinctions will be made among the different aIFN's.

aIFN is produced primarily by macrophages and B lymphocytes in response to a wide variety of stimuli which include DNA viruses, RNA viruses, virally infected cells, synthetic double-stranded RNA polymers, bacteria, and bacterial products (Capobianchi *et al.*, 1988; Mannering and Deloria, 1986). It is actively secreted by the cell producing it into the extracellular space where it diffuses until it binds to specific receptor molecules on the surfaces of adjacent cells (Rubinstein and Orchansky, 1986). The aIFN is then actively taken into the cell and transported to the nucleus where it triggers a variety of biochemical and physiological responses (Clemens and McNurlan, 1985; Smith-Johannsen *et al.*, 1984). The qualitative and quantitative nature of the response induced depend upon a variety of factors including the cell type involved, the genetic composition of the host organism, and, in the case of humans, sex and age. Males produce more aIFN than females, given the same *in vivo* stimulus (Bever *et al.*, 1985, 1988), and the amount of aIFN produced with an *in vitro* stimulus declines after the age of 50 (Abb *et al.*, 1984).

The magnitude of an organism's cellular response to aIFN is under direct genetic control by means of at least two separate mechanisms. First, the cell membrane receptor to which aIFN binds is encoded on human chromosome 21 (Epstein and Epstein, 1976), and it has been shown that cells trisomic for chromosome 21 have increased sensitivity to the effects of aIFN (Tan *et al.*, 1975; Epstein and Epstein, 1980). This increased sensitivity appears to be due to an increased density of receptors on the cell surface (Epstein *et al.*, 1982). Second, an autosomal dominant gene in mice that determines the ability of aIFN to inhibit the production of respiratory disease by influenza A virus has been identified and termed the Mx gene (Haller *et al.*, 1980, 1981). Specifically, animals expressing the Mx gene product in their cells are totally protected from influenza A virus challenge by levels of serum aIFN that have little or no effect in animals not expressing the gene. Recently, a human analogue of the murine Mx gene has been identified and shown to exert similar biological effects (Staeheli and Haller, 1985; Arnheiter and Haller, 1987).

As mentioned above, the classical and most widely recognized response of a cell to exposure to aIFN is the induction of an antiviral state (Toy, 1983). However, aIFN also induces a variety of other responses in cells and possesses a number of biological activities that can influence the functioning of the CNS and that are relevant to the hypothesis being presented. Specifically, aIFN can directly modify neural activity as well as interact more generally with cellular metabolic processes.

Exposure of neurons in cell culture to aIFN induces a state of hyperexcitability associated with high rates of spontaneous firing (Calvet and Gressor, 1979). Similar effects of aIFN on neuronal firing rates have also been shown *in vivo* upon microinjection into various regions of the CNS of rats (Dafny *et al.*, 1985). Neurons of the cerebral cortex, hippocampus, and thalamus showed marked increases of their firing rates, while those in the hypothalamus showed substantial decreases. Further, aIFN can interact with and modify the activities of neurotransmitter systems of the CNS. It shows high-affinity binding to opiate receptors and possesses opiate activity several times that of β-endorphin and morphine (Blalock and Smith, 1981). The physiological relevance of this property manifests in aIFN's abilities to influence opiate withdrawal (Lorenzo *et al.*, 1987; Dafny, 1985) and to induce a catatonic state in intracerebrally injected mice similar to that produced by endorphins (Blalock and Smith, 1981). Also, cleavage of aIFN by nonspecific proteases, such as would occur in typical catabolic processes, generates peptides that possess potent adrenocorticotropin (ACTH)-like activity (Blalock and Smith, 1980). Through this mechanism aIFN could influence, and possibly disrupt, the regulation of the opioid and dopamine transmitter systems since ACTH directly interacts with both (Springer *et al.*, 1983; Cools *et al.*, 1978).

Some of these properties of aIFN are probably involved in the neurotoxicity shown by aIFN in patients treated with high doses of it for cancer (Adams *et al.*, 1984; Smedley *et al.*, 1983), chronic hepatitis (McDonald *et al.*, 1987, Renault *et al.*, 1987), or amyotrophic lateral sclerosis (Farkkila *et al.*, 1984; Iivanainen *et al.*,

1985). The toxicity usually manifests as a syndrome of apathy, social withdrawal, paucity of speech, thought blocking, and irritability. EEG abnormalities are common (Mattson *et al.*, 1983; Suter *et al.*, 1984; Bottomley and Toy, 1985), and seizures (Bottomley and Toy, 1985) as well as precipitation of paranoid schizophrenia (Lok et al., 1988) have been reported. The syndrome is easily reversible, and the patients usually return to normal within 1 to 2 weeks of cessation of aIFN administration (Farkkila *et al.*, 1984; Smedley *et al.*, 1983). The physiological basis of this syndrome is not known. However, it is likely that it results from direct effects of aIFN on the CNS in spite of the general exclusion of aIFN by the blood-brain barrier (Smith *et al.*, 1985) since access of aIFN to the brain may be gained by penetration of those areas where the barrier is weak or nonexistent. An example of such an area is the anterior hypothalamus which allows entry of interleukin 1, a molecule very similar to aIFN, from the peripheral blood into the CNS in its role as an endogenous pyrogen (Rosendorff and Mooney, 1971).

The neurotoxicity of aIFN may also be involved in some of the neuropsychiatric clinical manifestations of certain forms of viral encephalitis. For example, infection of the CNS with rabies virus often leads to severe psychoticlike disease with little or no overt neuropathological changes being evident at the time of death (Perl, 1975; Johnson, 1982). The production of high levels of aIFN in the brains of patients with rabies (Merigan *et al.*, 1984) suggests that it may be involved in the loss of neural function underlying the clinical disease. Similarly, the relatively minor neuropathological changes observed in the brains of many patients with severe AIDS dementia complex (ADC) have led to the suggestion that a neurotoxic substance is produced by the infected cells within the CNS (Price *et al.*, 1988, Budka *et al.*, 1987). The pathologically high levels of aIFN present in the peripheral blood of patients with AIDS (Abb, 1985; Buimovici-Klein *et al.*, 1986) combined with the fact that the majority of infected cells within the CNS are macrophages or microglial cells (Vazeux *et al.*, 1987), which are the main producers of aIFN, suggest that aIFN may be the postulated neurotoxin involved. Of special importance relative to the schizophrenia hypothesis being proposed here are numerous reports of ADC manifesting as a disease clinically indistinguishable from schizophrenia (Buhrich *et al.*, 1988; Halevie-Goldman *et al.*, 1987; Thomas and Szabadi, 1987; Nurnberg *et al.*, 1984). The neurotoxicity of aIFN may be the factor that the two diseases share.

In addition to these neuronally specific effects, aIFN can influence the CNS in more general ways. Most importantly, aIFN is a potent inhibitor of cellular proliferation and differentiation (Clemens and McNurlan, 1985; Rossi, 1985). Not only can aIFN influence the differentiation and activation of lymphocytes and macrophages (Zarling, 1984), but it can also inhibit hematopoiesis (Martelly and Jullien, 1974), depress the expression of tyrosinase in differentiating melanocytes (Fisher *et al.*, 1981), and accelerate the formation of myotubules in maturing skeletal muscle cells (Fisher *et al.*, 1983). The anti-cell proliferative activity of aIFN provides much of the rationale for its use as a chemotherapeutic agent for several forms of cancer (Dunnick and Galasso, 1980), especially hairy cell leukemia (Quesada *et al.*, 1984).

In summary, aIFN is a physiologically powerful family of polypeptides produced by cells in response to viral infections. It possesses a wide range of biological activities and can clearly function as a potent neurotoxin capable of inducing clinically significant CNS dysfunction by a variety of mechanisms. The degree to which a cell, or an entire organism, is susceptible to the actions of aIFN is under direct genetic control. Therefore, it is possible that the focal induction of aIFN within the CNS in response to viral reactivation events could lead to a range of disorders of neural function. The degree of dysfunction and its clinical manifestations would depend upon the severity and anatomical location of the viral reactivation coupled with the genetically determined responsiveness of the individual toward aIFN. As detailed below, we postulate that such a disease mechanism may be involved in the etiology of schizophrenia.

A PERSPECTIVE ON THE SYMPTOMATOLOGY OF SCHIZOPHRENIA

A brief overview of the symptoms and course of illness in schizophrenia will orient the reader to concepts and terminology used to describe the clinical significance of the aIFN theory. The psychiatric manifestations and associated features of schizophrenia are diverse. The diagnosis presently has the status of a clinical syndrome, and many workers anticipate etiological heterogeneity and the presence of several disease entities within the syndrome (Kendell, 1975; McHugh and Slavney, 1983; Carpenter, 1987). In addition to symptomatic diversity, the course of schizophrenia is increasingly considered to have a dynamic nature of relapse and relative remission (Zubin *et al.*, 1983).

When originally defined, dementia praecox (i.e., schizophrenia), Kraepelin (1919) divided manifestations into two groups roughly corresponding to today's emphasis on positive and negative symptoms (Strauss *et al.*, 1974). Positive symptoms such as hallucinations, delusions, and thought disorder are essential for diagnosis and their fluctuations constitute what are commonly considered periods of relapse and relative remission in research (Falloon *et al.*, 1983). Negative symptoms, such as deficiencies in social drive and emotional range, as well as impoverishment of thought and speech content account for much of the long-term disability of schizophrenia (Carpenter *et al.*, 1987) and are not often considered in the context of states of relapse and relative remission. Negative symptoms do fluctuate in concert with positive symptoms (Goldberg, 1985). However, a subgroup of schizophrenic patients is considered to have negative symptoms that endure between episodes, constituting what is termed a deficit syndrome (Carpenter *et al.*, 1988).

Other domains of symptomatology such as neurological signs, inappropriate affect, and impairment in cognition contribute to the diversity of schizophrenia

(Carpenter and Buchanan, 1989). Furthermore, long-term follow-up studies reveal about eight distinct course types (Ciompi, 1980; Huber *et al.*, 1980; Carpenter and Kirkpatrick, 1989).

Subtyping of schizophrenia into what may be more etiologically homogeneous groups is a major focus of current psychiatric research (Keith and Matthews, 1988). It is possible, however, that the heterogeneity of manifestation belies a unifying causal mechanism. The present theory attempts to account for the observed diversity within the framework of a single pathogenesis.

THE aIFN THEORY OF SCHIZOPHRENIA

The fundamental components of the hypothesis are summarized in the following series of statements:

1. A variety of viral agents routinely establish latent infections in the human CNS, and these viruses are subject to periodic reactivations. These infections can be established at any time during the life of the individual, including *in utero*.
2. As part of the normal defensive response of the CNS to these viral reactivational events, aIFN is produced by cells (initially microglia and later lymphocytes and macrophages) in the immediate vicinity of the reactivation after being induced either by the virus itself or by virally infected cells.
3. This locally produced aIFN then interacts with the cells in and around the viral reactivation focus to induce an antiviral state and concurrently alters neuronal activity (both directly and through neurotransmitter interactions) and, in some instances, inhibits differentiation and proliferation of the surrounding cells.
4. This process continues until the viral reactivation event is terminated by specific antiviral immunological responses.
5. Acute neuronal dysfunction caused by the aIFN manifests as the positive and negative symptoms associated with relapses of disease in schizophrenic patients.
6. In CNS areas subject to repeated or long-lasting viral reactivations, the interference of aIFN with cellular differentiation and proliferation leads to minor structural abnormalities and to abnormal patterns of CNS development.
7. Over the young-adult life of the individual, when CNS development continues to be very active, these minor abnormalities accumulate which interact with aIFN behavioral toxicity, leading to a deficit syndrome in which increasingly large areas of normal life functioning are lost.
8. During the prenatal development of the schizophrenic individual, the

excess of aIFN creates a susceptibility to the occurrence of stigmata such as minor physical anomalies, abnormal nailfold capillary morphology, and dermatoglyphic abnormalities.

9. Clinical diversity is intrinsic to the theory in that different patients can have different degrees of excess of aIFN, different viruses that are reactivating, different anatomical locations of viral reactivation, and variability in the duration and extent of reactivations. Sameness in clinical manifestation is imparted by the personality characteristics of each individual patient and the constancy of CNS anatomy.
10. Long-term studies of schizophrenia have identified a sex difference with males faring worse and a general trend for all patients to have a lessening of positive symptoms in later years of the illness. The sex difference in severity is accounted for by the sex difference in aIFN production with males having a greater response to stimulation than females. The lessening of symptoms with age is accounted for by the decline in aIFN inducibility that is normally seen with age.

Several aspects of this scenario warrant special consideration, and these are discussed in the sections below.

Abnormalities of the Response of Schizophrenics to aIFN

Statements 1 and 2 reflect a process that probably occurs in the CNS of many, if not all, people, while the others refer to the postulated process in patients with schizophrenia. Implicit in this distinction is a major prediction of the hypothesis, namely that patients with schizophrenia have something inherently abnormal in their aIFN responses within the CNS. The precise nature of this abnormality is unclear; however, the final result of it is that pathological levels of aIFN activity are produced in response to viral reactivation events.

Two possible causes, either viral or immunological, can be proposed that can account for this abnormality. Patients with schizophrenia either may have increased levels of latent viruses within their CNS or the latent infections that they have may be subject to unusually severe reactivations. The large body of negative results concerning the presence of active viral replication in the CNS tissues of schizophrenics (DeLisi and Crow, 1986; Torrey and Kaufmann, 1986) combined with the failure of numerous studies to detect a consistent immunological abnormality in them (DeLisi, 1984; Schindler *et al.*, 1986) strongly suggest that this explanation is unlikely. The second possible explanation, and the one favored here, is that patients with schizophrenia have a genetically determined hyperresponsiveness toward aIFN, analogous to either the general hyperresponsiveness seen in Down's syndrome (Nurmi *et al.*, 1982; Epstein and Epstein, 1982) or a more circumscribed hyperresponsiveness in the case of mice carrying the Mx gene, as described previously (Haller *et al.*, 1980, 1981; Staeheli and Haller, 1985; Arnheiter and

Haller, 1987). Thus, levels of aIFN within the CNS that cause no significant problems in most individuals may be pathologically high, in terms of activity, in patients with schizophrenia.

This explanation is attractive for a variety of reasons. First, a genetically determined hyperresponsiveness toward aIFN may offer a significant selective advantage to the population carrying it since it would provide an increased resistance toward viral infections and cancer. There is a suggestion of such an increased resistance toward viruses for family members of schizophrenic patients (Carter and Watts, 1971). Further, an increased resistance toward viral infections may help to balance the reproductive disadvantage that has been associated with schizophrenia. This effect, termed heterozygote advantage, may help to account for the persistence of schizophrenia in the face of less efficient reproduction (Carter and Watts, 1971; Hammer and Zubin, 1968; Huxley *et al.*, 1964; Jarvik and Chadwick, 1973). Second, a hyperresponsiveness toward aIFN, as opposed to a hyperproduction of it, can account for many of the experimental results that have been reported concerning the role of IFN in schizophrenia.

Numerous studies have been done to analyze the serum and CSF of schizophrenic patients for the presence of IFN as an indirect measure of viral activity in the disease. In most instances the findings were negative (Roy *et al.*, 1985; Schindler *et al.*, 1986; Rimón *et al.*, 1985), but in a few studies IFN was detected (Preble and Torrey, 1985; Libikova *et al.*, 1977) and interpreted as suggesting an active viral infection within the CNS or an immunological abnormality. Hyperresponsiveness of patients toward aIFN would result in production of only low or "normal" levels of aIFN in the CSF with the result that schizophrenic patients would be indistinguishable from normal individuals. Further, the focal production of aIFN in direct association with a viral reactivation event would make detection of the aIFN produced in the CSF or serum very unlikely due to the large dilutional effects involved.

In other studies, the ability of peripheral blood mononuclear cells from schizophrenic patients to produce aIFN was examined (Moises *et al.*, 1985, 1986). Significantly lower levels of aIFN were produced by the patients' cells than by cells from normal individuals, and the conclusion was drawn that a defect in aIFN production exists in the patients and interpreted as supporting a model of increased susceptibility to viruses and viral etiology of schizophrenia. The postulated hyperresponsiveness of schizophrenic patients toward aIFN offers an alternate explanation for these results. It has been shown that repeated exposure of an animal to an inducer of aIFN (viral or otherwise) results in the formation of a transient refractive state in which aIFN production is substantially reduced (Stringfellow *et al.*, 1977; Borden and Murphy, 1971; Borden *et al.*, 1975). If schizophrenic patients are hyperresponsive toward aIFN, then a substantial percentage of the leukocytes in their peripheral blood may at any one time be in a refractory state due to exposure to routine environmental stimuli. This would result in an apparent "defect" of their aIFN response. This effect may be restricted to cells in the peripheral blood since, by their very nature, they would probably be exposed to stimuli irrespective of the tissue location. aIFN-producing cells within the brain, and possibly other organs, would not be expected to be exposed to such routine stimuli and would therefore remain completely reactive. This reasoning is supported by similar findings of decreased induced aIFN in Down's syndrome patients (Nair and Schwartz, 1984) whose cells are hypersensitive to aIFN (Tan *et al.*, 1975; Epstein and Epstein, 1980).

Heterogeneity of the Clinical Manifestations of Schizophrenia

It is probable that, in latently infected CNS tissues, viral foci are distributed randomly throughout the entire CNS since no particular site has been described as the location of measles virus RNA in normal brains (Haase *et al.*, 1981) and the distribution of latent HCMV in normal human brain tissue appears to show little specificity for anatomical regions (D. R. Carrigan, unpublished observation). If all such foci of latent infection are susceptible to reactivation, then a focus of aIFN production could be induced at any time in virtually any region of the brain. By analogy to the large percentage of CNS lesions in multiple sclerosis that fail to produce overt clinical disease (Drayer and Barrett, 1984; Poser, 1980), it might be expected that many of those foci would be clinically silent, i.e., not associated with overt signs or symptoms. Therefore, a degree of anatomical specificity of the symptoms induced may exist, especially if certain regions of the brain were particularly sensitive either to the direct neuronal effects of aIFN or to the disruption caused by aIFN of neurotransmitter regulation (e.g., dopamine metabolism). Anatomical differences in the effects of aIFN on the brain have been demonstrated (Dafny *et al.*, 1985). Further, it might be expected that even within these "sensitive" regions anatomic differences might exist with respect to the precise symptoms induced by aIFN production. Therefore, since each patient would undoubtedly have a unique combination of latently infected sites within these regions, reactivation of the virus within those sites would produce a unique and characteristic spectrum of symptoms. Each patient would in essence have a "unique" disease, and the psychotic relapses of any single patient would often resemble each other. At the same time, the existence of the specific aIFN-sensitive anatomical regions would provide a general consistency of disease among schizophrenic patients. This scenario closely resembles clinical observations that have been made with groups of schizophrenic patients.

Gender and Age Differences in Symptom Severity in Schizophrenia

Numerous studies of gender and age in schizophrenia have indicated that a large number of patients undergo a lessening of psychotic symptoms in later years (Huber *et al.*, 1980; Ciompi, 1980) and that males tend to fare worse with the disease (Seeman, 1986; Lewine, 1981; Watt *et al.*, 1983). These observations can provide a clue to pathophysiology. In the Bonn long-term follow-up study (Huber *et al.*, 1980), the stability of remission became associated with age only after age 50, a result consistent with similar work in the Lausanne study (Ciompi, 1980). The sex difference in severity is accounted for by the sex difference in aIFN production with males having a greater response to stimulation than females (Bever *et al.*, 1985, 1988). The lessening of symptoms with age is accounted for by the decline in aIFN inducibility that is seen with age (Abb *et al.*, 1984).

Role of Stress in Schizophrenic Relapse

Stress is thought to be a risk factor for the onset of the disease and for relapse in schizophrenic patients (Day, 1981). Studies of the family treatment of schizophrenia indicate that the frequency of relapse can be effectively modified by reducing certain types of environmental stress (Falloon, 1986; Leff *et al.*, 1982). The biological basis for these effects is not understood, but the aIFN theory being proposed here offers a possible explanation.

A large body of evidence accumulated over the past three decades indicates that reactivations of latent human herpesvirus infections may be triggered by stressful life events (Goldmeier and Johnson, 1982; Glaser *et al.*, 1985). In a study of military cadets, serious EBV-associated illness was positively correlated with several particular stress-related risk factors (Kasl *et al.*, 1979). In another similar study, serum antibody titers against HSV, EBV, and CMV were higher in medical students before or during final examinations than immediately after summer vacation (Glaser *et al.*, 1985). Therefore, it can be postulated that during periods of high personal stress the chance of a viral reactivation event occurring within the CNS is increased; and, as discussed above, in a specifically susceptible individual this reactivation may lead to the onset or relapse of schizophrenic symptoms by inducing a local production of aIFN within the CNS at or near the point of viral reactivation.

In addition to triggering the onset of psychotic symptoms, such a mechanism would also serve to begin a self-perpetuating cycle of disease. This possibility emerges from consideration of how stress probably leads to viral reactivation. In a wide variety of systems, both human and experimental, stress has been shown to depress immunological responses. For example, in humans bereavement from loss of a spouse is associated with a decrease in lymphocyte proliferative responses to mitogens (Bartrop *et al.*, 1977; Schleifer *et al.*, 1983). In animals a variety of acute stressors result in impairment of T-lymphocyte-mediated immunological parameters and alter susceptibility to experimental infectious and neoplastic diseases (Monjan, 1981). These observations coupled with the high rates of herpesvirus reactivations and diseases in immunocompromised patients (Engelhard *et al.*, 1986) suggest that stress-associated viral reactivations may result from the induced transient immunosuppression of the affected individual. In most people these viral reactivations are asymptomatic since the immune responses are capable of limiting the infection and eventually driving it back into the latent state (Klein, 1982). However, if the viral reactivation triggers an immunopathological response with resultant psychotic symptoms, such as that postulated here for patients with schizophrenia, the psychosis itself may serve as a potent new source of additional stress to the patient. This new stress would then serve to increase the degree of immunosuppression present which would hinder the limitation of the viral reactivation within the CNS. Thus, the induction of aIFN would be amplified in magnitude and extended in time. The resulting increase in the concentration of aIFN in the tissue would help to slow viral replication but probably would not terminate it since in all cases where it has been studied tissue IFN limits but does not prevent viral replication (Gresser *et al.*, 1976; Sekellick and Marcus, 1980) and immunocompromised individuals have normal or exaggerated IFN responses (Rhodes-Feuillette *et al.*, 1983; Buimovici-Klein *et al.*, 1986) and are still subject to severe, chronic viral infections (Engelhard *et al.*, 1986). These increases in aIFN concentration would, however, produce more profound CNS dysfunction which would amplify the psychotic symptoms, serving in turn to perpetuate the entire process.

Developmental Abnormalities in Schizophrenic Patients

As noted previously, aIFN is known to exert effects on cellular proliferation and differentiation (Clemens and McNurlan, 1985; Rossi, 1985). It has been suggested that aIFN can be considered as a hormone acting in concert with growth factors (Inglot, 1983; Smith and Blalock, 1981–82) and aIFN is normally present in human amniotic fluid, suggesting that it may have a role in normal development (Chany *et al.*, 1982; Tan and Inoue, 1982; Lebon *et al.*, 1982). These factors, combined with the postulated hyperresponsiveness of schizophrenics to aIFN, may help to explain the origin of many of the developmental abnormalities that have been described in patients with schizophrenia. Another developmental effect in addition to that imposed by the simple aIFN excess in schizophrenic patients is the possibility of *in utero* establishment of latent infections in both the CNS and peripheral organs. Several types of observations suggest that such a process may be operative in patients with schizophrenia since several types of physical abnormalities have been described in them that appear to be due to abnormalities of development.

Several authors have put forth CNS developmental theories of schizophrenia (Weinberger, 1987; Haracz, 1984, 1985; Feinberg, 1982/3; Gattaz *et al.*, 1987; Conrad and Scheibel, 1987). The substrate for these theories is based on the prolonged nature of CNS development and the widespread neuroanatomical and functional neurological abnormalities seen in schizophrenia. The human CNS undergoes a prolonged period of maturation and is presumably vulnerable, until young adulthood, to insults such as aIFN would provide, i.e., inhibition of cellular differentiation and proliferation. More specifically, CNS organizational events, including synaptic development, synaptic pruning, and glial proliferation and differentiation, occur from gestation to several years of age (Volpe, 1987). The frontal cortex has a prolonged period of maturation, and cell differentiation and development of the cortical sublayers continue to the age of puberty (Orzhekhovskaya, 1981). Further, the frontal cortical neurons undergo extensive elaboration after birth (Goldman-Rakic *et al.*, 1983), and the synaptic density changes from birth to adolescence (Huttenlocher, 1979). Using a variety of techniques, abnormalities have been found in most areas of the CNS of schizophrenic patients. These include ventricular enlargement and sulcal widening (reviewed in Shelton and Weinberger, 1986), decreased size of medial limbic structures (Bogerts *et al.*, 1985), disorientation of hippocampal pyramidal cells (Scheibel and Kovelman, 1981; Kovelman and Scheibel, 1986; Altshuler *et al.*, 1987), and a variable incidence of cerebellar vermis atrophy (reviewed in Weinberger *et al.*, 1983). The variety of findings as well as the type of findings generally leads to the conclusion that there is an influence on CNS development in schizophrenic patients.

The aforementioned developmental theories came to differing conclusions about the most likely time period of a developmental insult with the extremes being Weinberger (1987) arguing for an intrauterine lesion that interacts with subsequent development while Feinberg (1982/3) argues for a developmental process, possibly a slow virus, that interferes with the normal decrease in synaptic density during adolescence. It is beyond the scope of this chapter to critically review the evidence in support of an earlier versus later CNS developmental influence or for an underlying pattern in the reported abnormalities. The aIFN theory provides a framework to account for early as well as ongoing developmental abnormalities because of aIFN's effects on cellular proliferation and differentiation. In the situation of excessive aIFN effect, early development would be influenced when aIFN may be playing a role as a growth factor in the intrauterine environment. Developmental abnormalities during the extensive synaptic remodeling of adolescence would also be expected because of aIFN's action as a cell cycle inhibitor.

With respect to the periphery, it has been observed that patients with schizophrenia have an excess of physical abnormalities compared with normal controls. Most of these abnormalities are of types thought to be associated with developmental processes and, because of the extra-CNS location, imply a systemic process. These include increased numbers of dermatoglyphic abnormalities (Mellor, 1968; Polednak, 1972), minor physical anomalies (Guy *et al.*, 1983; Green *et al.*, 1987; Gualtieri *et al.*, 1982), and abnormal nailfold capillary morphology (Maricq, 1966a, b; Buchanan and Jones, 1969). Similar minor physical anomalies are also relatively common in individuals with mental retardation (Firestone *et al.*, 1978), hyperactivity (Gualtieri *et al.*, 1982; Firestone *et al.*, 1978; Waldrop *et al.*, 1968; Quinn and Rapoport, 1974), and in children having experienced *in utero* viral infections (Wright *et al.*, 1972). Of special interest in this context is the fact that abnormal dermatoglyphics and nailfold capillary morphology, similar to those seen in schizophrenic patients, are common in individuals with trisomy of chromosome 21 or Down's syndrome (Fang, 1950; Higashino and Moss, 1967). The development of the Waldrop scale for measurement of minor physical anomalies was based on anomalies that are common in Down's syndrome (Waldrop *et al.*, 1968). Further, the receptor for aIFN is located on the distal half of the long arm of chromosome 21 (21q22) (Epstein and Epstein, 1976) and trisomy of this area is reported to be sufficient to result in the intellectual deficits, facial abnormalities, and cardiac anomalies of Down's syndrome (Rethore, 1981). Also, as noted previously, cell lines that are trisomic for chromosome 21 have increased sensitivity to aIFN (Tan *et al.*, 1975; Epstein and Epstein, 1980) as have individuals with Down's syndrome (Nurmi *et al.*, 1982; Epstein and Epstein, 1982). Thus, schizophrenic patients may share a hyperresponsiveness to aIFN with individuals having Down's syndrome, and this may explain the occurrence of minor physical abnormalities in both. However, the similarities probably end there because the mechanisms of aIFN hypersensitivity are likely different in the two groups, with the Down's syndrome patients having many additional abnormalities of the CNS and other organ systems.

Many viruses are able to invade the developing human fetus, and viral teratology is a well-known phenomenon (Overall, 1981; Sever, 1982). However, many viral infections of the fetus and newborn are acutely asymptomatic and do not appear to produce serious sequelae. Perhaps the best example of this phenomenon is intrauterine or neonatal HCMV infection (Monif *et al.*, 1972). In the United States, approximately 1% of all neonates are congenitally infected with HCMV and are actively secreting the virus at birth (Nankervis and Kumar, 1978; Hanshaw, 1971). Of these children, approximately 10% have clinically apparent infections with signs and symptoms ranging from petechiae to full cytomegalic inclusion disease which includes microcephaly, hepatosplenomegaly, and chorioretinitis, and is fatal in a substantial proportion of the affected infants (Dorfman, 1978). Of the remaining 90% of the infected children, most will remain asymptomatic although many of them will develop learning disabilities, demonstrate mental retardation, or be found to have sensorineural hearing losses as they grow older (Stagno *et al.*, 1984; Reynolds *et al.*, 1974; Yow *et al.*, 1988). Based upon the recent identification of latent HCMV in the brains of normal individuals (Toorkey and Carrigan, 1989), it is likely that latent virus is present in the CNS and other organs of many, if not all, of these congenitally infected children. Similar latent infections may also be established by a number of other viruses, especially ones that cause few symptomatic acute infections in the newborns since they would escape notice and any relationship to diseases occurring later in life would be very difficult to establish.

Therefore, periodic reactivations of these latent viruses within the CNS and other organs may begin before birth and, if so, would occur during fetal growth and development as well as during the rapid growth period following birth. These reactivations would periodically expose developing CNS and other tissues to aIFN since the capacity to produce it is established early in embryonic development in mammals (Greene *et al.*, 1984). In most instances the damage caused by this process would probably be minor; however, in individuals hyperresponsive to aIFN the cumulative effects could lead to a wide variety of physical defects.

Thus, within the context of the proposed model, two factors may be interactively operative to produce the spectrum of findings in schizophrenia: (1) an excess of aIFN during development as it functions as a normal developmental modulator, and (2) the establishment of intrauterine and postnatal viral infections. Since development of the CNS extends well into adult life, the defects induced would accumulate over a long period of time and may contribute to the chronic negative symptoms and neuropsychological deficits seen in many patients. Since psychosis is postulated to result from viral reactivation, the full expression of schizophrenia would require both the aIFN defect and a reactivating viral flora. Schizophrenia spectrum disorders, such as schizotypal personality or Crow's pure type II syndrome (Crow *et al.*, 1986), may require only the aIFN defect.

RESEARCH DIRECTIONS

The aIFN theory proposed here suggests future research in two ways. First, the hypothesis is focused upon a few components of several complex biological systems, i.e., viral latency, biological response modifiers, regulation of the immune response, and the physiology of the CNS in schizophrenics. By creating a context in which other components of these systems can be viewed, the theory suggests ways in which its own conceptual base can be expanded. For example, we have thus far focused our attention on the possible role of aIFN in schizophrenia. However, there are several other cytokines, such as the interleukins and tumor necrosis factors, that may also be involved since they are produced concurrently with aIFN during immune responses. These cytokines have received less study in terms of their effects on the nervous system and are not as readily formulated into formal hypotheses related to schizophrenia.

Ongoing Theory Development

As is the case with aIFN, both macrophage-derived tumor necrosis factor-alpha (TNF-a) and interleukin 1 (IL-1) have a large spectrum of biological effects and may be quite active within the nervous system. For example, the presence of IL-1-immunoreactive neurons in brain has recently been reported (Breder *et al.*, 1988), suggesting a broader role for this particular mediator within the CNS than its known property of fever induction (Dinarello, 1985). Thus, the effects of IL-1 and TNF-a on neurons in cell culture and in the CNS itself should be studied using procedures already applied to aIFN. The possibility that each mediator may cause a distinctive change in the physiology of neurons, or selectively affect different regions of the CNS is intriguing and would yield information that is valuable for understanding the pathophysiology of encephalitides and possibly other CNS diseases of putative viral or immune etiology, such as schizophrenia and multiple sclerosis.

The postulated role of stress in the initiation and perpetuation of schizophrenic relapse provides another example of how the aIFN theory can help to structure future research. It is proposed that stress-induced immunosuppression leads to viral reactivation within the CNS and that this can lead to the onset of disease appearance or relapse. Since the basic components of this mechanism, such as stress predisposing to immunosuppression and to viral reactivation, have been demonstrated in experimental and clinical studies, it is important now to study whether stress-induced immunosuppression predisposes to schizophrenic relapse. This work will require prospective longitudinal designs, standardized definition of relapse and serial assessment of immune parameters to place the evidence of immune suppression causally distal to the stressor and proximal to the manifestations of relapse.

The second type of future research involves the direct testing of theory predictions.

Direct Testing of Theory Predictions

Excessive aIFN Responsiveness

If schizophrenia is caused by a genetically influenced, pathological production of aIFN or responsiveness toward it by schizophrenic patients, then these abnormalities should be demonstrable in patients with schizophrenia. The testing of this prediction will be complicated by the possible down-regulation of aIFN responses in the periphery of schizophrenic patients, as discussed above, and by the fact that serum and CSF levels of aIFN are not likely to be elevated during focal CNS viral reactivation due to dilutional factors. However, studies could be structured in either of two ways. First, an excessive production of aIFN by peripheral blood mononuclear cells from schizophrenic patients could be studied by using any of the many known aIFN inducers. Careful selection of controls would be necessary in order to assure interpretability of the results. For example, patients would have to be screened to exclude those with recent or current infections (e.g., fevers, systemic symptoms), and a protocol to induce aIFN in a standard fashion that yielded stable repeatable results (test-retest reliability) would have to be developed. Sex and age would have to be carefully controlled, since both are related to aIFN production (Bever *et al.*, 1985, 1988; Abb *et al.*, 1984). Also, careful consideration would have to be given to the clinical status of the patients since their aIFN responsiveness might be expected to vary with their relapse and remission status.

The responsiveness hypothesis could be tested by inducing aIFN production *in vivo* by use of inducing agents such as poly-IC since such studies have been reported in normal individuals as well as those with various diseases (Bever *et al.*, 1985, 1988). Quantification of the aIFN responses induced in the subjects could rely both on the direct measurement of serum aIFN and on the measurement of one or more intracellular proteins induced by aIFN. 2′, 5′-Oligoadenylate synthetase and protein kinase C are two of the intracellular proteins that have received study in this regard and have been used to monitor experimental (Barouki *et al.*, 1987) and therapeutic administration of aIFN (Furuta *et al.*, 1987) as well as viral infections (Williams *et al.*, 1982). The simultaneous measurement of both serum aIFN levels and aIFN-induced intracellular proteins would also provide a quantitative assessment of the responsiveness of the patients toward aIFN. Confirmation of the data obtained could be accomplished by the exogenous administration of aIFN to the subjects followed by measurement of the induced intracellular proteins.

Developmental and Symptomatic Aspects of Schizophrenia

The aIFN hypothesis allows several predictions to be made concerning the relationships between schizophrenia and developmental abnormalities such as minor physical anomalies, capillary nailfold abnormalities, dermatoglyphic abnormalities, negative and deficit symptoms, and CNS morphological abnormalities. aIFN is normally found in amniotic fluid in humans (Chany *et al.*, 1982; Tan and Inoue, 1982; Lebon *et al.*, 1982) and thought to play a role in normal development. aIFN is also produced constitutively in the normal adult (Mannering and Deloria, 1986). Severe dysregulation in aIFN sensitivity would be expected to be associated with effects on development occurring *in utero* and postnatally. Abnormal sensitivity may result in low-grade aIFN behavioral toxicity from the constitutively produced aIFN (Waltrip *et al.*, 1990).

The population of patients with developmental stigmata would, in general, be expected to contain the patients with the most severe dysregulation of aIFN as well as patients with both a lesser degree of aIFN sensitivity and viral exposure *in utero*. Patients with the most severe aIFN dysregulation may, however, not have the most severe course of positive symptoms in all cases because they may not happen to have a CNS viral flora that is reactivating to provide the driving force for psychotic exacerbation. As explained earlier, it may be that patients with a relatively large constitutional defect in aIFN sensitivity and no reactivating viral flora are those patients who have schizophrenia spectrum disorders, such as schizotypal personality features or a more pure negative symptom picture (Crow's type II) (Crow *et al.*, 1986) resulting from CNS hypersensitivity to constitutively produced aIFN. Thus, associations between developmental stigmata and (1) negative symptoms, (2) schizophrenia-spectrum personality features, and (3) CNS morphological abnormalities are predicted.

EPILOGUE

In closing, the primary benefit that a detailed theoretical construction such as the one presented here provides is a rationale to bring areas of science together that do not usually interact. The organizing framework provided helps to focus and give direction to new areas of investigation and facilitates reevaluation of past studies from a fresh perspective. Since our hypothesis is based on a limited number of assumptions about subtle deviations from normal conditions, the research emanating from this theory is quite likely to yield information of fundamental relevance to the various disciplinary fields involved and suggest areas of further work and other disease conditions to which the ideas may apply.

ACKNOWLEDGMENTS. This work was supported by the following grants: NARSAD Award, MH09595-02, MH00814-01A1, MH40279-03, NS24665-03.

REFERENCES

Abb, J., 1985, Serum interferon and clinical manifestations of infection with human T-lymphotropic virus type III, *Med. Microbiol. Immunol.* **174**:205–210.

Abb, J., Abb, H., and Deinhardt, F., 1984, Age-related decline of human interferon alpha and interferon gamma production, *Blut* **48**:285–289.

Adams, F., Quesada, J. R., and Gutterman, J. U., 1984, Neuropsychiatric manifestations of human leukocyte interferon therapy in patients with cancer, *J. Am. Med. Assoc.* **252**:938–941.

Ahokas, A., Rimon, R., Koskiniemi, M., Vaheri, A., Julkunen, I., and Sarna, S., 1987, Viral antibodies and interferon in acute psychiatric disorders, *J. Clin. Psychiatry* **48**:194–196.

Albrecht, P., Boone, E., Torrey, E. F., Hicks, J. T., and Daniel, N., 1980b, Raised cytomegalovirus-antibody level in cerebrospinal fluid of schizophrenic patients, *Lancet* **2**:769–772.

Altshuler, L. L., Conrad, A., Kovelman, J. A., and Scheibel, A., 1987, Hippocampal pyramidal cell orientation in schizophrenia, *Arch. Gen. Psychiatry* **44**:1094–1098.

Arnheiter, E. R. H., and Haller, O., 1987. Microinjection of an antibody to the interferon induced Mx protein inhibits the establishment of an antiviral state, *Experientia* **43**:690.

Baker, H. F., Bloxham, C., Crow, T. J., Davies, H., Ferrier, I. N., Johnstone, E. C., Parry, R. P., Ridley, R. M., Taylor, G. R., and Tyrrell, D. A. J., 1983, The viral hypothesis of schizophrenia: Some experimental approaches, in: *Research on the Viral Hypothesis of Mental Disorders*, (P. V. Morozov, ed.), Karger, Basel, pp. 1–19.

Baringer, J. R., 1975, Herpes simplex virus infection of nervous tissue in animals and man, *Prog. Med. Virol.* **20**:1–26.

Barouki, F. M., Witter, F. R., Griffin, D. E., Nadler, P. I., Woods, A., Wood, D. L., and Lietman, P. S., 1987, Time course of interferon levels, antiviral state, 2′,5′-oligoadenylate synthetase and side effects in healthy men, *J. Interferon Res.* **7**:29–39.

Bartrop, R. W., Luckhurst, E., Lazarus, L., Kiloh, L. G., and Penny, R., 1977, Depressed lymphocyte function after bereavement, *Lancet* **1**:834–836.

Bever, C. T., McFarlin, D. E., and Levy, H. B., 1985, A comparison of interferon responses to poly ICLC in males and females, *J. Interferon Res.* **5**:423–428.

Bever, C. T., McFarland, H. F., McFarlin, D. E., and Levy, H. B., 1988, The kinetics of interferon induction by poly ICLC in humans, *J. Interferon Res.* **8**:419–425.

Blalock, J. E., and Smith, E. M., 1980, Human leukocyte interferon: Structural and biological relatedness to adrenocorticotropic hormone and endorphins, *Proc. Natl. Acad. Sci. USA* **77**:5972–5974.

Blalock, J. E., and Smith, E. M., 1981, Human leukocyte interferon (HuIFN-a): Potent endorphin-like opioid activity, *Biochem. Biophys. Res. Commun.* **101**:472–478.

Bogerts, B., Meertz, E., and Schonfeldt-Bausch, R., 1985, Basal ganglia and limbic system pathology in schizophrenia, *Arch. Gen. Psychiatry* **42**:784–791.

Borden, E. C., and Murphy, F. A., 1971, The interferon refractory state: In vivo and in vitro studies of its mechanism, *J. Immunol.* **106**:134–142.

Borden, E. C., Prochowinik, E. V., and Carter, W. A., 1975, The interferon refractory state: II. Biological characterization of a refractoriness-inducing protein, *J. Immunol.* **114**:752–756.

Bottomley, J. M., and Toy, J. L., 1985, Clinical side effects and toxicities of interferon, in: *Interferon 4: In Vivo and Clinical Studies*, (N. B. Finter and R. K. Oldham, eds.), Amsterdam, Elsevier, pp. 155–180.

Brahic, M., Smith, R. A., Gibbs, C. J., Jr., Garruto, R. M., Tourtellotte, W. W., and Cash, E., 1985, Detection of picornavirus sequences in nervous tissue of amyotrophic lateral sclerosis and control patients, *Ann. Neurol.* **18**:337–343.

Breder, C. D., Dinarello, C. A., and Saper, C. B., 1988, Interleukin-1 immunoreactive innervation of the human hypothalamus, *Science* **240**:321–324.

Buchanan, C. E., and Jones, M. B., 1969, A within family study of schizophrenia and a visible subpapillary plexus in the nailfold, *Schizophrenia* **1**:61–75.

Budka, H., Costanzi, G., Cristina, S., Lechi, A., Parravicini, C., Trabattoni, R., and Vago, L., 1987, Brain pathology induced by infection with the human immunodeficiency virus (HIV): A histological, immunocytochemical, and electron microscopical study of 100 autopsy cases, *Acta Neuropathol.* **75**:185–198.

Buhrich, N., Cooper, D. A., and Freed, E., 1988, HIV infection associated with symptoms indistinguishable from functional psychosis, *Br. J. Psychiatry* **152**:649–653.

Buimovici-Klein, E., Lange, M., Klein, R. J., Grieco, M. H., and Cooper, L. Z., 1986, Long-term follow-up of serum-interferon and its acid-stability in a group of homosexual men, *AIDS Res.* **2(2)**:99–108.

Calvet, M., and Gressor, I., 1979, Interferon enhances the excitability of cultured neurones, *Nature* **278**:558–560.

Capobianchi, M. R., DeMarco, F., DiMarco, P., and Dianzani, F., 1988, Acid-labile human interferon alpha production by peripheral blood mononuclear cells stimulated by HIV-infected cells, *Arch. Virol.* **99**:9–19.

Carpenter, W. T., 1987, Approaches to knowledge and understanding of schizophrenia, *Schiz. Bull.* **13**:1–8.

Carpenter, W. T., and Buchanan, R. W., 1989, Domains of psychopathology relevant to the study of etiology and treatment of schizophrenia, in: *Schizophrenia: Scientific Progress* (S. C. Schultz, and C. T. Tamminga, eds.), Oxford University Press, London, pp. 13–23.

Carpenter, W. T., and Kirkpatrick, B., 1989, The heterogeneity of longterm course schizophrenia: Implications for future research, *Schiz. Bull.* **14:**645–652.

Carpenter, W. T., Heinrichs, D. W., and Hanlon, T. E., 1987, A comparative trial of pharmacologic strategies in schizophrenia, *Am. J. Psychiatry* **144:**1466–1470.

Carpenter, W. T., Heinrichs, D. W., and Wagman, A. M. I., 1988, Deficit and nondeficit forms of schizophrenia: The concept, *Am. J. Psychiatry* **145:**578–583.

Carter, M., and Watts, C. A. H., 1971, Possible biological advantages among schizophrenics' relatives, *Br. J. Psychiatry* **118:**453–460.

Chany, C., Duc-Goiran, P., Robert-Galliot, B., Chudzio, T., and Lebon, P., 1982, Study of human amniotic interferon, in: *Interferons* (T. C. Merigan and R. M. Friedman, eds.), Academic Press, New York, pp. 241–248.

Ciompi, L., 1980, Catamnestic long-term study on the course of life and aging of schizophrenics, *Schiz. Bull.* **6:**606–618.

Clemens, M. J., and McNurlan, M. A., 1985, Regulation of cell proliferation and differentiation by interferons, *Biochem. J.* **226:**345–360.

Conrad, A. J., and Scheibel, A. B., 1987, Schizophrenia and the hippocampus: The embryological hypothesis extended, *Schiz. Bull.* **13:**577–587.

Cools, A. R., Wiegant, V. M., and Gispen, W. H., 1978, Distinct dopaminergic systems in ACTH-induced grooming, *Eur. J. Pharmacol.* **50:**265–268.

Creasey, A. A., Vitt, C. R., Herst, C., O'Rourke, E., Doyle, L., Innis, M. A., McCabe, P. C., McCormick, F., Milley, R., Lin, L. S., and White, T. J., 1988, Functional properties of proteins coded by three human a-interferon genes and a pseudogene, *Cancer Res.* **48:**1763–1770.

Crow, T. J., 1984, A re-evaluation of the viral hypothesis: Is psychosis the result of retroviral integration at a site close to the cerebral dominance gene? *Br. J. Psychiatry* **145:**243–253.

Crow, T. J., 1986, The continuum of psychosis and its implication for the structure of the gene, *Br. J. Psychiatry* **149:**419–429.

Crow, T. J., 1987a, A pseudoautosomal locus for psychosis?*Lancet* **2:**1532.

Crow, T. J., 1987b, Genes and viruses in schizophrenia: The retrovirus transposon hypothesis, in: *Viruses, Immunity, and Mental Disorders* (E. Kurstak, Z. J. Lipowski, and P. V. Morozov, eds.), Plenum Press, New York, pp. 125–134.

Crow, T. J., Taylor, G. R., and Tyrrell, D. A. J., 1986, Two syndromes in schizophrenia and the viral hypothesis, *Prog. Brain Res.* **65:**17–27.

Dafny, N., 1983, Modification of morphine withdrawal by interferon, *Life Sciences* **32:**303–305.

Dafny, N., Prieto-Gomez, B., and Reyes-Vazquez, C., 1985, Does the immune system communicate with the central nervous system? Interferon modifies central nervous activity, *J. Neuroimmunol.* **9:**1–12.

Day, R., 1981, Life events and schizophrenia: The "triggering" hypothesis, *Acta Psychiatr. Scand.* **64:**97–122.

DeLisi, L. E., 1984, Is immune dysfunction associated with schizophrenia? A review of the data, *Psychopharmacol. Bull.* **20:**509–513.

DeLisi, L. E., and Crow, T. J., 1986, Is schizophrenia a viral or immunologic disorder? *Psychiatr. Clin. North Am.* **9:**115–132.

Dinarello, C. A., 1985, An update on human interleukin-1: From molecular biology to clinical relevance, *J. Clin. Immunol.* **5:**287–297.

Dorfman, L. J., 1978, Cytomegalic inclusion disease, in: *Infections of the Nervous System* (P. F. Vinken and G. W. Bruyn, eds.), North-Holland, Amsterdam, pp. 209–233.

Drayer, B. P., and Barrett, L., 1984, Magnetic resonance imaging and CT scanning in multiple sclerosis, *Ann. N.Y. Acad. Sci.* **436:**294–314.

Dunnick, J. K., and Galasso, G. J., 1980, Update on clinical trials with exogenous interferon, *J. Infect. Dis.* **142:**293–299.

Elder, G. A., and Sever, J. L., 1988, Neurologic disorders associated with AIDS retroviral infection, *Rev. Infect. Dis.* **10**:286–295.

Engelhard, D., Marks, M. I., and Good, R. A., 1986, Infections in bone marrow transplant recipients, *J. Pediatr.* **108**:335–346.

Epstein, C. J., and Epstein, L. B., 1982, Genetic control of the response to interferon, *Tex. Rep. Biol. Med.* **41**:324–331.

Epstein, C. J., McManus, N. H., Epstein, L. B., Branaca, A. A., D'Alessandro, S. B., and Baglione, C., 1982, Evidence that the gene product of the human chromosome 21 locus, IFRC, is the interferon-alpha receptor, *Biochem. Biophys. Res. Commun.* **107**:1060–1066.

Epstein, L. B., and Epstein, C. J., 1976, Localization of the gene AVG for the antiviral expression of immune and classical interferon to the distal portion of the long arm of chromosome 21, *J. Infect. Dis.* **133(Suppl)**:A56–A62.

Epstein, L. B., and Epstein, C. J., 1980, T lymphocyte function and sensitivity to interferon in trisomy 21, *Cell Immunol.* **51**:303–318.

Falloon, I. R. H., 1986, Family stress and schizophrenia, *Psychiatr. Clin. North Am.* **9**:165–182.

Falloon, I. R. H., Marshall, G. N., Boyd, J. L., Razani, J., and Wood-Severio, C., 1983, Relapse in schizophrenia: A review of the concept and its definitions, *Psychol. Med.* **13**:469–477.

Fang, T. C., 1950, The third interdigital patterns on the palms of the general British population, mongoloid and non-mongoloid mental defectives, *J. Ment. Sci.* **96**:780–787.

Farkkila, M., Iivanainen, M., Roine, R., Bergstrom, L., Laaksonen, R., Niemi, M. L., and Cantell, K., 1984, Neurotoxic and other side effects of high-dose interferon in amyotrophic lateral sclerosis, *Acta Neurol. Scand.* **69**:42–46.

Feinberg, I., 1982/3, Schizophrenia: Caused by a fault in programmed synaptic elimination during adolescence? *J. Psychiatr. Res.* **17**:319–334.

Firestone, P., Peters, S., and Rivier, M., 1978, Minor physical anomalies in hyperactive, retarded and normal children and their families, *Child Psychol. Psychiatry* **19**:155–160.

Fisher, P. B., Mufson, R. A., and Weinstein, I. B., 1981, Interferon inhibits melanogenesis in B-16 mouse melanoma cells, *Biochem. Biophys. Res. Commun.* **100**:823–830.

Fisher, P. B., Miranda, A. F., Babiss, L. E., Pestka, S., and Weinstein, I. B., 1983, Opposing effects of interferon produced in bacteria and of tumor promoters on myogenesis in human myoblast cultures, *Proc. Natl. Acad. Sci. USA* **80**:2961–2965.

Fraser, N. W., Lawrence, W. C., Wroblewska, Z., Gilden, D. H., and Koprowski, H., 1981, Herpes simplex type 1 DNA in human brain tissue, *Proc. Natl. Acad. Sci. USA* **78**:6461–6465.

Furuta, M., Akashi, K., Nakamura, Y., Matsumoto, K., Yamaguchi, H., Takamatsu, S., and Shimizu, T., 1987, 2', 5'-oligoadenylate synthetase activity in peripheral blood lymphocytes as a clinical marker in interferon therapy for chronic hepatitis B, *J. Interferon Res.* **7**:111–119.

Gajdusek, D. C., 1985, Unconventional viruses causing subacute spongiform encephalopathies, in: *Virology* (B. N. Fields, D. M. Knipe, R. M. Chanock, J. L. Melnick, B. Roizman, and R. E. Shope, eds.), Raven Press, New York, pp. 1519–1557.

Gattaz, W. F., Kohlmeyer, K., and Gasser, T., 1987, Structural brain abnormalities in schizophrenia, in: *Search for the Causes of Schizophrenia* (H. Hafner, W. F. Gattaz, and W. Janzarik, eds.), Springer-Verlag, Berlin, pp. 250–259.

Giulian D., Baker, T. J., Shih, L. N., and Lachman, L. B., 1986, Interleukin 1 of the central nervous system is produced by ameboid microglia, *J. Exp. Med.* **164**:594–604.

Glaser, R., Kiecolt-Glaser, J. K., Speicher, C. E., and Holliday, J. E., 1985, Stress, loneliness, and changes in herpesvirus latency, *J. Behav. Med.* **8**:249–260.

Goldberg, S. C., 1985, Negative and deficit symptoms do respond to neuroleptics, *Schiz. Bull.* **11**:453–456.

Goldman-Rakic, P. S., Isseroff, A., Schwartz, M. L., and Bugbee, N. N., 1983, The neurobiology of cognitive development, in: *Handbook of Child Psychology, Biology and Infancy Development* (P. Mussen, ed.), Wiley, New York, pp. 281–344.

Goldmeier, D., and Johnson, A., 1982, Does psychiatric illness affect the recurrence rate of genital herpes? *Br. J. Vener. Dis.* **58**:40–43.

Gotlieb-Stematsky, T., Floru, S., Becker, D., Kritchman, E., and Leventon-Kriss, S., 1987, Antibody and cell-mediated immunity to herpes simplex and Epstein-Barr viruses in psychotic patients, in: *Viruses, Immunity, and Mental Disorders* (E. Kurstak, Z. J. Lipowski, and P. V. Morozov, eds.), Plenum Press, New york, pp. 173–177.

Green, M. F., Satz, P., Soper, H. V., and Kharabi, F., 1987, Relationship between physical anomalies and age at onset of schizophrenia, *Am J. Psychiatry* **144**:666–667.

Greene, J. J., Dyer, R. H., Yang, L. C., and Ts'o, P. O. P., 1984, Developmentally regulated expression of the interferon system during Syrian hamster embryogenesis, *J. Interferon Res.* **4**:517–527.

Gresser, I., Tovey, M. G., Bandu, M. T., Maury, C., and Brouty-Boye, D., 1976, Role of interferon in the pathogenesis of virus disease in mice as demonstrated by the use of anti-interferon serum: I. Rapid evolution of encephalomyocarditis virus infection, *J. Exp. Med.* **144**:1305–1323.

Gualtieri, C. T., Adams, A., Shen, C. D., and Loiselle, D., 1982, Minor physical anomalies in alcoholic and schizophrenic adults and hyperactive and autistic children, *Am. J. Psychiatry* **139**:640–643.

Guy, J. D., Majorski, L. V., Wallace, C. J., and Guy, M. P., 1983, The incidence of minor physical anomalies in adult male schizophrenics, *Schiz. Bull.* **9**:571–582.

Haase, A. T., Ventura, P., Gibbs, C. J., and Tourtellotte, W. W., 1981, Measles virus nucleotide sequences: Detection by hybridization in situ, *Science* **212**:672–675.

Haase, A. T., Stowring, L., Ventura, P., Burks, J., Ebers, G., Tourtellotte, W., and Warren K., 1984, Detection by hybridization of viral infection of the human central nervous system, *Ann. N.Y. Acad. Sci.* **436**:103–108.

Halevie-Goldman, B. D., Potkin, S. G., and Poyourow, P., 1987, AIDS-related complex presenting as psychosis, *Am. J. Psychiatry* **144**:964.

Haller, O., Arnheiter, H., Lindenmann, J., and Gresser, I., 1980, Host gene influences sensitivity to interferon action selectively for influenza virus, *Nature* **283**:660–662.

Haller, O., Arnheiter, H., Gresser, I., and Lindenmann, J., 1981, Virus-specific interferon action: Protection of newborn Mx carriers against lethal infection with influenza virus, *J. Exp. Med.* **154**:199–203.

Hammer, M., and Zubin, J., 1968, Evolution, culture, and psychopathology, *J. Gen. Psychol.* **78**: 151–164.

Hanninen, P., Arstila, P., Lang, H., Salmi, A., and Panelius, M., 1980, Involvement of the central nervous system in acute, uncomplicated measles virus infection, *J. Clin. Microbiol.* **11**:610–613.

Hanshaw, J. B., 1971, Congenital cytomegalovirus infection: A fifteen year perspective, *J. Infect. Dis.* **123**:555–561.

Haracz, J. L., 1984, Neural plasticity hypothesis of schizophrenia, *Neurosci. Biobehav. Rev.* **8**:55–71.

Haracz, J. L., 1985, Neural plasticity in schizophrenia, *Schiz. Bull.* **11**:191–229.

Hendrick, I., 1928, Encephalitis lethargica and the interpretation of mental disease, *Am. J. Psychiatry* **7**:989–1014.

Higashino, S. M., and Moss, A. J., 1967, Capillary microscopy: Abnormalities in cystic fibrosis, congenital heart disease, and mongolism, *Am. J. Dis. Child.* **113**:439–443.

Huber, G., Gross, G., Schuttler, R., and Linz, M., 1980, Longitudinal studies of schizophrenic patients, *Schiz. Bull.* **6**:592–605.

Huttenlocher, P. R., 1979, Synaptic density in human frontal cortex—Developmental changes and effects of aging, *Brain Res.* **163**:195–205.

Huxley, J., Mayr, E., Osmond, H., and Hoffer, A., 1964, Schizophrenia as a genetic morphism, *Nature* **204**:220–221.

Iivanainen, M., Laaksonen, R., Niemi, M. L., Farkkila, M., Bergstrom, L., Mattson, K., Niiranen, A., and Cantell, K., 1985, Memory and psychomotor impairment following high-dose interferon treatment in amyotrophic lateral sclerosis, *Acta Neurol. Scand.* **72**:475–480.

Inglot, A. D., 1983, The hormonal concept of interferon, *Arch. Virol.* **76**:1–13.

Jarvik, L. F., and Chadwick, S. B., 1973, Schizophrenia and survival, in: *Psychopathology: Contributions from the Social, Behavioral, and Biological Sciences* (M. Hammer, K. Salzinger, and S. Sutton, eds.), Wiley, New York, pp. 57–73.

Johnson, K. P., and Carrigan, D. R., 1981, Neurologic diseases caused by measles virus, *Neurology* International Congress Series No. 568: 404–415.

Johnson, R. T., 1982, *Viral Infections of the Nervous System*, Raven Press, New York.

Jordan, M. C., 1983, Latent infection and the elusive cytomegalovirus, *Rev. Infect. Dis.* **5**:205–215.

Kasl, S. V., Evans, A. S., and Niederman, J. C., 1979, Psychosocial risk factors in the development of infectious mononucleosis, *Psychosom. Med.* **41**:445–466.

Kaufmann, C. A., Weinberger, D. R., Yolken, R. H., Torrey, E. F., and Potkin, S. G., 1983, Viruses and schizophrenia, *Lancet* **2**:1136–1137.

Keith, S. J., and Matthews, S. M., eds., 1988, Issue theme: A national plan for schizophrenia research, *Schiz. Bull.* **14**.

Kendell, R. E., 1975, *The Role of Diagnosis in Psychiatry*, Blackwell, Oxford.

King, D. J., Cooper, S. J., Earle, J. A. P., Martin, S. J., McFerran, N. V., Rima, B. K., and Wisdom, G. B., 1985a, A survey of serum antibodies to eight common viruses in psychiatric patients, *Br. J. Psychiatry* **147**:137–144.

King, D. J., Cooper, S. J., Earle, J. A. P., Martin, S. J., McFerran, N. V., and Wisdom, G. B., 1985b, Serum and CSF antibody titres to seven common viruses in schizophrenic patients, *Br. J. Psychiatry* **147**:145–149.

Klein, R. J., 1982, The pathogenesis of acute, latent and recurrent herpes simplex virus infections, *Arch. Virol.* **72**:143–168.

Kovelman, J. A., and Scheibel, A. B., 1986, A neurohistological correlate of schizophrenia, *Biol. Psychiatry* **19**:1601–1621.

Kraepelin, E., 1919, *Dementia Praecox and Paraphrenia*, Livingstone, Edinburgh.

Larsson, I., Landstrom, L., Larner, E., Lundgren, E., Miorner, H., and Strannegard, O., 1978, Interferon production in glia and glioma cell lines, *Infect. Immun.* **22**:786–789.

Lebon, P., Girard, S., Thepot, F., and Chany, C., 1982, The presence of alpha-interferon in human amniotic fluid, *J. Gen. Virol.* **59**:393–396.

Leff, J., Kuipers, L., Berkowitz, R., Eberlein-Vries, R., and Sturgeon, D., 1982, A controlled trial of social intervention in the families of schizophrenic patients, *Br. J. Psychiatry* **141**:121–134.

Lewine, R. R. J., 1981, Sex differences in schizophrenia: Timing or subtypes? *Psychol. Bull.* **90**: 432–444.

Libikova, H., Stancek, D., Wiedermann, V., Hasto, J., and Breier, S., 1977, Psychopharmaca and electroconvulsive therapy in relation to viral antibodies and interferon. Experimental and clinical study, *Arch. Immunol. Ther. Exp.* **25**:641–649.

Libikova, H., Breier, S., Kocisova, M., Pagady, J., Stunzner, D., and Ujhazyova, D., 1979, Assay of interferon and viral antibodies in the cerebrospinal fluid in clinical neurology and psychiatry, *Acta Biol. Med. Ger.* **38**:879–893.

Lok, A. S. F., Wu, P., Lai, C., and Leung, E. K. Y., 1988, Long-term follow-up in a randomised controlled trial of recombinant $alpha_2$-interferon in Chinese patients with chronic hepatitis B infection, *Lancet* **2**:298–302.

Lorenzo, P., Portoles, A., Jr., Beneit, J. V., Ronda, E., and Portoles, A., 1987, Physical dependence to morphine diminishes the interferon response in mice, *Immunopharmacology* **14**:93–100.

McCowan, P. K., and Cook, L. C., 1928, The mental aspect of chronic epidemic encephalitis, *Lancet* **1**:1316–1320.

McDonald, E. M., Mann, A. H., and Thomas, H. C., 1987, Interferons as mediators of psychiatric morbidity: An investigation in a trial of recombinant a-interferon in hepatitis-B carriers, *Lancet* **2**:1175–1178.

McHugh, P. R., and Slavney, P. R., 1983, *The Perspectives of Psychiatry*, The Johns Hopkins University Press, Baltimore.

McKinney, R. E., Jr., Katz, S. L., and Wilfert, C. M., 1987, Chronic enteroviral meningoencephalitis in agammaglobulinemic patients, *Rev. Infect. Dis.* **9**:334–356.

Mannering, G. J., and Deloria, L. B., 1986, The pharmacology and toxicology of the interferons: An overview, *Annu. Rev. Pharmacol. Toxicol.* **26**:455–515.

Maricq, H. R., 1966a, Familial schizophrenia as defined by nailfold capillary pattern and selected psychiatric traits, *J. Nerv. Ment. Dis.* **142**:369–375.

Maricq, H. R., 1966b, Capillary morphology and the course of illness in schizophrenic patients, *J. Nerv. Ment. Dis.* **142**:66–71.

Martelly, I., and Jullien, P., 1974, Effect of repeated injections of polyriboinosinic-polyribocytidylic acid on mouse hematopoietic stem cells, *J. Natl. Cancer Inst.* **53**:1021–1025.

Masdeu, J. C., Small, C. B., Weiss, L., Elkin, C. M., Llena, J., and Mesa-Tejada, R., 1988, Multifocal cytomegalovirus encephalitis in AIDS, *Ann. Neurol.* **23**:97–99.

Mattson, K., Niiranen, A., Iivanainen, M., Farkkilia, M., Bergstrom, I., Holsti, L. R., Kauppinen, H. L., and Cantell, K., 1983, Neurotoxicity of interferon, *Cancer Treat. Rep.* **67**:958–961.

Mellor, C. S., 1968, Dermatoglyphics in schizophrenia, *Br. J. Psychiatry* **114**:1387–1397.

Melnick, J. L., 1985, Enteroviruses: Polioviruses, coxsackieviruses, echoviruses, and newer enteroviruses, in: *Virology* (B. N. Fields, D. M. Knipe, R. M. Chanock, J. L. Melnick, B. Roizman, and R. E. Shope, eds.), Raven Press, New York, pp. 739–794.

Menninger, K., 1926, Influenza and schizophrenia, *Am. J. Psychiatry* **5**:469–529.

Menninger, K., 1928, The schizophrenic syndrome as a product of acute infectious disease, *Arch. Neurol. Psychiatry* **20**:464–481.

Merigan, T. C., Baer, G. M., Winkler, W. G., Bernard, K. W., Gibert, C. G., Chany, C., Veronesi, R., and the collaborative group, 1984, Human leukocyte interferon administration to patients with symptomatic and suspected rabies, *Ann. Neurol.* **16**:82–87.

Moises, H. W., Schindler, L., Lerous, M., and Kirchner, H., 1985, Decreased production of interferon alpha and interferon gamma in leucocyte cultures of schizophrenic patients, *Acta Psychiatr. Scand.* **72**:45–50.

Moises, H. W., Beck, H., Schindler, L., and Kirchner, H., 1986, Interferon production in schizophrenic patients, in: *Biological Psychiatry 1985* (C. H. Shagass, R. C. Josiassen, W. H. Bridger, K. J. Weiss, D. Stoff, and G. M. Simpson eds.), Elsevier, Amsterdam, pp. 1098–1100.

Monif, G. R. G., Egan, E. A., II, Held, B., and Eitzman, D. V., 1972, The correlation of maternal cytomegalovirus infection during varying stages in gestation with neonatal involvement, *J. Pediatr.* **80**:17–20.

Monjan, A. A., 1981, Stress and immunologic competence: Studies in animals, in: *Psychoneuroimmunology* (R. Ader, ed.), Academic Press, New York, pp. 185–228.

Murray, R. M., and Reveley, A. M., 1983, Schizophrenia as an infection, *Lancet* **I**:583.

Nair, M. P., and Schwartz, S. A., 1984, Association of decreased T-cell-mediated natural cytotoxicity and interferon production in Down's syndrome, *Clin. Immunol. Immunopathol.* **33**:412–424.

Nankervis, G. A., and Kumar, M. L., 1978, Diseases produced by cytomegaloviruses, *Med. Clin. North Am.* **62**:1021–1035.

Nurmi, T., Huttunen, K., Lassila, O., Henttonen, M., Sakkinen, A., Linna, S. L., and Tiilikainen, A., 1982, Natural killer cell function in trisomy-21 (Down's syndrome), *Clin. Exp. Immunol.* **47**: 735–741.

Nurnberg, H. G., Prudic, J., Fiori, M., and Freedman, E. P., 1984, Psychopathology complicating acquired immune deficiency syndrome (AIDS), *Am. J. Psychiatry* **141**:95–96.

Orzhekhovskaya, N. S., 1981, Frontal-striatal relationships in primate ontogeny, *Neurosci. Behav. Physiol.* **11**:379–385.

Overall, J. C., 1981, Viral infections of the fetus and newborn, in: *Textbook of Pediatric Infectious Diseases* (R. D. Feigin and J. D. Cherry, eds.), Saunders, Philadelphia, pp. 684–721.

Perl, D. P., 1975, The pathology of rabies in the central nervous system, in: *The Natural History of Rabies* (G. M. Baer, ed.), Academic Press, New York, pp. 235–272.

Polednak, A. P., 1972, Dermatoglyphics of Negro schizophrenic males, *Br. J. Psychiatry* **120**:397–398.

Poser, C. M., 1980, Exacerbations, activity, and progression in multiple sclerosis, *Arch. Neurol.* **37**:471–474.

Preble, O. T., and Torrey, E. F., 1985, Serum interferon in patients with psychosis, *Am. J. Psychiatry* **142**:1184–1186.

Prentice, R. L., Dalgleish, A. G., Gatenby, P. A., Loblay, R. H., Wade, S., Kappagoda, N., and Basten, A., 1985, Central nervous system echovirus infection in Bruton's x-linked hypogammaglobulinemia, *Aust. N.Z. J. Med.* **15**:443–445.

Price, R. W., Brew, B., Sidtis, J., Rosenblum, M., Scheck, A. C., and Cleary, P., 1988, The brain in AIDS: Central nervous system HIV-1 infection and AIDS dementia complex, *Science* **239**: 586–592.

Quesada, J. R., Reuben, J., Manning, J. T., Hersh, E. M., and Gutterman, J. U., 1984, Alpha interferon for induction of remission in hairy cell leukemia, *N. Engl. J. Med.* **310**:15–18.

Quinn, P. O., and Rapoport, J. L., 1974, Minor physical anomalies and neurologic status in hyperactive boys, *Pediatrics* **53**:742–747.

Reinicke, V., Mordhorst, C. H., and Ingerslev, N., 1974, Central nervous system affection in connection with "ordinary" measles, *Scand. J. Infect. Dis.* **6**:131–135.

Reiss-Levy, E., Baker, A., Don, N., and Caldwell, G., 1986, Two concurrent epidemics of enteroviral meningitis in an obstetric neonatal unit, *Aust. N.Z. J. Med.* **16**:365–372.

Renault, P. F., Hoofnagle, J. H., Park, Y., Mullen, K. D., Peters, M., Jones, D. B., Rustgi, V., and Jones, E. A., 1987, Psychiatric complications of long-term interferon alfa therapy, *Ann. Intern. Med.* **147**:1577–1580.

Rethore, M., 1981, Structural variation of chromosome 21 and symptoms of Down's syndrome, *Hum. Genet.* **2**(Suppl):173–182.

Reynolds, D. W., Stagno, S., Stubbs, K. G., Dahle, A. J., Livingston, M. M., Saxon, S. S., and Alford, C. A., 1974, Inapparent congenital cytomegalovirus infection with elevated cord IgM levels, *N. Engl. J. Med.* **290**:291–296.

Rhodes-Feuillette, A., Canivet, M., Champsaur, H., Gluckman, E., Mazeron, M. C., and Peries, J., 1983, Circulating interferon in cytomegalovirus infected bone-marrow-transplant recipients and in infants with congenital cytomegalovirus disease, *J. Interferon Res.* **3**:45–52.

Rimón, R., Nishmi, M., and Halonen, P., 1978, Serum and CSF antibody levels to herpes simplex type I, measles, and rubella viruses in patients with schizophrenia, *Ann. Clin. Res.* **10**:291–293.

Rimón, R., Ahokas, A., Hintikka, J., and Heikkila, L., 1985, Serum interferon in schizophrenia, *Ann. Clin. Res.* **17**:139–140.

Robert-Guroff, M., Torrey, E. F., and Brown, M., 1985, Retroviruses and schizophrenia, *Br. J. Psychiatry* **146**:326.

Rodriguez, M., Leibowitz, J. L., and Lampert, P. W., 1983, Persistent infection of oligodendrocytes in Theiler's virus-induced encephalomyelitis, *Ann. Neurol.* **13**:426–433.

Roizman, B., and Sears, A. E., 1987, An inquiry into the mechanisms of herpes simplex virus latency, *Annu. Rev. Microbiol.* **41**:543–571.

Rosendorff, C., and Mooney, J. J., 1971, Central nervous system sites of action of purified leucocyte pyrogen, *Am. J. Physiol.* **220**:597–603.

Rossi, G. B., 1985, Interferons and cell differentiation, *Interferon* **6**:31–68.

Roy, A., Pickar, D., Ninan, P., Hooks, J., and Paul, S., 1985, A search for interferon in the CSF of chronic schizophrenic patients, *Am. J. Psychiatry* **142**:269.

Rubinstein, M., and Orchansky, P., 1986, The interferon receptors, *CRC Crit. Rev. Biochem.* **21:** 249–275.

Sands, I. J., 1928, The acute psychiatric type of epidemic encephalitis, *Am. J. Psychiatry* **7:**975–987.

Scheibel, A. B., and Kovelman, J. A., 1981, Disorientation of the hippocampal pyramidal cell and its processes in the schizophrenic patient, *Biol. Psychiatry* **16:**101–102.

Schindler, L., Leroux, M., Beck, J., Moises, H. W., and Kirchner, H., 1986, Studies of cellular immunity, serum interferon titers, and natural killer cell activity in schizophrenic patients, *Acta Psychiatr. Scand.* **73:**651–657.

Schleifer, S. J., Keller, S. E., Camerino, M., Thornton, C. J., and Stein, M., 1983, Suppression of lymphocyte stimulation following bereavement, *J. Am. Med. Assoc.* **250:**374–377.

Seeman, M. V., 1986, Current outcome in schizophrenia: Women vs. men, *Acta Psychiatr. Scand.* **73:**609–617.

Sekellick, M. J., and Marcus, P. I., 1980, The interferon system as a regulator of persistent infection, *Ann. N.Y. Acad. Sci.* **350:**545–557.

Sequiera, L. W., Carrasco, L. H., Curry, A., Jennings, L. C., Lord, M. A., and Sutton, R. N. P., 1979, Detection of herpes-simplex viral genome in brain tissue, *Lancet* **2:**609–612.

Sever, J. L., 1982, Infections in pregnancy, highlights from the collaborative perinatal project, *Teratology* **25:**227–237.

Shelton, R. C., and Weinberger, D. R., 1986, X-Ray computerized tomography studies of schizophrenia: A review and synthesis, in: *The Neurology of Schizophrenia* (H. A. Nasrallah, and D. R. Weinberger, eds.), Elsevier, Amsterdam, pp. 207–250.

Shrikhande, S., Hirsch, S. R., Coleman, J. C., Reveley, M. A., and Dayton, R., 1985, Cytomegalovirus and schizophrenia: A test of a viral hypothesis, *Br. J. Psychiatry* **146:**503–506.

Smedley, H., Katrak, M., Sikora, K., and Wheeler, T., 1983, Neurological effects of recombinant human interferon, *Br. Med. J.* **286:**262–264.

Smith, E. M., and Blalock, J. E., 1981–82, The hormonal nature of the interferon system, *Tex. Rep. Biol. Med.* **41:**350–358.

Smith, R. A., Norris, F., Palmer, D., Bernhardt, L., and Wills, R. J., 1985, Distribution of alpha interferon in serum and cerebrospinal fluid after systemic administration, *Clin. Pharmacol. Ther.* **37:**85–88.

Smith-Johannsen, H., Hou, Y.-T., Liu, X.-Y., and Tan, Y.-H., 1984, Regulatory control of interferon synthesis and action, *Handb. Exp. Pharmacol.* **71:**101–135.

Snyder, S. H., 1973, Amphetamine psychosis: A "model" schizophrenia mediated by catecholamines, *Am. J. Psychiatry* **130:**61–67.

Springer, J. E., Isaacson, R. L., Ryan, J. P., and Hannigan, J. H., Jr., 1983, Dopamine depletion in nucleus accumbens reduces $ACTH_{1-24}$-induced excessive grooming, *Life Sci.* **33:**207–211.

Staeheli, P., and Haller, O., 1985, Interferon-induced human protein with homology to protein Mx of influenza virus-resistant mice, *Mol. Cell. Biol.* **5:**2150–2153.

Stagno, S., Pass, R. F., Dworsky, M. E., Britt, W. J., and Alford, C. A., 1984, Congenital and perinatal cytomegalovirus infections: Clinical characteristics and pathogenic factors, *Birth Defects: Orig. Artic. Ser.* **20:**65–85.

Stevens, J. R., 1988, Schizophrenia and multiple sclerosis, *Schiz. Bull.* **14:**231–241.

Stevens, J. R., Langloss, J. M., Albrecht, P., Yolken, R., and Wang, Y.-N., 1984, A search for cytomegalovirus and herpes viral antigen in brains of schizophrenic patients, *Arch. Gen. Psychiatry* **41:**795–801.

Strauss, J. S., Carpenter, W. T., and Bartko, J. J., 1974, Towards an understanding of the symptom picture considered characteristic of schizophrenia: Its description, precursors and outcome, *Schiz. Bull.* **Winter:**61–69.

Stringfellow, D. A., Kern, E. R., Kelsey, D. K., and Glasgow, L. A., 1977, Suppressed response to interferon induction in mice infected with encephalomyocarditis virus, Semliki forest virus, influenza A2 virus, herpesvirus hominis type 2, or murine cytomegalovirus, *J. Infect. Dis.* **135**:540–551.

Suter, C. C., Westmoreland, B. F., Sharbrough, F. W., and Hermann, R. C., 1984, Electroencephalographic abnormalities in interferon encephalopathy: A preliminary report, *Mayo Clin. Proc.* **59**:847–850.

Tan, Y. H., and Inoue, M., 1982, The detection of interferon activity in human amniotic fluid, in: *Interferons* (T. C. Merigan and R. M. Friedman, eds.), Academic Press, New York, pp. 249–252.

Tan, Y. H., Chou, E. L., and Lundh, N., 1975, Regulation of chromosome 21-directed anti-viral gene(s) as a consequence of age, *Nature* **257**:310–312.

Taylor, G. R., Crow, T. J., Higgins, T., and Reynolds, G., 1985, Search for cytomegalovirus in postmortem brain tissue from patients with Huntington's chorea and other psychiatric disease by molecular hybridization using cloned DNA, *J. Neuropathol. Exp. Neurol.* **44**:176–184.

Thomas, C. S., and Szabadi, E., 1987, Paranoid psychosis as the first presentation of a fulminating lethal case of AIDS, *Br. J. Psychiatry* **151**:693–695.

Toorkey, C. B., and Carrigan, D. R., 1989, Immunohistochemical detection of an immediate early antigen of human cytomegalovirus in normal tissues, *J. Infect. Dis.* **160**:741–751.

Torrey, E. F., and Kaufmann, C. A., 1986, Schizophrenia and neuroviruses, in: *Handbook of Schizophrenia*, Volume 1 (H. A. Nasrallah and D. R. Weinberger, eds.), Elsevier, Amsterdam, pp. 361–376.

Torrey, E. F., Yolken, R. H., and Winfrey, C. J., 1982, Cytomegalovirus antibody in cerebrospinal fluid of schizophrenic patients detected by enzyme immunoassay, *Science* **216**:892–894.

Torrey, E. F., Rawlings, R., and Waldman, I. N., 1988, Schizophrenia births and viral diseases in two states, *Schiz. Res.* **1**:73–77.

Toy, J. L., 1983, The interferons, *Clin. Exp. Immunol.* **54**:1–13.

Traugott, U., and Lebon, P., 1988, Multiple sclerosis: Involvement of interferons in lesion pathogenesis, *Ann. Neurol.* **24**:243–251.

Vafai, A., Murray, R. S., Wellish, M., Devlin, M., and Gilden, D. H., 1988, Expression of varicella-zoster virus and herpes simplex virus in normal human trigeminal ganglia, *Proc. Natl. Acad. Sci. USA* **85**:2362–2366.

Vazeux, R., Brousse, N., Jarry, A., Henin, D., Marche, C., Vedrenne, C., Mikol, J., Wolff, M., Michon, C., Rozenbaum, W., Bureau, J. F., Montagnier, L., and Brahic, M., 1987, AIDS subacute encephalitis: Identification of HIV-infected cells, *Am. J. Pathol.* **126**:403–410.

Volpe, J. J., 1987, *The Neurology of the Newborn*, Saunders, Philadelphia, pp. 33–68.

Waldrop, M. F., Pedersen, F. A., and Bell, R. Q., 1968, Minor physical anomalies and behavior in preschool children, *Child Dev.* **39**:391–400.

Waltrip, R. W., Carrigan, D. R., Carpenter, W. T., 1990, Immunopathology and viral reactivation: A general theory of schizophrenia, *J. Nerv. Ment. Dis.* **178**:729–738.

Watt, D. C., Katz, K., and Shepherd, M., 1983, The natural history of schizophrenia: A 5-year prospective follow-up of a representative sample of schizophrenics by means of a standardized clinical and social assessment, *Psychol. Med.* **13**:663–670.

Weinberger, D. R., 1987, Implications of normal brain development for the pathogenesis of schizophrenia, *Arch. Gen. Psychiatry* **44**:660–669.

Weinberger, D. R., Wagner, R. L., and Wyatt, R. J., 1983, Neuropathological studies of schizophrenia: A selective review, *Schiz. Bull.* **9**:193–212.

Williams, B. R. G., Read, S. E., Freedman, M. H., Carver, D. H., and Gelfand, E. W., 1982, The assay of 2′–5′A synthetase as an indicator of interferon activity and virus infection *in vivo*, in: *Interferons* (T. C. Merrigan and R. M. Friedman, eds.), Academic Press, New York, pp. 253–267.

Winston, D. J., Huang, E.-S., Miller, M. J., Lin, C.-H., Ho, W. G., Gale, R. P., and Champlin, R. E., 1985, Molecular epidemiology of cytomegalovirus infections associated with bone marrow transplantation, *Ann. Intern. Med.* **102**:16–20.

Wright, H. T., Parker, C. E., and Mavalwala, J., 1972, Unusual dermatoglyphic findings associated with cytomegalic inclusion disease of infancy—A first report and practical review, *Calif. Med.* **116:** 14–20.
Yow, M. D., Williamson, D. W., Leeds, L. J., Thompson, P., Woodward, R. M., Walmus, B. F., Lester, J. W., Six, H. R., and Griffiths, P. D., 1988, Epidemiologic characteristics of cytomegalovirus infection in mothers and their infants, *Am. J. Obstet. Gynecol.* **158:**1189–1195.
Zarling, J. M., 1984, Effects of interferon and its inducers on leucocytes and their immunologic functions, in: *Interferons and Their Applications* (P. E. Came and W. A. Carter, eds.), Springer-Verlag, Berlin, pp. 403–431.
Zubin, J., Magaziner, J., and Steinhauer, S. R., 1983, The metamorphosis of schizophrenia: From chronicity to vulnerability, *Psychol. Med.* **13:**551–571.

Chapter 3

Herpes Simplex Virus Type 1 DNA in Human Brain Tissue

Any Association with Mental Disease?

J. Rajčáni, M. Murányiová, M. Kúdelová, J. Pogády, V. Mucha, and P. Babál

INTRODUCTION

The putative role of viruses, especially of herpes simplex virus (HSV), in the etiology of schizophrenia and related mental disorders has been discussed since the finding of elevated antibody levels to HSV type 1 in psychiatric patients (Rimón and Halonen, 1969). Líbiková (1983) found that the geometric mean titer of neutralizing antibodies (NA) to HSV type 1 was higher in each age group of schizophrenic (SCH) patients as compared to controls. The hemagglutination inhibition antibodies to measles virus and the complement fixation antibodies to varicella–zoster virus were not increased when tested in the same sera. Repeated

J. Rajčáni, M. Kúdelová, and V. Mucha • *Institute of Virology, Slovak Academy of Sciences, Bratislava, Czechoslovakia.* M. Murányiová and J. Pogády • *Mental Research Laboratory, Institute of Medical Bionics, Bratislava, Czechoslovakia.* P. Babál • *Department of Pathology, Medical Faculty, Bratislava, Czechoslovakia.*

serologic investigation with a great number of sera from SCH patients and controls confirmed the elevated NA titers in the presence and absence of complement in the sera of domestic SCH patients but not in those obtained from abroad (Rajčáni *et al.*, 1987). Using ELISA and a sensitive neutralization test in the presence of complement, we found that both tests were positive in 42 of 262 (16%) CSF samples from SCH patients. The NA titered ≥ 4 and the ELISA ≥ 128 (Bártová *et al.*, 1987). For this reason we decided to compare the results of both tests in a further representative group of SCH patients.

Another approach is the examination of brain biopsy specimens obtained at curative stereotactic surgery (Pogády and Nádvorník, 1982). Electron microscopy showed in the cytoplasm of some neurons herpesvirus nucleocapsid-like structures, but no virus assembly, budding, or maturation: we concluded that the observed structures were dense-core vesicles (Rajčáni *et al.*, 1987). This interpretation was further strengthened by the absence of reactivation of any infectious virus when the biopsy specimens were cultured for 10 days and then assayed in Vero cells, human diploid cells, and suckling mice. Promising seemed, however, the finding of HSV-1 DNA sequences in the right *nc. amygdalae* of three out of ten patients with paranoid SCH, imbecility, and aggressive behavior (Kúdelová *et al.*, 1988). Therefore, we extended our investigations to necropsy samples from the brains of mentally healthy subjects showing no histopathologic changes.

MATERIALS AND METHODS

Sera and Patients

Sera were obtained from 725 subjects: 233 SCH patients (paranoid SCH, catatonic SCH, hebephrenic SCH), 277 chronic alcoholics, and 215 controls (Table 1).

Serologic Tests

For neutralization, 100 PFU of HSV-1 strain KOS was mixed with serial twofold serum dilutions (previously inactivated at 56°C for 30 min) and incubated for 2 hr in the presence and absence of complement. The virus-serum mixture was inoculated into Vero cells and the cytopathic effect (CPE) was read on days 3–4 postinoculation. The results were evaluated independently by two investigators.

ELISA was performed according to standard protocols (Hsiung, 1982). The antigen was prepared from KOS-infected human lung embryo (HLE) cells. At a concentration of 5 μg/ml, the antigen-coated wells of domestic microplates (Koh-I-Noor, Dalečín, ČSFR) reacted with the ascitic fluid containing a reference anti-gB monoclonal antibody to dilution 64,000. Control wells were coated with a

Table 1. Age Distribution of Serum Donors and the Number of Sera Tested

Diagnosis (patients)	Age decade (years)	Neutralization test Total	A[a]	B[a]	ELISA	Total NA + ELISA	NA
Schizophrenics	20–29	27	10	17	27		
	30–39	48	28	20	48		
	40–49	47	30	17	47		
	50–59	47	35	12	47		
	⩾ 60	64	48	16	64	233	233
Alcoholics		277	228	49	277	277	277
Controls	20–29	101	62	39	39		
	30–39	84	38	46	83		
	40–49	19	8	11	11		
	50–59	11	6	5	5	138	215
	⩾ 60		0	0	0		
Total						648	725

[a]Two independent investigators.

similarly prepared extract of noninfected cells. The domestic conjugate (anti-human IgG/Px) reacted with the monoclonal antibody up to a dilution of 2000, but it was used at a dilution of 400; the antigen for coating was used at a protein concentration of 10 μg/ml. Endpoints read at OD_{492} were calculated to achieve a ratio ⩾ 2.1.

Brain Biopsy Specimens

Biopsy specimens were obtained from patients with paranoid SCH, imbecility, and mental retardation with aggressive behavior who underwent curative stereotactic surgery (Clinical Stereotaxy, Regional Psychiatry Hospital, Pezinok) as previously described (Kúdelová *et al.*, 1988). Necropsy specimens of the trigeminal ganglion (TG), brain stem (BS), hypothalamus (Hy), *nc. amygdalae* (Amg), *gyrus hippocampi* (GH), *gyrus dentatus* (GD), and *bulbus olfactorius* (BO) were obtained from mentally healthy subjects autopsied 3½–8 hr after death (Department of Pathology, Medical Faculty, Bratislava).

Latent Infection in Rabbits

Albino rabbits were infected in the right scarified cornea with 2×10^6 PFU of the Kupka strain of HSV-1 as described (Rajčáni *et al.*, 1977). Both trigeminal ganglia, brain stem at both sides, and the right cornea were removed, immersed in sterile saline containing 3% fetal calf serum, and used for explantation as well as DNA extraction.

Explantation Procedure

The tissue specimens were minced and cultured for 10 days in medium CMRL-1415 containing 10% fetal calf serum and antibiotics. The medium was exchanged on days 4 and 7 in culture. The last medium sample was obtained on day 10. All three samples were assayed for the presence of virus. The fragments from the same tissue were collected on day 10 and either used for DNA extraction or assayed for the presence of virus (Table 6).

DNA Extraction

The samples were treated with a lytic buffer (O.2 M Tris-HCl, pH 7.9, 0.5 M EDTA, and 0.5% SDS), proteinase K (100 μg/ml, 2 hr, 65°C), and further extracted with phenol-saturated buffer (0.01 M Tris-HCl, pH 7.5, 0.15 M NaCl, 1 mM EDTA). After RNase treatment and chloroform-isoamyl alcohol extraction the DNA was precipitated with a threefold volume of alcohol. (For details see Maniatis *et al.*, 1982.)

Preparation of HSV DNA, Labeling of the Probes, and Hybridization

HSV-1 DNA was isolated from the nucleocapsids sedimented by differential centrifugation (Kúdelová *et al.*, 1988). The HSV-1 DNA fragments *Kpn*I *i*, *d*, and *h* from strain 17 were kindly provided by Dr. V. Preston, MRC Virology Unit, Institute of Virology, Glasgow; they were cloned in the plasmid pAT 153. The purified HSV-1 as well as the fragments were nick-translated according to Rigby *et al.* (1977) using [α-^{32}P]-dCTP and [α-^{32}P]-dGTP (specific activity 110 TBq/mmole, IZINTA, Budapest, Hungary). The specific activity of the labeled DNA ranged from 2 to 4×10^7 cpm/μg.

Spot blot hybridization was performed as described by Fraser *et al.*(1981). The DNA extracted from the CNS and ganglion specimens was denatured by heating (5 min, 95°C) and spotted on a nylon filter (Hybond N, Amersham). The filters were treated according to the protocols of the manufacturer, cross-linked by UV irradiation on a standard UV-transilluminator for 5 min. The filters were prehybridized in 2 × SSC containing 50% formamide, 0.5% SDS, 2.5 × Denhardt's solution (for details see Membrane transfer and detection methods, Amersham protocol 1985) in the presence of 100 μg/ml salmon sperm DNA (at 42°C overnight), hybridized in the same solution containing nick-translated probe (minimally 5×10^5 cpm/ml) at 42°C overnight. After repeated washings (2 × SSC, 2 × SSC with 0.1% SDS, and 0.1 × SSC at 65°C) the filters were wrapped with Saran Wrap and autoradiographed with X-ray film (Medix Rapid) for 2–3 days at −70°C.

Statistical Analysis

The NA titers and the ELISA titers in individual groups (SCH patients, chronic alcoholics, control subjects) were compared by determining the mean $\log_2$ values in individual groups and evaluating the differences by t test. Negative titers were not included in the test.

RESULTS

Serologic Investigations

For the first calculations, ELISA results of 183 serum samples from SCH patients were compared with the results of 100 serum samples from control subjects (Table 2). Statistical analysis showed no significant difference in the mean ELISA titer of HSV-1 antibodies between the SCH patients and age-matched controls. Later, a total of 233 serum samples from SCH patients was compared with 215 control serum samples. All sera were examined in ELISA and in neutralization test in the presence and absence of complement with the exception of 79 control sera examined by neutralization test only (Table 1). In addition, sera from 277 chronic alcoholics were examined by neutralization test. The number of seropositive SCH patients was 215 (92.3%), that of alcoholics 267 (96.4%), and that of controls 204 (91%). Table 3 shows that the mean NA titers were higher in SCH patients than in controls when examined in the presence or absence of complement ($p = 0.001$). In contrast, no such difference was found when comparing the ELISA titers. Chronic alcoholics showed higher NA titers as compared to controls in the absence of complement. However, the latter difference diminished (Table 4) when 157 positive sera read by investigator A only and taken from the patients of age groups 20–49 were compared with the sera of age-matched controls read by the same investigator (compare Table 1). This calculation showed no significant difference (at $p = 0.05$) between the NA serum levels in alcoholics and controls either in the presence or in the absence of complement.

Hybridization with the Brain Necropsy Specimens

The DNA extracts from the necropsy specimens were hybridized with a mixture of the *Kpn*I fragments *h* and *i*. Strong hybridization was seen with a single trigeminal ganglion and one brain stem sample (Fig. 1A). The two positive *nc. amygdalae* samples showed spots of medium intensity corresponding to that of the extract of 10^4 KOS-infected HLE cells (Fig. 1B). The positive hybridization rate with the DNA extract from *nc. amygdalae* obtained from biopsy specimens was

Table 2. ELISA with HSV-1 Antigen in the Sera of Schizophrenic Patients and Corresponding Controls

Log_2 of the titer	Titer (dilution reciprocal)	Age groups (schizophrenics)					
		20–29	30–39	40–49	50–59	≥ 60	Total
10	1,024	5	4	2	4	2	17
11.3	2,560	2	2	—	1	1	6
12.3	5,120						
13.3	10,240	1	3	2	—	—	6
14.3	20,480	1	11	5	3	7	27
15.3	40,960	6	13	15	8	13	55
16.3	81,920	3	9	12	8	16	48
17.3	162,840	1	5	6	4	8	24
	Total	19	47	42	28	47	183
		$\bar{x}$ = 14.893[b]	$\bar{x}$ = 15.182	$\bar{x}$ = 15.697			$\bar{x}$ = 15.47
		S.D. = 1.720	S.D. = 1.391	S.D. = 1.041			S.D. = 1.469
		Age groups (controls)					
10	1,024	3	3				6
11.3	2,560	3	2		1		6
12.3	5,120						
13.3	10,240	1	3				4
14.3	20,480	4	2	2			8
15.3	40,960	10	12	2			24
16.3	81,920	12	16	5	4		37
17.3	162,840	5	8	2			15
	Total	38	46	11	5		100
		$\bar{x}$ = 15.436	$\bar{x}$ = 15.504	$\bar{x}$ = 15.958			$\bar{x}$ = 15.543
		S.D. = 1.581	S.D. = 1.749	S.D. = 0.979			S.D. = 1.617

[a]Number of serum samples in the corresponding age group revealing the given titer.
[b]$\bar{x}$ = average (geometric mean) titer (log_2).

Table 3. Comparison of Mean NA and ELISA titers in SCH Patients, Chronic Alcoholics, and Control Subjects

	Control subjects			SCH patients			Chronic alcoholics	
	NA(C+)[a]	NA(C−)	ELISA	NA(C+)	NA(C−)	ELISA	NA(C+)	NA(C−)
Sample *N*	204	204	125	215	215	215	267	267
Mean titer	765	128	41,765	1201	242	44,146	662	201
Log_2 of mean	9.58	7.00	15.35	10.23	7.92	15.43	9.37	7.65
S.D.	1.88	1.56	1.88	2.17	1.95	1.82	2.25	1.83
Group[b]	1	2	3	4	5	6	7	8

[a]C+, C−: presence or absence of complement.
[b]Significant differences: 4 > 1 ($p = 0.002$); 5 > 2 ($p = 0.001$); 8 > 2 ($p = 0.001$).

Table 4. Neutralizing Antibodies to HSV-1 in Chronic Alcoholics[a]

Group	Neutralizing antibodies (mean titer)	
	C+	C−
Alcoholics (157 positive sera)	10.2 ± 1.9	7.15 ± 1.78[b]
Control subjects (108 sera)	10.4 ± 1.9	7.45 ± 1.54[b]

[a]For explanations see Tables 2 and 3.
[b]No significant difference at $p \leq 0.05$.

slightly higher than with the DNA extract from necropsy specimens (Table 5). The positive hybridization rate with the trigeminal ganglion samples (used as positive controls) seemed relevant if it is considered that at least 40% of human trigeminal ganglia are expected to carry the latent genome (Baringer and Swoveland, 1973). To avoid the scoring of nonspecific hybridization and to eliminate false-positive results, extracts from noninfected and infected HLE cells were included for each membrane. A hybridization intensity corresponding to that of 10^3 KOS-infected

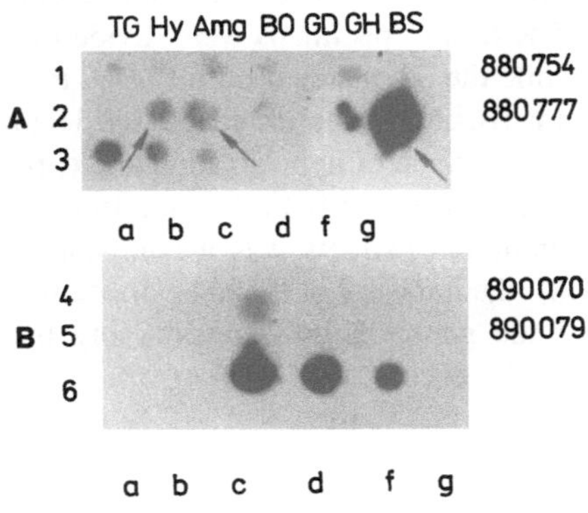

Figure 1. Hybridization of the labeled *Kpn*I fragments *h* and *i* with the deproteinized extract of necropsied brain samples. (1) Autopsy protocol No. 880 754; (2) autopsy protocol No. 880 777; (3)KOS-infected HLE cells (a = 10^6, b = 10^5, c = 10^4, d = 10^3, f = 10^2) and noninfected HLE cells (g = 10^6); (4) autopsy protocol No. 890 070; (5) autopsy protocol No. 890 079; (6) noninfected HLE cells (10^6) at a, b; KOS-infected HLE cells (c = 10^6, d = 10^5, f = 10^4, g = 10^3).

TG, trigeminal ganglion; Hy, hypothalamus; Amg, nc. amygdalae, BO, bulbus olfactorius; GD, gyrus dentatus; GH, gyrus hippocampi; BS, brain stem.

The two slightly positive spots are indicated by arrows; an extremely large spot spilled is the brain stem from 880 777.

No background hybridization was seen with other brain specimens.

Table 5. Spot Blot Hybridization of Necropsied Human Brain DNA Extracts with the HSV-1 DNA Probes

Tissue	Necropsy[a]	Biopsy[b]	Total	
			PNS	CNS
Trigeminal ganglion	11/21 (52.4%)		11/21 (52.4%)	
Brain stem	2/12 (16.7%)			14/94 (14.8%)
Hypothalamus	2/21 (9.5%)			
Nc. amygdalae	4/26 (15.4%)	3/18 (16.6%)		
Gyrus hippocampi	1/17 (5.8%)			
Olfactory bulb	5/18 (27.8%)			

[a]Hybridized with *Kpn*I fragments *h* and *i* strain 17.
[b]Hybridized with total HSV-1 DNA (domestic strain HSZP).

HLE cells was regarded for negative background when the total DNA in the deproteinized brain extract reached the limit of 5 μg per spot (Fig. 2).

Hybridization with the Neural Tissues of HSV-Infected Rabbits

Eleven rabbits were inoculated with the Kupka strain in the right scarified cornea. By 207–479 days later the right cornea, both trigeminal ganglia, and brain stem were removed. The tissue specimens were divided into two parts: one was cultured for 10 days while the other was used for DNA extraction. The explanted fragments from the same tissue were collected and used either for DNA extraction or for virus titration. Comparison of hybridization and explantation results (Table 6) showed the following: (1) Positive hybridization in the noncultured as well as cultured homolateral ganglion extracts was accompanied by virus reactivation (rabbits Nos. 13 and 18): the intensity of the hybridization spot with the extract of the explanted part of the ganglion was considerably increased. (2) Negative

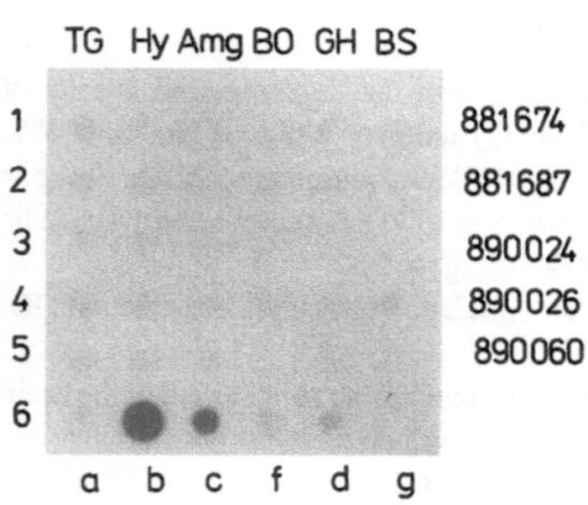

Figure 2. Negative hybridization of the labeled *Kpn*I probes *h* and *i* with the deproteinized extract of necropsied brain samples. (1) Autopsy protocol No. 881 674; (2) No. 881 687; (3) No. 890 024; (4) No. 890 026; (5) No. 890 060; (6) noninfected HLE cells (10^6) at a; KOS-infected HLE cells (b = 10^6, c = 10^5, f = 10^4, d = 10^3, g = 10^2). For abbreviations see Fig. 1.

Table 6. Comparison of HSV-1 Latency in Rabbits by Hybridization and Explantation Techniques

Rabbit	Virus	RTG[a]			LTG			RBS			LBS			Co			Autopsy	DNA probe
No.	strain	H	HE	IE	H	HE	IE	H	HE	IE	H	HE	IE	H	HE	IE	(days p.i.)	(*Kpn*I fragments)
13	Kupka	+	+	+	–	–	–	+	–	–	+	–	–	–	–	–	207	*i*
15	Kupka	+	–	–	+	–	–	+	–	–	+	–	–	+	–	–	209	*i*
11	Kupka	+	–	–	–	–	–	–	–	–	–	–	–	–	–	–	207	*d*+*i*
14	Kupka	+	–	–	–	–	–	–	–	–	–	–	–	–	–	–	209	*d*+*i*
17	Kupka	+	–	–	+	–	–	+	–	–	–	–	–	–	–	–	216	*d*+*i*
18	Kupka	+	+	+	–	–	–	–	–	–	–	–	–	–	–	–	216	*d*+*i*
19	Kupka	–	+	+	–	–	–	–	–	–	–	–	–	–	–	–	221	*h*+*i*
20	Kupka	–	+	+	–	+	+	–	–	–	–	–	–	–	–	–	221	*h*+*i*
22	Kupka	–	Nd	+	–	Nd	+	–	Nd	–	–	Nd	–	–	Nd	–	482	*h*+*i*
24	Kupka	+	Nd	+	–	Nd	–	–	Nd	–	–	Nd	–	–	Nd	–	479	*h*+*i*
25	Kupka	–	Nd	+	–	Nd	–	+	Nd	–	–	Nd	–	–	Nd	–	479	*h*+*i*
Total	H	7/11			2/11			4/11			2/11			1/11				
	HE		4/8			1/8			0/8			0/8			0/8			
	IE			7/11			2/11			0/11			0/11			0/11		

[a]RTG, LTG, right or left trigeminal ganglion; RBS, LBS, right or left brain stem, Co, cornea. H, hybridization (with the DNA extract of noncultured tissue); HE, hybridization with the explant; IE, virus isolation during explantation. Nd, hybridization not done: infectivity assay with the suspension of explants was in each case in accord with the hybridization result.

hybridization with the noncultured ganglion extracts was followed by strongly positive hybridization of the cultured ganglion extracts (rabbits Nos. 19 and 20, Fig. 3) or by positive infectivity assay of the cultured ganglion suspension (rabbits Nos. 22 and 25); in all of these cases the virus was isolated also from medium fluid at the second or third exchange. (3) Slight positive hybridization with the noncultured ganglion extract was completely negative with the cultured ganglion extract: the same was true with four right and two left brain stem extracts (Fig. 4). No virus was isolated.

The simplest interpretation of the results given under point 3 would be a false-positive hybridization. However, all controls including noninfected rabbit tissue were completely negative: neither hybridized infected rabbit cells to the labeled pAT 153 DNA (results not shown). The small amount of HSV DNA detectable in the noncultured ganglion or brain stem extracts probably underwent DNase digestion in culture. It seems unlikely that the cellular DNA, if responsible for a false-positive hybridization, would be self-digested in the surviving explants. We believe that some human as well as rabbit specimens contained HSV DNA sequences which did not reactivate in culture.

DISCUSSION

The elevated NA titers to HSV-1 in the sera of SCH patients were not confirmed by ELISA: similar results with ELISA had been reported by Jorgensen *et al.* (1982). In addition, the geometric mean titer of NA in the sera of chronic alcoholics was influenced by the selection of data for statistical calculations. Furthermore, the number of sera, the selection of patients, the storage and shipment of sera, the conditions and type of the test may influence the serologic results. We earlier reported (Rajčáni *et al.*, 1987) that elevated NA to HSV-1 were found only in the sera of domestic SCH patients but not in those coming from abroad. Obviously many variables may influence the different results reported by different

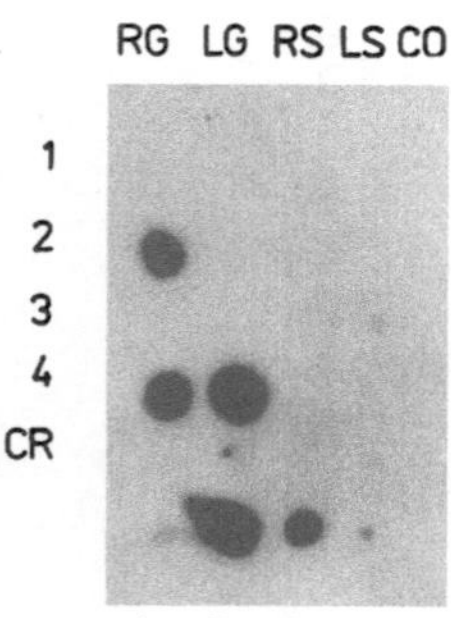

Figure 3. Spot blot hybridization of the DNA extracts from neural tissues of rabbits with established HSV latency using the labeled *Kpn*I fragments *h* and *i*. Abbreviations: RG, right trigeminal ganglion; LG, left trigeminal ganglion; RS, right brain stem; LS, left brain stem; Co, cornea.

1, rabbit No. 19, not cultured; 2, rabbit No. 19, after 10 days in culture; 3, rabbit No. 20, not cultured; 4, rabbit No. 20, after 10 days in culture; CR, control rabbit tissues.

A, 10^6 noninfected REF cells; B, 10^6 infected REF cells harvested at 20 hr p.i.; C, 10^5 infected REF cells; D, 10^4 infected REF cells; E, 10^3 infected REF cells.

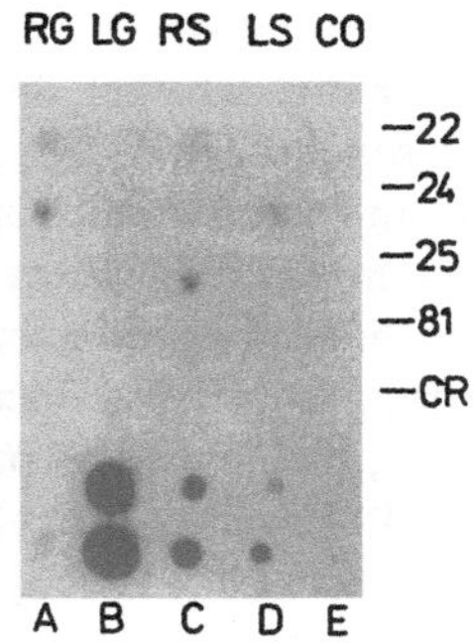

Figure 4. Spot blot hybridization of the DNA extracts from neural tissues of rabbits with established HSV latency using a mixture of labeled *KpnI* fragments *h* and *i*. For abbreviations see Fig. 3.

Rabbit numbers 22, 24, 25, 81; CR, control rabbit (noninfected). A, control REF cells. B, 10^6 infected REF cells (above: harvested 20 hr p.i.; below: harvested 12 hr p.i.). C, 10^5 infected REF cells (harvested 20 and 12 hr p.i.). D, 10^4 infected REF cells (harvested 20 and 12 hr p.i.). E, 10^3 infected REF cells (harvested 20 and 12 hr p.i.).

investigators. While some studies (Halonen *et al.*, 1974; Lycke *et al.*, 1974; Cappel and Sprecher, 1983; Cappel *et al.*, 1978) confirmed the possible role of herpesviruses in the etiology of mental disease, others found no relationship (Pokorný *et al.*, 1973; Rimón *et al.*, 1978, 1979; Rimón, 1983; Gotlieb-Stematsky *et al.*, 1987).

HSV-1 antibodies were found in the CSF of SCH patients (Gotlieb-Stematsky *et al.*, 1981; Bártová *et al.*, 1987). Using both ELISA and neutralization test in the presence of complement, we found antibodies to HSV-1 in at least 16% of the 262 CSF samples. Albrecht *et al.* (1980) and Torrey *et al.* (1982, 1983) found IgM class antibody to CMV in the CSF of 11% of SCH patients and NA antibodies in 32% of these samples. In contrast, Rimón *et al.* (1986) found no IgM class antibody to CMV in the CSF of their SCH patients: the authors have doubted the association of CMV antibody in the CSF with SCH although 17% of their CSF samples exhibited a serum-to-CSF ratio ≥ 20. It should be mentioned in this context that in a proportion of senile dementia cases the CSF may contain a small amount of antibodies to viruses such as HSV, CMV, or hepatitis B (results not shown). It can be assumed, however, that the presence of virus-antibody complexes in the CSF may precipitate or worsen the clinical symptoms in a nonspecific manner.

The presence of HSV DNA sequences in the human brain in psychiatric illness was first described by *in situ* hybridization (Sequeira *et al.*, 1979). Fraser *et al.*, (1981) reported HSV-1 DNA not only in the extract of 6 of 11 human brain samples in the frontal and parietal cortex in multiple sclerosis but also in the brain stem of normal CNS. Gannacliffe *et al.* (1985) detected HSV-1 DNA in the temporal lobe of epileptic patients. We detected the HSV-1 DNA sequences not only in the *nc. amygdalae* of mentally ill patients but also in that of mentally healthy subjects. The brain stem and trigeminal ganglion were sampled as potentially positive brain areas where HSV DNA was anticipated to be present at least in some of the samples. Indeed, despite the subsequent autolysis (extraction at 3.5–8 hr postmortem), extremely intensive hybridization was seen with one trigeminal ganglion and one brain stem sample. The presence of HSV DNA in the hypothalamus and *nc. amygdalae* of brains from mentally healthy subjects weakens the significance of the biopsy findings in the etiology of SCH. It is difficult to predict whether the HSV DNA carriers are at risk of brain pathology: the presence of HSV DNA is relatively frequent at least in the trigeminal ganglion. The latent genome in the ganglion is certainly the source of recurrent cutaneous herpes (Baringer, 1975; Stevens, 1975; Klein, 1982) but nothing is known about the mechanism of occurrence of herpetic encephalitis. The presence of HSV-1 DNA during latency was documented along the whole sensory pathway, i.e., in the brain stem, thalamus, and parietal cortex of mice (Cabrera *et al.*, 1980; Stroop *et al.*, 1984). Recently, using DNA complementary to the latency-associated mRNAs the presence of the HSV genome was confirmed in the terminal nucleus of trigeminal root in the brain stem (Deatly *et al.*, 1988). Our experimental data in rabbits with established latency seem to confirm this notion. The lack of strong correlation between explantation and hybridization results showed on one hand the absence of positive hybridization in some noncultured samples which yielded virus in culture (the amount of viral DNA was below the sensitivity of the test), and on the other hand it points to the presence of spontaneously noninducible HSV genome in the ganglion and brain stem. The reactivation rate of latent virus in culture can be enhanced using hypomethylating compounds such as 5-azacytidine (Whitby *et al.*, 1987). We found this comparing the frequency at which the reactivation occurred in cultured ganglion fragments from DBA-2 mice previously infected with different HSV strains (Rajčáni *et al.*, 1990). Spontaneously noninducible HSV-1 genome was described by Brown *et al.* (1979) and by Lewis *et al.* (1984) who superinfected the ganglion explants with a ts mutant at supraoptimal temperature and rescued the endogenous virus. Thomas *et al.* (1985) showed that upon reinfection with an HSV-2 strain this virus acted in *trans* to reactivate the previously introduced HSV-1 genome. The above-mentioned data seem to support the assumption that the endogenous uninducible HSV genome may be reactivated by recombination with the DNA of a second HSV strain introduced at reinfection (Stroop, 1986).

CONCLUSIONS

Serologic investigations performed over nearly a decade (as reported here and in the previous volume) included more than 1000 serum samples and about 300 CSF samples from SCH patients, chronic alcoholics, and other psychiatric patients as well as age-matched controls from a hematologic department. No unequivocal statements could be drawn except that the NA antibody titers were elevated in the SCH patients and that 16% of these patients had antibodies to HSV-1 in the CSF in low titers. A more fruitful area of research seems to be the investigation of the presence of HSV-1 and CMV DNA sequences in the brain biopsy and necropsy samples. Preliminary results showed that in man as well as in rabbits with established latent infection, the brain stem and *nc. amygdalae* contained HSV-1 DNA sequences which did not spontaneously reactivate in culture. The significance of noninducible viral DNA sequences for the brain pathology may represent an interesting field for future research.

REFERENCES

Albrecht, P., Torrey, E. F., Boone, E., and Hicks, J. T., 1980, Raised cytomegalovirus antibody level in cerebrospinal fluid of schizophrenic patients, *Lancet* **2**:769–772.

Baringer, J. R., 1975, Herpes simplex virus infection of nervous tissue in animals and man, *Prog. Med. Virol.* **20**:1–16.

Baringer, J. R., and Swoveland, P., 1973, Recovery of herpes simplex virus from human trigeminal ganglions, *N. Engl. J. Med.* **288**:648–650.

Bártová, Ľ., Rajčáni, J., and Pogády, J., 1987, Herpes simplex virus antibodies in the cerebrospinal fluid of schizophrenic patients, *Acta Virol.* **31**:443–446.

Brown, S. M., Shbak-Sharpe, J. H., Warren, K. G., Wroblewska, Z., and Koprowski, H., 1979, Detection by complementation of defective or uninducible herpes simplex type 1 virus genomes latent in human ganglia, *Proc. Natl. Acad. Sci USA* **76**:2364–2368.

Cabrera, C. V., Wohlenberg, C., Openshaw, H., Rey-Mendez, M., Puga, A., and Notkins, L., 1980, Herpes simplex virus DNA sequences in the CNS of latently infected mice, *Nature* **288**:288–290.

Cappel, R., and Sprecher, S., 1983, Are herpes simplex virus responsible for neuropsychiatric diseases? in: *Research on the Viral Hypothesis of Mental Disorders* (P. V. Morozov, ed.), *Adv. Biol. Psychiatry* **12**:168–173.

Cappel, R., Gregoire, F., Thirty, L., and Sprecher, S., 1978, Antibody and cell mediated immunity to herpes simplex virus in psychotic depression, *J. Clin. Psychiatry* **39**:266–268.

Deatly, A. M., Spisack, J. D., Lavi, E., O'Boyle, D. R., and Fraser, N. W., 1988, Latent herpes simplex virus type 1 transcripts in peripheral and central nervous system tissues of mice map to similar regions of the viral genome, *J. Virol.* **62**:749–756.

Fraser, N., Lawrence, N. C., Wroblewska, Z., Gilden, D. H., and Koprowski, H., 1981, Herpes simplex type 1 DNA in human brain tissue, *Proc. Natl. Acad. Sci. USA* **78**:6461–6465.

Gannacliffe, A., Saldanka, J. A., Itzhaki, R. F., and Sutton, R. N. P., 1985, Herpes simplex viral DNA in temporal lobe epilepsy, *Lancet* **1**:214–215.

Gotlieb-Stematsky, T., Zonis, J., Arlazoroff, A., Mozes, T., Sigal, M., and Szekely, A. G., 1981, Antibodies to Epstein-Barr virus, herpes simplex type 1, cytomegalovirus and measles virus in psychiatric patients, *Arch. Virol.* **67**:333–339.

Gotlieb-Stematsky, T., Floru, S., Becker, D., Kritchman, E., and Leventon-Kriss, S., 1987, Antibody and cell mediated immunity to herpes simplex and Epstein-Barr viruses in psychotic patients, in: *Viruses, Immunity and Mental Disorders* (E. Kurstak, Z. J. Lipowski, and P. V. Morozov, eds.), Plenum Medical, New York, pp. 173–178.

Halonen, P. E., Rimón, R., Arohonka, K., and Jantti, V., 1974, Antibody levels to herpes simplex type 1, measles and rubella viruses in psychiatric patients, *Br. J. Psychiatry* **125**:461–465.

Hsiung, G. D., 1982, *Diagnostic Virology*, 3rd ed., Yale University Press, New Haven, Conn.

Jorgensen, S. O., Goldschmidt, V. V., and Vestergaard, B. F., 1982, Herpes simplex virus antibodies in child psychiatric patients and normal children, *Acta Psychiatr. Scand.* **66**:42–49.

Klein, R. J., 1982, The pathogenesis of acute, latent and recurrent herpes simplex virus infections, *Arch. Virol.* **72**:143–168.

Kúdelová, M., Rajčáni, J., Pogády, J., and Šramka, M., 1988, Herpes simplex virus DNA in the brain of psychotic patients, *Acta Virol.* **32**:455–460.

Lewis, M. E., Brown, S. M., Warren, K. G., and Subak-Sharpe, J. H., 1984, Recovery of herpes simplex virus genetic information from human trigeminal ganglion cells following superinfection with herpes simplex type 2 temperature sensitive mutants, *J. Gen. Virol.* **65**:215–219.

Líbiková, H., 1983, Schizophrenia and viruses: Principles of etiologic studies, in: *Advances in Biological Psychiatry*, Volume 12 (P. V. Morozov, ed.), Karger, Basel, pp. 20–51.

Lycke, E., Norrby, E., and Roos, B. E., 1974, Serological study of mentally ill patients with particular reference to the prevalence of herpes simplex virus infections, *Br. J. Psychiatry* **124**:273–279.

Maniatis, T., Fritsch, E. F., and Sambrook, J., 1982, *Molecular Cloning: A Laboratory Manual*, Cold Spring Harbor Laboratory, Cold Spring Harbor, N.Y., pp. 84–94.

Pogády, J., and Nádvorník, P., 1982, Psychosurgery: Critical survey of hitherto experience, *Cs. Psychiatr.* **78**:3–16 [in Slovak].

Pokorný, A., Rawls, W., Adam, E., and Mefferd, R., 1973, Depression, psychopathy and herpes virus type 1 antibodies. Lack of relationship, *Arch. Gen. Psychiatry* **29**:820–822.

Rajčáni, J., Čiampor, F., Sabó, A., Líbiková, H., and Rosenbergová, M., 1977, Activation of latent herpesvirus hominis in explants: Influence of immune serum, *Arch. Virol.* **54**:55–69.

Rajčáni, J., Líbiková, H., Smereková, J., Mucha, V., Kúdelová, M., Pogády, J., Breier, Š., and Škodáček, I., 1987, Investigations on the possible role of viruses affecting the CNS in the etiology of schizophrenia and related mental disorders, in: *Viruses, Immunity and Mental Disorders* (E. Kurstak, Z. J. Lipowski, and P. V. Morozov, eds.), Plenum Medical, New York, pp. 135–148.

Rajčáni, J., Herget, U., Koštál, M., and Kaerner, H. C., 1990, Latency competence of herpes simplex virus strains ANG, ANGpath and its gC and gE minus mutants. *Acta Virol.* **34**:477–486.

Rigby, P. W. J., Dickmann, M., Rhodes, C., and Berg, P., 1977, Labelling deoxyribonucleic acid to high specific activity by in vitro nick translation with DNA polymerase I, *J. Mol. Biol.* **113**:237–251.

Rimón, R., 1983, Viral aetiology of schizophrenia? *Ann. Clin. Res.* **15**:1–3.

Rimón, R., and Halonen, P., 1969, Herpes simplex virus infection and depressive illness, *Dis. Nerv. Syst.* **30**:338–340.

Rimón, R., Nishuri, M., and Halonen, P., 1978, Serum and CSF antibody levels to herpes simplex type 1, measles and rubella viruses in patients with schizophrenia, *Ann. Clin. Res.* **10**:291–293.

Rimón, R., Halonen, P., Puhakka, P., Laitinen, L., Marttila, R., and Salmela, L., 1979, Immunoglobulin G antibodies to herpes simplex virus detected by radioimmunoassay in serum and cerebrospinal fluid of patients with schizophrenia, *J. Clin. Psychiatry* **64**:241–243.

Rimón, R., Ahokas, A., and Palo, J., 1986, Serum and cerebrospinal fluid antibodies to cytomegalovirus in schizophrenia, *Acta Psychiatr. Scand.* **73**:642–644.

Sequeira, L. W., Jenninys, L. C., Carraseo, L. H., Lord, M. A., Curry, A., and Sutton, R. N. P., 1979, Detection of herpes simplex viral genome in brain tissue, *Lancet* **2**:609–612.

Stevens, J. G., 1975, Latent herpes simplex virus and the nervous system, *Curr. Top. Microbiol. Immunol.* **70**:31–50.

Stroop, W. G., 1986, Herpes simplex virus encephalitis of the adult: Reactivation of latent brain infection, *Pathol. Immunopathol. Res.* **5**:156–169.

Stroop, W. G., Rock, D. L., and Fraser, N. W., 1984, Localization of herpes simplex virus in the trigeminal and olfactory system of the mouse CNS during acute and latent infections by in situ hybridization, *Lab. Invest.* **51**:27–38.

Thomas, E., Lycke, E., and Vahlne, A., 1985, Retrieval of latent herpes simplex type 1 genetic information from murine trigeminal ganglia by superinfection with heterotypic virus in vivo, *J. Gen. Virol.* **66**:1763–1770.

Torrey, E., Yolken, R., and Winfrey, C., 1982, Cytomegalovirus antibody in CSF of schizophrenic patients detected by enzyme immunoassay, *Science* **216**:892–894.

Torrey, E., Yolken, R. H., and Albrecht, P., 1983, Cytomegalovirus as a possible etiological agent in schizophrenia, in: *Research on the Viral Hypothesis of Mental Disorders*, *Adv. Biol. Psychiatry* **12**:150–160.

Whitby, A. J., Blyth, W. A., and Hill, T. J., 1987, The effect of DNA hypomethylating agents on the reactivation of herpes simplex virus from latently infected mouse ganglia in vitro, *Arch. Virol.* **97**:137–144.

Chapter 4

Genetic Sequences of Influenza Virus in Children with Congenital CNS Pathology

Y. Y. Tentsov, V. A. Zuev, A. M. Shevchenko,
A. A. Rzhaninova, N. B. Nefedova, and N. G. Ignatova

Early experiments demonstrated that as a result of intranasal inoculation of pregnant mice with influenza A virus, individual offspring could be found 3 weeks after birth with signs of a slowly running infectious process manifested as progressive retardation in weight and body size, and disorders in movement coordination and gait. Such a slow influenza infection in animals is characterized by marked immune deficiency, long-term influenza virus persistence, and progressive degenerative changes in different organs and tissues, among them the brain and spinal cord and the neuroendocrine system. The disease was invariably fatal within 2–3 months (Zuev *et al.*, 1983; Zuev, 1988).

Proceeding from these experiments, a study was made of experimental and

Y. Y. Tentsov and A. A. Rzhaninova • *D. I. Ivanovsky Institute of Virology of the USSR Academy of Medical Sciences, 123098 Moscow, USSR.* V. A. Zuev, N. B. Nefedova, and N. G. Ignatova • *N. F. Gamaleya Institute of Epidemiology and Microbiology of the USSR Academy of Medical Sciences, 123098 Moscow, USSR.* A. M. Shevchenko • *The Chair of Childhood Neuropathology of the Bielorussian State Institute for Advanced Medical Training, 220714 Minsk, USSR.*

clinical correlations in 40 young infants with CNS involvement whose mothers had a history of influenza or influenza-like diseases at various periods of their pregnancy. This study of the CNS involvement in such infants, the time course of changes in body weight and growth, certain immunological parameters, and catamnesis revealed significant coincidences between clinical and experimental data (Zuev and Shevchenko, 1986; Shevchenko, 1986, 1987). Therefore, our present study was aimed at virological, serological, and molecular-biological examinations of three infants with congenital pathology of the CNS born to mothers who had had influenza during pregnancy.

MATERIALS AND METHODS

Children

Specimens from two groups of children were examined. The control group comprised four children from 1 to 3 years of age with diagnoses of dyskinesia of biliary tracts (I-v, P-o), diabetes mellitus (K-va), and gastroduodenitis (T-v). No influenza or influenza-like diseases had been recorded in their mothers during pregnancy.

The study group included three infants of different ages with signs of congenital CNS involvement of progressive course. All were born to mothers who had had influenza (clinical diagnosis) at various periods of their pregnancy. Postnatally the infants had no cases of acute respiratory diseases and received no vaccinations against influenza. Some excerpts from their case histories follow.

Sch-o. A boy of 2½ years. His mother had had influenza in the 20th week of pregnancy. The diagnosis: congenital (influenza?) encephalomyelopathy of progressive course. Objectively: retardation of psychomotor development; tetraparesis, predominantly flaccid, of the spinal type; neuroendocrine syndrome (hypophysial nanism and hypogonadism); state of immune deficiency. Blood for the study was collected three times within 83 days.

A-va. A girl of 7 months. Her mother had had influenza in the 20th week of pregnancy. The diagnosis: congenital progressive hydrocephaly (of influenza etiology?). Objectively: head circumference 56 cm; retardation of psychomotor development. The baby died at age 14 months with occlusive-hypertensive crisis. Blood specimens for the study were collected at 7 months of age.

A-k, under observation since the age of 2 weeks. The mother had had influenza in the 38th week of pregnancy (14 days before delivery). The diagnosis: congenital (influenza?) encephalopathy of progressive course, congenital bronchopneumonia. Objectively (at age 3 months): retardation of psychomotor development; spastic tetraparesis; hypertension syndrome, neurotrophic syndrome with cachexia. The baby died at 4 months of age. No autopsy was done. Blood and CSF specimens were collected at 1½ months of age.

Virological Studies

For isolation of infectious influenza virus, clinical specimens (CSF, blood serum, blood cell homogenates) were inoculated into 9-day-old chicken embryonated eggs which were incubated at 36°C for 48–72 hr, after which the presence of hemagglutinating activity was determined in the allantoic fluid. Human antiglobulin serum (Pavlenko and Mirchink, 1977) was added to some clinical specimens before inoculation into chick embryos. When negative results were obtained after the first inoculation, at least four "blind" passages were carried out.

Immunoblotting

Purified influenza A/USSR/90/77 virus was electrophoresed in 10% polyacrylamide gel according to the method of Laemmli (1970). The immune blots were prepared by the method of Towbin *et al.* (1979), blocked in 5% skimmed milk with 10% bovine serum in PBS (0.14 M sodium chloride, 0.01 M sodium phosphate, pH 7.4). The immune blots were incubated with serum or plasma from the sick children, washed, and treated according to the method of Johnson *et al.* (1984).

Serological Tests

Titers of antibody to influenza virus in sera or plasma were determined by the conventional hemagglutination-inhibition test. To remove nonspecific inhibitors, the sera or plasma were heated at 56°C for 30 min and treated with potassium *m*-periodate.

MOLECULAR-BIOLOGICAL STUDIES

Isolation of RNA from Clinical Specimens

Heparinized blood cells (approximately 10^6) were pelleted by centrifugation and resuspended in STE (0.1 M sodium chloride, 0.01 M Tris-HCl, pH 7.5, and 0.001 M EDTA). The blood cells, plasma, and CSF were incubated with proteinase K at a concentration of 200 μg/ml in the presence of 0.5% sodium dodecyl sulfate (SDS) for 1 hr at 37°C. RNA was sequentially extracted with phenol, phenol-chloroform (1:1), and chloroform, precipitated with 2.5 volumes of ethanol, and the precipitate was washed twice with 70% ethanol.

DNA Probes

Recombinant plasmids containing full-length cDNA genes of influenza virus were supplied by: plasmid pYHA12 containing HA gene of influenza A/Udorn/307/72

(H3N2) virus (Yuferov *et al.*, 1984) from V. P. Yuferov, D. I. Ivanovsky Institute of Virology; plasmid pIM[25] containing M gene of influenza A/USSR/90/77 (H1N1) (Samokhvalov *et al.*, 1985) from E. I. Samokhvalov, D. I. Ivanovsky Institute of Virology; plasmid pNP with NP gene of influenza A/PR/8/34 (H1N1) (Beklemishev *et al.*, 1985) from N. A. Petrov, Institute of Molecular Biology; plasmid pHAI containing HA gene of influenza A/USSR/90/77 (H1N1) from A. A. Shilov, D. I. Ivanovsky Institute of Virology. The plasmids were grown and purified by the alkaline method (Birnboim and Doly, 1979). cDNA genes of influenza virus were excised from plasmid vectors with the appropriate restriction endonucleases, separated from vector sequence by agarose electrophoresis, electroeluted from the agarose (Maniatis *et al.*, 1982), and radiolabeled with [α-^{32}P]-deoxytriphosphate by "nick" translation (Rigby *et al.*, 1977).

Hybridization

RNA from clinical specimens was denatured as described previously (Baurin *et al.*, 1985; Bukrinskaya *et al.*, 1986), spotted on nylon membrane filter Biodyne A (Pall, USA), dried at room temperature, and immobilized at 80°C for 1 hr. Prehybridization was carried out for 1 hr at 42°C in a solution containing 50% formamide 4 × SSC (1 × SSC—0.15 M sodium chloride, 0.015 M sodium citrate), 50 mM sodium phosphate, pH 7.7; 5 × Denhardt solution (0.2 mg/ml each of Ficoll, polyvinylpyrrolidone, and fraction V of bovine serum albumin) (Denhardt, 1966), 0.2% SDS, 0.2 mg/ml denatured salmon sperm DNA. Hybridization was done under the same conditions in the presence of ^{32}P-labeled DNA probe denatured for 5 min at 100°C, and for 12–15 hr at 42°C. After hybridization the blots were washed three times in a solution of 2 × SSC and 0.1% SDS (10 min at 25°C) and three times in 0.1 × SSC and 0.1% SDS (20 min at 56°C each). Autoradiography was carried out at −70°C overnight with intensifying screens EUI-I and X-ray film.

RESULTS

Serum, blood cells, and CSF specimens from the sick children A-k, A-va, and Sch-o, as well as serum and blood cell specimens from the mothers of A-k and A-va were tested for the presence of infectious influenza virus by inoculation into the allantoic cavity of developing chick embryos (Table 1). As shown in Table 1, no infectious influenza virus could be isolated from any of the specimens. The concentration of antibody to influenza virus in the children's sera was not high, with the exception of the serum from Sch-o, in which antihemagglutinin titers were slightly higher and present to two influenza A virus subtypes. The negative results of the virological studies and, at the same time, serological evidence of the

Table 1. Virological and Serological Examinations of Specimens, Collected from Mothers and Infants with Signs of Congenital CNS Pathology

The patient	Titer of influenza virus (EID_{50}/0.2 ml)[a]	Titer of antihemagglutinin in serum		
		H1N1	H2N2	H3N3
A-k (infant)	0	1:16	<1:8	<1:8
A-k (mother)[b]	0	1:16	<1:8	1:32
A-va (infant)	0	<1:16	<1:16	<1:16
A-va (mother)[b]	0	1:64	<1:8	1:16
Sch-o (infant)	0	1:32	1:8	1:64

[a]Fifty percent infectious dose, calculated by inoculation of 9-day-old chicken embryonated eggs.
[b]Mother's blood was collected during period of baby's examination.

influenza infection in the mothers in combination with clinical signs of congenital progressive pathology in children prompted the search for molecular structures of influenza virus in these children.

For the detection of genetic sequences of influenza virus, RNA was isolated from clinical specimens and hybridized with ^{32}P-labeled cNDA probes. Two probes, labeled cDNAs of NP and M genes, were used to prove the presence of specific influenza A virus sequences because of their known conservatism (Stuart-Harris *et al.*, 1985). The antigenic subtype was determined with two other probes—labeled cDNA genes of H1 and H3 hemagglutinins.

With the first two sick children (A-k and A-va), genetic sequences of influenza virus were sought only in the blood serum and in one case (A-k) in the CSF (Fig. 1

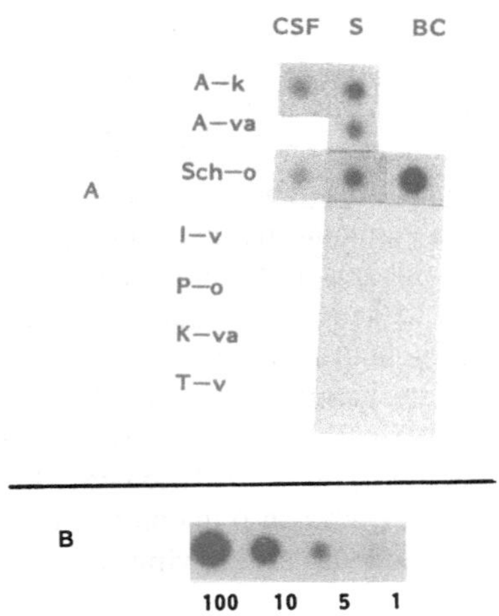

Figure 1. Detection of genetic sequences of influenza A virus in clinical materials by hybridization with ^{32}P-labeled probe of NP gene. (A) Clinical materials from the study and control groups of children; (B) control of hybridization method's sensitiveness (in picograms). CSF, cerebrospinal liquid; S, serum; BC, blood cells.

Table 2. Genetic Sequences of Influenza A Virus in Children with Congenital CNS Pathology

	Clinical Materials		
Group of children	CSF	Serum	Blood cells
The study group:			
A-k	+[a]	++	ND[b]
A-va	ND	++	ND
Sch-o (26.8.88)	+	++	++++
(8.9.88)	ND	++	++++
(17.11.88)	ND	++	++++
The control group			
I-v	ND	−[c]	−
P-o	ND	−	−
K-va	ND	−	−
T-v	ND	−	−

[a]Positive result.
[b]ND, not done.
[c]Negative result.

and Table 2). It will be seen from the data in Fig. 1 and Table 2 that serum specimens from both children contained genetic sequences of influenza A virus, and in A-k's specimens virus-specific sequences were also found in small amount in the CSF specimen. In the control group of children without signs of congenital CNS pathology, no genetic sequences of influenza virus were found in any of the specimens tested (Fig. 1, Table 2).

For the third child of the study group, Sch-o, one CSF specimen and three blood specimens collected within 83 days—at a 13-day interval between the first and second specimens and at a 70-day interval between the second and third specimens—were used for these tests (Table 2, Figs. 1 and 2). It will be seen in Table 2 that genetic sequences of influenza A virus were detected in the CSF in a small amount, in the serum in a larger amount, but the main portion of the virus-specific material was contained in the blood cells. As seen in Figs. 1 and 2, H1, NP, and M genes of influenza A virus could be detected in the blood cells of Sch-o throughout the entire observation period. The immunoblotting technique was used to detect antibody to individual viral proteins in the serum of this child. Influenza A/USSR/90/77 (H1N1) virus was used as the antigen (Fig. 3). It will be seen from Fig. 3 that no antibody to viral M, HA2, and HA0 proteins could be detected in the serum from Sch-o in contrast to a positive serum (positive control) in which the antibodies to all the viral proteins were present.

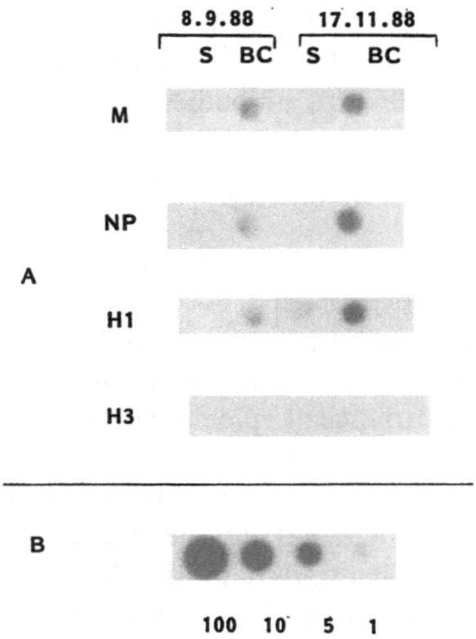

Figure 2. Detection of gene sequences M, NP, and H1 of influenza A viruses in blood specimens of sick infant Sch-o. (A) Hybridization of clinical specimens with probes to different genes; (B) control of hybridization method's sensitiveness (in picograms). S, serum; BC, blood cells.

DISCUSSION

Acute influenza infection in man and animals is characterized by a short incubation period and rapid appearance of signs of the disease in uncomplicated cases during no more than 7–10 days (Stuart-Harris *et al.*, 1985). Such a time course reflects intensive reproduction of the infectious virus in sensitive cells of the upper respiratory tract, a short period of viremia, and subsequent rapid decline of virus concentration in the host due to which no infectious virus can be found within 3–5 days after the onset of the disease using routine methods. It is for this reason that the possibility of detecting persisting influenza virus in the host has long been

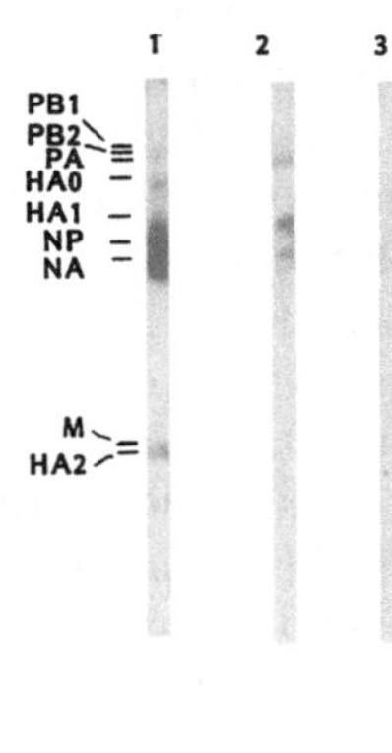

Figure 3. Immunoblotting of serum of sick infant Sch-o. 1, positive serum (positive control); 2, serum of sick infant Sch-o in dilution 1:100; 3, negative serum (negative control).

debated and only in recent years it has been shown that such persisting influenza virus can be detected in the host by special methods including careful elimination of influenza antibodies, disruption of immune complexes, and so forth (Pavlenko and Mirchink, 1977; Zuev, 1988). Persisting influenza virus may also be isolated from human beings suffering from congenital immune deficiency (Harrison *et al.*, 1985).

In our study, the mothers of all three children with congenital CNS pathology had experienced, according to the anamnestic data, influenza disease at different periods of pregnancy. And although the diagnosis of "influenza" had not been verified virologically, the diseases in all these mothers coincided in time with the occurrence of epidemic influenza outbreaks in the regions and in two cases (A-k's and A-va's mother) were confirmed serologically.

In our materials, the probability of transplacental transmission of influenza virus and intrauterine infection of the fetuses is substantiated by the lack of postnatal signs of the development of acute influenza infection in all babies and the simultaneous development in all three babies of the clinical picture of congenital CNS pathology of progressive course. To this, low titers of antibody to influenza virus in the babies' sera should be added which, at the same time, confirms their exposure to the virus.

Finally, direct evidence of infection of these children with influenza virus is the detection of significant amounts of genetic sequences of influenza A virus in their blood cells which had been demonstrated by means of three probes to NP, M, and H1 genes used in the study.

In one of the infants (Sch-o) with signs of congenital CNS pathology, the picture of which most exactly corresponded to the symptom complex of experimental slow influenza infection (Zuev *et al.*, 1983; Mirchink *et al.*, 1984; Zuev, 1988), three examinations of blood demonstrated in blood cells the persistence of at least three detectable genes, NP, M, and H1, throughout the observation period of 83 days. The results of immunoblotting tests revealed in this child a certain defectiveness of the persisting influenza virus which can be judged by the lack in his serum of antibodies to M, HA0, and HA2 proteins. The lack of antibodies to M protein appears to indicate disorders in its synthesis. In this connection it should be mentioned that disorders in M protein synthesis in influenza virus lead to the development of an abortive form of infection in inoculated cell cultures (Bukrinskaya *et al.*, 1981; Frielle *et al.*, 1984). Moreover, it is also known that disorders in M protein synthesis in reproduction of paramyxoviruses, for example, are typical of the development of such a well-known slow virus infection as subacute sclerosing panencephalitis (Hall and Choppin, 1981).

It cannot be ruled out that the failure to detect serum antibodies to HA0 and HA2 proteins may mean not the lack of their synthesis and cleavage, since serum antibodies to HA1 protein are detectable, but be due to disorders in the processing of HA0 and HA2 proteins.

In recent years, the use of molecular hybridization of nucleic acids as a method for rapid diagnosis of viral infections opens special avenues for the detection of persisting viruses characterized by a certain degree of defectiveness. At the same time, it should be noted that our detection of persisting defective influenza virus in a child with signs of congenital CNS pathology does not present absolute proof of the cause of the disease but suggests such an association and the necessity of further studies in this field.

REFERENCES

Baurin, V. V., Tentsov, Y. Y., Ivanova, L. A., and Bukrinskaya, A. G., 1985, Molecular hybridization of nucleic acids in rapid diagnosis of influenza, *Vopr. Virusol.* **5**:540–544 [in Russian].

Beklemishev, A. B., Blinov, V. M., Vasilenko, S. K., Golovin, S. Y., Karginov, V. A., Mamaev, L. V., Mikriukov, N. N., Netesov, S. V., Petrenko, V. A., Petrov, N. A., and Frolov, I. V., 1985, Synthesis, cloning and sequencing of a full-length DNA copy of NP gene of the influenza virus A, *Bioorg. Chem.* **11**:636–640 [in Russian].

Birnboim, H. C., and Doly, J., 1979, A rapid alkaline extraction procedure for screening recombinant plasmid DNA, *Nucleic Acids Res.* **7**:1513–1518.

Bukrinskaya, A. G., Starov, A. I., and Isaeva, K. A., 1981, Influenza viruses assembly and its defects, *Biosystems* **13**:157–161.

Bukrinskaya, A. G., Tentsov, Y. Y., Vorkunova, G. K., Tabachnikov, B. I., and Tyasto, E. A., 1986, Rapid diagnosis of influenza: Comparative evaluation of different methods, *Vopr. Virusol.* **3**:280–283 [in Russian].

Denhardt, D. T., 1966, A membrane-filter technique for the detection of complementary DNA, *Biochem. Biophys. Res. Commun.* **23**:641–646.

Frielle, D. W., Huang, D. D., and Youngner, J. S., 1984, Persistent infection with influenza A virus: Evolution of virus mutants, *Virology* **138**:103–117.

Hall, W. W., and Choppin, P. W., 1981, Measles-virus proteins in the brain tissue of patients with subacute sclerosing panencephalitis. Absence of the M protein, *N. Engl. J. Med.* **304**:1152–1155.

Harrison, C. J., Jenski, L. J., Sketch, T., and Gilchrist, M. J., 1985, Onset of cell-mediated immune function (CMI) after bone marrow transplant coincides with cessation of chronic shedding of influenza A virus (Flu A), *J. Cell. Biochem. Suppl.* **9C**:283.

Johnson, D. A., Gautsch, J. W., Sportman, J. R., and Elder, J. R., 1984, Improved technique utilizing nonfat dry milk for analysis of proteins and nucleic acids transferred to nitrocellulose, *Gene Anal. Tech.* **1**:3–8.

Laemmli, U. K., 1970, Cleavage of structural proteins during the assembly of the head of bacteriophage T4, *Nature* **227**:680–685.

Maniatis, T., Fritsch, E. F., and Sambrook, J., 1982, *Molecular Cloning: A Laboratory Manual*, Cold Spring Harbor Laboratory, Cold Spring Harbor, N.Y., p. 162.

Mirchink, E. P., Zuev, V. A., and Miroshina, E. K., 1984, Slow influenza infection developing in the progeny of female mice infected during pregnancy, *Vopr. Virusol.* **1**:32–35 [in Russian].

Pavlenko, R. G., and Mirchink, E. P., 1977, Persistence of influenza virus in the organism of the sensitive animals infected with different doses of the virus, *Vestn. Akad. Med. Nauk SSSR* **7**:16–21 [in Russian].

Rigby, P. W., Dieckman, W., Rhodes, C., and Berg, P., 1977, Labeling deoxyribonucleic acid to high specific activity in vitro by nick-translation with DNA polymerase I, *J. Mol. Biol.* **113**:237–251.

Samokhvalov, E. I., Karginov, V. A., Chizhikov, V. E., and Blinov, V. M., 1985, Primary structure of RNA segment 7 of the influenza virus A/USSR/90/77 (H1N1), *Bioorg. Chem.* **11**:1080–1085 [in Russian].

Shevchenko, A. M., 1986, Retardation in weight and body size of children, which were born to women who had a history of influenza or influenza-like diseases at period of pregnancy, *Regulatorno-prisposobitelnie mechanismi v norme i patologii*, Leningrad, pp. 189–191 [in Russian].

Shevchenko, A. M., 1987, Characteristics of neurological disturbances of children, whose mothers had a history of influenza or influenza-like diseases at period of pregnancy, *Regulatorno-prisposobitelnie mechanismi v norme i patologii*, Leningrad, pp. 172–174 [in Russian].

Stuart-Harris, C. H., Schild, G. C., and Oxford, J. S., 1985, *Influenza*, Arnold, London.

Towbin, H. T., Staehlin, T., and Gardon, J., 1979, Electrophoresis transfer of protein from polyacrylamide gels to nitrocellulose sheets: Procedure and some applications, *Proc. Natl. Acad. Sci. USA* **76**:4350–4355.

Yuferov, V. P., Karginov, V. A., Samokhvalov, E. I., Chizhikov, V. E., Vasilenko, S. K., Urivaev, L. V., and Zhdanov, V. M., 1984, Nucleotide sequence of the haemagglutinin gene of influenza virus A A/Udorn/307/72 (H3N2), *Dokl. Akad. Nauk SSSR* **287**:738–742 [in Russian].

Zuev, V. A., 1988, Slow virus infections in man and animals, *Meditsina*, Moscow, pp. 115–136 [in Russian].

Zuev, V. A., and Shevchenko, A. M., 1986, Congenital influenza infection in experiment and in childhood neurological clinic, *Materiali III syezda nevropatologov i psichiatrov Belorussii*, Minsk, pp. 318–320 [in Russian].

Zuev, V. A., Mirchink, E. P., and Kharitonova, A. M., 1983, Experimental slow influenza infection in mice, *Vopr. Virusol.* **1**:24–29 [in Russian].

Chapter **5**

Prognostic Markers of Human Immunodeficiency Virus-Associated Neurologic Symptoms in Patients with AIDS

Suraiya Rasheed

INTRODUCTION

Epidemiologic, virologic, and immunologic evidence strongly suggest that the acquired immune deficiency syndrome (AIDS) is caused by a retrovirus called the human immunodeficiency virus (HIV) (Barre-Sinoussi *et al.*, 1983; Popovic *et al.*, 1984; Levy *et al.*, 1984; Rasheed *et al.*, 1986a). The virus primarily infects human cells bearing CD4 receptors, including T4 lymphocytes, monocytes, macrophages, endothelial cells, Langerhans cells, epithelial cells, neuronal cells, and some B lymphocytes (Dalgleish *et al.*, 1984; Maddon *et al.*, 1986; Cheng-Mayer *et al.*, 1987; Wiley *et al.*, 1986; Rasheed *et al.*, 1989).

As a general rule, viruses that infect macrophages or lymphoid tissues are particularly responsible for the immunosuppression of the host. Since both the cellular and humoral immune systems of HIV-infected individuals are depressed,

Suraiya Rasheed • *Laboratory of Viral Oncology and AIDS Research, University of Southern California, Los Angeles, California 90032-3626.*

they also exhibit reduced responses to various non-HIV antigens and other environmental factors. Thus, HIV-infected individuals become susceptible to infections with other microorganisms and succumb to opportunistic pathogens including bacteria, protozoa, fungi and viruses [e.g., Epstein-Barr virus (EBV), cytomegalovirus (CMV), herpesviruses (HSV)]. The clinical consequences of HIV infections therefore range from prolonged asymptomatic states to severe depletion of CD4-positive T-helper lymphocytes, Kaposi's sarcoma, non-Hodgkin's lymphoma, and profound degeneration of the central nervous system (CNS).

NEUROLOGIC SYMPTOMS IN AIDS

Patients with AIDS show a broad range of neuropathologic dysfunctions. Early clinical neurologic manifestations in HIV-infected individuals include cognitive psychomotor dysfunctions, forgetfulness, poor concentration, and hallucinations (Price *et al.*, 1988; Navia *et al.*, 1986; De la Monte *et al.*, 1987; Piette *et al.*, 1986). Some of these symptoms precede the diagnosis of AIDS and may include subacute encephalitis, aseptic meningitis, and peripheral neuropathies.

CNS lymphoma and infection of the CNS by *Toxoplasma*, *Cryptococcus*, neurosyphilis, CMV, or other pathogens have been associated with various neurologic symptoms (Levine *et al.*, 1987; Levy *et al.*, 1988; Petito *et al.*, 1985). However, these agents have not been detected in all HIV-infected individuals (Rasheed *et al.*, 1988). In some cases, the acute fatal encephalitis was the only disease presented by HIV-infected individuals, suggesting that HIV may be the primary cause of CNS neuropathy that may not be related to secondary opportunistic infections of the CNS in these individuals (Rasheed *et al.*, 1988).

Entry of HIV into the CNS

Although several cell types have been shown to serve as reservoirs for the dissemination of HIV throughout the body, the predominant cell type in the brain that is infected by HIV is a cell of macrophage/monocyte lineage (Koenig *et al.*, 1986). However, cell-free virus can also reach the CNS by traversing the blood-brain barrier, or can leak through the endothelial lining of capillaries in the choroid plexus which is fenestrated. This is particularly true when large quantities of virus are present in the blood and with the flow of fluids the virus can reach the brain within a short time after infection. Entry of HIV from cerebrospinal fluid (CSF) to neuronal cells that bear CD4-like receptors may also be facilitated by receptor-mediated endocytosis of HIV particles complexed to antibodies, nonspecific phagocytosis of the virus, or entry via a non-CD4 or Fc-like receptor (Homsy *et al.*, 1989).

Virus Replication

Reports of active replication of HIV in glial or neuronal cells *in vitro* have been rare (Cheng-Mayer *et al.*, 1987). However, the virus has been isolated from the brain *in vitro* (Levy *et al.*, 1985; Gartner *et al.*, 1986; Rasheed *et al.*, 1987; Ho *et al.*, 1985) and HIV-like particles have been seen by electron microscopy (Epstein *et al.*, 1984).

Exposure of CD4-positive lymphocytes to high multiplicity of infection *in vitro* causes an acute infection which destroys more than 50% of infected cells due to polykaryon formation (Rasheed *et al.*, 1986b). This phase of infection is followed by a short period of recovery when approximately 30% of cells begin to proliferate and become persistently infected leading to a steady state in which virus is produced without any cytopathic effects (productive infection) (Rasheed *et al.*, 1986b). The persistently infected cells may enter a nonproductive (latent) stage and the integrated proviral genome persists as long as the cell is alive. Thus, HIV can cause productive, nonproductive cytopathic or noncytopathic infection in the same cell type.

In certain cells that may be permissive for virus replication, HIV produces its progeny or simply integrates, alters cell membranes and induces giant multinucleated syncytial cells. Since the permeability of the plasma membranes also increases after virus infection, the cells swell due to an influx of water into the cytoplasm. This ballooning of the cellular membrane facilitates cell fusion with other infected or uninfected CD4-bearing cells and induces classical HIV-induced cytopathology (Rasheed *et al.*, 1987a). These syncytial cells die eventually because they cannot sustain normal cellular functions. Thus, replication of virus in the CNS tissue *per se* may not be essential for the development of neurologic symptoms and the presence of cell-free virus or HIV-infected monocytes/macrophages in the vicinity of neuronal or glial cells may induce formation of multinucleated giant cells or gliomesenchymal nodules so frequently observed in patients with AIDS.

Immune Response

The HIV-encoded structural proteins and some regulatory proteins that are expressed in infected cells are antigenic. Although specific antibodies are produced in most HIV infections (Rasheed *et al.*, 1987b), the magnitude and the quality of the response depend on the virus load, antigenicity of viral proteins, host genetic factors as well as immunoregulatory responses. Further, both T and B cells cooperate with macrophages in recognizing the antigen and initiating immune responses. However, since macrophages control the rate and type of antigen delivery, they influence the quality and quantity of antibody produced in the host.

The nervous system has a unique antigenic constituent which stimulates the production of antibodies against HIV (Resnick *et al.*, 1985; Resnick and Shapshak, 1987). Recently we reported that approximately 92% of CSF from HIV-infected individuals with CNS symptoms produced HIV-related intrathecal antibodies indicating that these antibodies were made in CSF by the polyclonal immune cells (Rasheed *et al.*, 1988). Immunoblot (Western blot) analysis of CSF indicated that antibodies reactive with major HIV structural proteins, gp41, p65, p55, p31, and p24, were predominantly present in most samples tested. However, the amount of antibodies varied and there was no correlation between the presence or absence of HIV antibodies and CNS disease.

PERSISTENCE OF HIV INFECTION

Persistent infections are caused by antigenic variation, immunologic tolerance of the host, reduction in the specific immune responses to particular strains of HIV, presence of defective interfering particles, and lack of host-cellular factors that are essential for virus packaging, assembly, or exit from the cell (Clements *et al.*, 1980; Gendelman *et al.*, 1985; Huang and Baltimore, 1970). Host tolerance to HIV infections may also be due to the presence of large amounts of viral antigens or antigen-antibody complexes in the circulating body fluids. This may result in "desensitization" of immune responses and persistence of infection.

Since HIV persists for long periods of time, it is difficult to eliminate infected cells, particularly those present in the brain because they are protected by the immune surveillance. Further, since the virus is not killed in the macrophage/monocyte cells, it is possible that other lymphokines can activate macrophages in a manner such that instead of destroying the virus by lysosomal enzymes, they become resistant to killing and thus become carriers of virus infections. Moreover, any negative modulation of the immune responses or the endocrine system can impact in such a way that the virus can become latent or be activated from the latently infected cells.

Persistence of virus infection could also be due to the presence of different HIV strains. A heterogeneous population of viral strains exists in HIV-infected individuals (Wong-Staal *et al.*, 1985). Since the most variable region of the HIV genome is its envelope glycoprotein (Starich *et al.*, 1986) which is directly involved in immune selection, many strains escape immunity and continue to exist as productive or nonproductive infection simultaneously in the same individual. The process of persistence is facilitated because the virus has a high mutation rate due to errors in reverse transcription, and also due to the release of large amounts of antigenic material after death of syncytial cells.

Although genetically distinct, HIV is closely related to the lentivirus family of animal retroviruses including the Visna virus of sheep, the equine infectious anemia virus of horses, and the caprine anemia encephalitis virus of goats (Gonda *et al.*, 1985; Narayan and Cork, 1985; Gendelman *et al.*, 1985; Stephens *et al.*, 1986). These viruses have been shown to cause persistent neurologic diseases in animals that they infect. The symptoms are also similar to those produced by HIV with a long latent period and a slow onset of the disease (Narayan and Cork, 1985).

HIV-RELATED MARKERS OF CNS DISEASE IN ADULTS

Depletion of CD4-positive T-helper cells has been shown to be an important indicator of progression to AIDS (Fahey *et al.*, 1984; Fauci, 1988). However, the number of these cells fluctuates and no consensus pattern has been established for various disease states. We and others have previously shown that HIV-p24 antigenemia in blood of HIV-infected individuals is strongly associated with the development of symptomatic illness and this phenomenon is independent of the absolute number of T-helper cells in the blood (Eyter *et al.*, 1987; Polk *et al.*, 1987; Rasheed *et al.*, 1987).

To identify specific viral markers associated with CNS symptoms, we have recently evaluated 36 patients with neurologic symptoms and analyzed CSF and blood of both HIV-seropositive and HIV-seronegative individuals with CNS diseases (Rasheed *et al.*, 1988). Our results indicate that when all CNS infections were combined (i.e., those associated with HIV alone or in combination with infections with *Cryptococcus*, herpes zoster, CMV, and others), HIV could be isolated from 50% of HIV-seropositive patients (Rasheed *et al.*, 1988). However, HIV was isolated from 32% of CSF samples from HIV-seropositive individuals who exhibited CNS symptoms due to microbial or yeast infections (Rasheed *et al.*, 1988). In contrast, patients with encephalitis in which HIV was the primary infection associated with neurologic symptoms (i.e., no other pathogens identified), had a high (80%) virus isolation rate from the CSF (Rasheed *et al.*, 1988).

Comparison of HIV-seropositive individuals with and without CNS symptoms indicated that a higher level of virus load was present in the CSF of patients with neurologic diseases than in those without these symptoms. Although the quantity of HIV-p24 antigen in serum or CSF of patients with neurologic symptoms was not significantly different within this particular group of individuals, 80% of patients with encephalitis had p24 antigenemia compared to only 24% with other neurologic symptoms (Rasheed *et al.*, 1988).

One of the interesting findings of our study was the presence of cell-free HIV-gp120 in three of four CSF samples from HIV-seropositive patients with encephalitis (Rasheed, unpublished data). Because of the structural similarities between CD4-like receptors in the brain and HIV-envelope glycoprotein gp120, this antigen has a high binding affinity to neuronal cells (Maddon *et al.*, 1986; Pert *et al.*, 1986; Funke *et al.*, 1987). It is therefore possible that binding of the shed envelope proteins to areas of brain that are important for memory, learning, and so forth may play an important role in causing abnormalities in CNS functions. Alternatively, the shed viral envelope proteins gp120 and gp41 may bind to brain cells in a manner that induces them to produce cytopathic factors. Further, a common antigen or peptide may be responsible for viral pathology, because neuropeptidelike "transducing signals" can influence immune and brain functions through receptors similar to those used for HIV entry. To define the significance of envelope glycoproteins in encephalitis, we are currently analyzing a large number of CSF samples at different stages of CNS disease. It is possible that these antigens may be useful markers for the prognosis of neurologic symptoms in HIV-infected individuals.

PROGNOSTIC MARKERS OF HIV IN CHILDREN WITH NEUROLOGIC SYMPTOMS

Infants born to HIV-seropositive women have a 50% chance of carrying the virus (Nicholas *et al.*, 1989). Although most children born to HIV-infected mothers are positive for antibodies at birth, in a few cases no antibody was detected in the presence of virus infection (Nicholas *et al.*, 1989). The loss of antibody may be due to passive transfer of mother's antibody which is eliminated around 6 months of age or due to latent infection. The inability of these infants to produce antibodies could also be due to loss of cells that are necessary for immune stimulation of lymphocytes. Thus, infants exposed to HIV *in utero* may be symptomatic in the presence or absence of a productive HIV infection. Further, infection of immature cells results in a more severe disease in children than observed in adults (Epstein *et al.*, 1986; Khanani *et al.*, 1988).

Infants born to HIV-seropositive women manifest loss of developmental milestones and deterioration of motor functions (Epstein *et al.*, 1986; Khanani *et al.*, 1988). Presence of microcephaly in HIV-infected children in the absence of other CNS infections (e.g., CMV, *Toxoplasma*) suggests that HIV infection may solely be responsible for neurological manifestations in these children (Epstein *et al.*, 1986).

In a study of five cases, we have evaluated HIV markers in children with neurologic symptoms and found that the presence of HIV-p24 antigenemia in CSF was associated with dementia and progressive encephalopathy (Rasheed *et al.*, unpublished data). The total HIV antigen levels were also higher in CSF than in serum of children with neurologic deficits. Our data also indicate that HIV antigens may be detectable in CSF earlier than in serum of some immune-suppressed children, suggesting that measurement of HIV antigenemia may be a useful prognostic marker of CNS disease in HIV-infected children. In this respect the consequences of HIV infection differ markedly between adults and children.

Mechanisms of HIV-Related CNS Diseases

The mechanism(s) by which HIV kills or damages CNS cells is not clear. However, the brain, endocrine systems, hormones, and receptors on the surface of lymphocytes, all can modulate or regulate cellular immunity, induce new receptors, alter immune responses, increase susceptibility to virus infections, and control the recurrence of latency by a variety of mechanisms. Moreover, the cells of the immune system and the brain share some common antigenic determinants which are highly conserved (Pert *et al.*, 1986). The CD4-like molecules that are present in high densities in certain areas of the brain (e.g., hippocampus, cortex) become targets for HIV infection or binding of cell-free antigen to cellular membranes. This phenomenon leads to cell fusion and destruction of cells by polykaryon formation (Lifson *et al.*, 1986). In addition, specific brain cells may allow HIV to integrate in the chromosomal DNA which may interfere with expression of specific cellular gene(s) that may be responsible for neuropathologic changes observed in individuals infected by HIV.

The virulence of different HIV strains may influence clinical and pathologic manifestations of the disease. A nonvirulent strain may induce a milder disease due to the initial production of neutralizing antibodies. However, since a heterogeneous population of HIV strains exists in most infected individuals, the neutralizing antibodies, if produced, are diluted out or are unable to protect the individuals and the virus continues to replicate (Rasheed *et al.*, 1986a and 1987b).

It is also possible that biologic and biochemical differences between HIV strains might influence neurotropism of these viruses (Starich *et al.*, 1986; Shaw *et al.*, 1985; Anand *et al.*, 1989; Terwilliger *et al.*, 1986). These HIV strains may have preferential access to certain neuronal cells which may induce characteristic giant cells present in the brains of patients with subacute encephalitis. Further, the extent and severity of the neurologic disease may depend largely on the properties of HIV strains, the virus load that has been transferred from the periphery to the brain, the age of exposure, the genetic susceptibility, and the immunologic status of the individual. However, these mechanisms have not been clearly defined and it is not clear if mutation, deletion, or acquisition of a particular sequence in the HIV genome is responsible for a specific clinical entity.

Differences in HIV envelope sequences may affect the configuration of gp120 or gp41 which are essential for the interaction with the receptors in the brain cells (Rasheed, unpublished data). Thus, whether the virus replicates in monocytes/macrophages present in the brain or whether it enters directly into the CNS through the blood-brain barrier, the tissue damage due to cytopathic or cytotoxic effects may be directly related to HIV present in the brain.

Similar to other retroviruses, HIV also matures by budding from the plasma membrane. It is therefore possible that the viral envelope lipids which are derived from the host cells and carbohydrate moieties of the envelope glycoproteins which serve as antigenic determinants, may have specific affinity with neuronal cells. Further, as evidenced by our studies (Rasheed *et al.*, 1988), the viral envelope antigens that are shed in the plasma or CSF of HIV-infected individuals may bind directly to receptors in the brain cells and destroy target cells or change cellular functions. Thus, accumulation of viral proteins and the presence of high levels of intrathecal HIV antibodies in the CSF all favor the possibility of a more direct etiologic role of HIV in the development of encephalitis than previously envisioned.

It has been speculated that since monocytes/macrophages are the primary source of HIV in the brains of infected individuals, the HIV strains isolated from brain may have a preferential growth advantage in these cells. However, our studies indicate that this is not a universal phenomenon (Rasheed *et al.*, 1988). Isolation of HIV from 36 patients with CNS symptoms indicates that all CSF viruses could be isolated in normal phytohemagglutinin (PHA)-stimulated PBMCs. Host range study of randomly selected viruses from five patients with CNS diseases indicated that all strains tested replicated well in the U937 promonocyte cells and three of the five strains tested replicated both in the macrophages and in the CEM T4-cell line. Further, among the T-cell lines tested CEM cells showed higher titers and cytopathic effects than observed in HUT-78 or RH9 cells (Rasheed, unpublished data). These data suggest that mechanisms other than growth potential in monocytes are involved in the neurotropism and/or pathogenesis of the brain cells.

One of the important properties of HIV-related viruses that distinguishes these from other known retroviruses is the presence of several regulatory genes in addition to the structural genes, *gag*, *pol*, and *env*, present in most replication-competent retroviruses. The products of these genes modulate cellular functions and regulate molecular pathways involved in replication, packaging, and assembly of these viruses. Since some of the regulatory proteins are also antigenic, the up-regulation or down-regulation of these genes affects virus expression, antibody production, cytopathology, and/or virus persistence in various cells. Further, changes in the positive regulator of HIV (*tat*), differential regulator (*rev*), negative regulator (*nef*), virion infectivity factor (*vif*), or possibly the *cis*- or *trans*-acting elements essential for the regulation of these genes may all induce changes both in the HIV genome and in the infected cells (Haseltine and Wong-Staal, 1988). It is therefore possible that the presence of virus in the brain cells may produce lower levels of enzymes or proteins necessary for normal functions than those present in healthy cells. Alternatively, cellular functions may differ because of changes in the enzyme structure or functions. Characterization of HIV-gene products produced in the infected brain cells and identification of factors produced by macrophages or glial cells which affect neuronal cell functions may lead to a better understanding of mechanisms involved in the development of encephalitis or other neurologic symptoms in patients with AIDS.

CHARACTERISTICS OF HIV-INFECTION

1. Macrophages/monocytes traveling from periphery to CNS are primary carriers of HIV to the brain.
2. Direct infection of neuronal cells by cell-free HIV is rare but possible.
3. Virus heterogeneity, evasion of immune response, viral latency, and persistence of infection, all contribute to enhanced immune suppression and facilitate opportunistic infections.
4. Alterations in the expression of HIV-regulatory proteins or mutations in genetic sequences may affect viral replication in the neuronal cells.
5. Both cell-free and cell-associated virus present in the CSF may damage neuronal cells and induce giant multinucleated cells by binding to the CD4-like receptors in the brain cells.
6. Shed HIV-gp120 and gp41 may bind to CD4-like receptors in the brain, alter cellular functions, and destroy target cells by fusion of cellular membranes.
7. Lack of LTR-mediated transcription in resting cells may cause latency in neuronal cells bearing CD4-like receptors.
8. Activation of latent virus due to enzymes, proteins, or factors that may induce transcriptional changes in neuronal cells may also produce functional changes in these cells.
9. Integration of HIV provirus into chromosomal DNA may cause dysregulation of cellular gene functions and may influence production of altered or abnormal amounts of normal gene products in these cells.
10. Antigenic drift, hypervariability, and neurotropism of HIV may also destroy specialized functions of nerve cells or produce lower levels of specific enzymes or proteins necessary for normal cellular functions.
11. Production of intrathecal HIV antibodies may bind to hormone receptors and inhibit production of specific hormones necessary for normal brain functions.

REFERENCES

Anand, R., Srinivasan, A., Gardner, M., Luciw, P., and Dandekar, S., 1989, Biological and molecular characterization of human immunodeficiency virus (HIV-1) from the brain of a patient with progressive dementia, *Virology* **168**:79–89.

Barre-Sinoussi, F., Chermainn, J. C., Nageyre, M. T., Chamaret, S., Gruest, J., Daugeut, S., Anler-Blin, C., Vezinet-Brun, F., Rouzivux, C., Roxenbaum, W., and Montagnier, L., 1983, Isolation of a T-lymphotropic retrovirus from a patient at risk for acquired immune deficiency syndrome (AIDS), *Science* **220**:868–871.

Cheng-Mayer, C., Rutka, J. T., Rosenblum, M. L., McHugh, T., Sites, D. P., and Levy, J. A., 1987, Human immunodeficiency virus can productively infect cultured human glial cells, *Proc. Natl. Acad. Sci. USA* **84**:3526–3530.

Clements, J. E., Pedersen, F. S., Narayan, O., and Haseltine, W. A., 1980, Genomic changes associated with antigenemic variation of visna virus during persistent infection, *Proc. Natl. Acad. Sci USA* **77**:4454–4458.

Dalgleish, A. G., Beverly, P. C., Clapham, P. R., Crawford, D. H., Greaves, M. F., and Weiss, R. A., 1984, The CD4 (TC4) antigen is an essential component of the receptor for the AIDS retrovirus, *Nature* **312**:763–767.

De la Monte, S. M., Ho, D. D., Schooley, R. T., Hirsch, M. S., and Richardson, E. P., Jr., 1987, Subacute encephalomyelitis of AIDS and its reaction to HTLV-III infection, *Neurology* **37**:562–569.

Epstein, L. G., Sharer, L. R., and Cho, E. S., 1984, HTLV-III/LAV-like retrovirus particles in the brain of patients with AIDS encephalopathy, *AIDS Res.* **1**:447–457.

Epstein, L. G., Sharer, L. R., Oleske, J. M., Connor, E. M., Goudsmit, J., Bagdon, L., Robert-Guroff, M., and Koenigsberger, M. R., 1986, Neurologic manifestations of HIV infection in children, *Pediatrics* **78**:678–687.

Eyter, M. E., Ballard, J. O., Gail, M. H., Drummond, J. E., and Goedert, J. J., 1987, Predictive markers for the acquired immunodeficiency syndrome (AIDS) in hemophiliacs: Persistence of p24 antigen and low T4 cell count, *Ann. Intern. Med.* **107**:1–6.

Fahey, J. L., Prince, H., Weaver, M., Groopman, J., Visscher, B., Schwartz, K., and Detels, R., 1984, Quantitative changes in T helper or T suppressor/cytotoxic lymphocyte subsets that distinguish AIDS from other immune subset disorders, *Am. J. Med.* **76**:95–100.

Fauci, A. S., 1988, The human immunodeficiency virus: Infectivity and mechanisms of pathogenesis, *Science* **239**:617–622.

Funke, I., Hahn, A., Rieber, E. P., Weiss, E., and Reithmuller, G., 1987, The cellular receptor (CD4) of the human immunodeficiency virus is expressed on neurons and glial cells in human brain, *J. Exp. Med.* **165**:1230–1235.

Gartner, S., Markovits, P., and Markovitz, D. M., 1986, Virus isolation from and identification of HTLV-III/LAV-producing cells in brain tissue from a patient with AIDS, *J. Am. Med. Assoc.* **256**:2365–2371.

Gendelman, H. E., Narayan, O., Molineaux, S., Clements, J. E., and Ghotbi, Z., 1985, Slow, persistent replication of lentiviruses: Role of tissue macrophages and macrophage precursors in bone marrow, *Proc. Natl. Acad. Sci. USA* **82**:7086–7090.

Gonda, M. A., Wong-Staal, F., and Gallo, R. C., 1985, Sequence homology and morphology and morphologic similarity of HTLV-III and visna virus, a pathogenic lentivirus, *Science* **227**: 173–177.

Haseltine, W. A., and Wong-Staal, F., 1988, The molecular biology of the AIDS virus, *Sci. Am.* **259**:52–63.

Ho, D. D., Rota, T. R., Schooley, R. T., Kaplan, J. C., Allan, J. D., Groopman, J. E., Resnik, L., Feinstein, D., Andrews, C. A., and Hirsch, M. S., 1985, Isolation of HTLV-III from cerebrospinal fluid and neural tissues of patients with neurologic syndromes related to the acquired immunodeficiency syndrome, *N. Engl. J. Med.* **313**:1493–1497.

Homsy, J., Meyer, M., Tateno, M., Clarkson, S. J., and Leve, A., 1989, The Fc and not CD4 receptor mediates antibody enhancement of HIV infection in human cells, *Science* **244**:1357–1360.

Huang, A. S., and Baltimore, D., 1970, Defective viral particles and viral disease process, *Nature* **226**:325–327.

Khanani, R. M., Hafeez, A., Rab, S. M., and Rasheed, S., 1988, Human immunodeficiency virus-associated disorders in Pakistan, *AIDS Res. Hum. Retroviruses* **4**(2):149–154.

Koenig, S., Gendelman, H. E., Orenstein, J. M., DalCanto, M.C., Pezeshkpour, G. H., Yungbluth, M., Janotta, F., Aksamit, A., Martin, M. A., and Fauci A. S., 1986, Detection of AIDS virus in macrophages in brain tissue from AIDS patients with encephalopathy, *Science* **233**:1089–1093.

Levine, A. M., Gill, P. S., and Rasheed, S., 1987, AIDS-related malignant B-cell lymphomas, in: *AIDS Modern Concepts and Therapeutic Challenges* (S. Broder, ed.), M. Dekker, New York, pp. 233–244.

Levy, J. A., Hoffman, A. D., Kramer, S. M., Landis, J. A., Shimabukuro, J. M., and Oshiro, L. S., 1984, Isolation of lymphocytotropic retroviruses from San Francisco patients with AIDS, *Science* **225**:840–842.

Levy, J. A., Shimabukuro, J., Hollander, H., Mills, J., and Kaminsky, L., 1985, Isolation of AIDS-associated retroviruses from cerebrospinal fluid and brain of patients with neurological symptoms, *Lancet* **2**:586–588.

Levy, R. M., Bredesen, D. E., and Rosenblum, M. L., 1988, Opportunistic central nervous system pathology in patients with AIDS, *Ann. Neurol.* **23**:S7–S12.

Lifson, J. D., Feinberg, M. B., Reyes, G. R., Rabin, L., Banapour, B., Chakrabati, S., Wong-Staal, F., Steimer, K. S., and Engleman, E. G., 1986, Induction of CD4-dependent cell fusion by the HTLV-III/LAV envelope glycoprotein, *Nature* **323**:725–728.

Maddon, P. J., Dalgleish, A. G., McDougal, J. S., Clapham, P. R., Weiss, R. A., and Axel, R., 1986, The T4 gene encodes the AIDS virus receptor and is expressed in the immune system and the brain, *Cell* **47**:333–348.

Narayan, O., and Cork, L. C., 1985, Lentiviral diseases of sheep and goat: Chronic pneumonia leukencephalomyelitis and arthritis, *Rev. Infect. Dis.* **7**:89–98.

Navia, B. A., Cho, E.-S., Petito, C. K., and Price, R. W., 1986, The AIDS dementia complex. II. Neuropathology, *Ann. Neurol.* **19**:525–535.

Nicholas, S. W., Sondheimer, D. L., Willoughby, A. D., Yaffe, S. J., and Katz, S. L., 1989, Human immunodeficiency virus infection in childhood, adolescence and pregnancy: A status report and maternal research agenda, *Pediatrics* **83**:293–308.

Pert, C. B., Hill, J. M., and Ruff, M. R., 1986, Octapeptides deducted from the neuropeptide receptor-like pattern of antigen T4 in brain potently inhibit human immunodeficiency virus receptor binding and T-cell infectivity, *Proc. Natl. Acad. Sci. USA* **23**:9254–9258.

Petito, C. K., Navia, B. A., Cho, E.-S., Jordan, B. D., George, D. C., and Price, R. W., 1985, Vacuolar myelopathy pathologically resembling subacute combined degeneration in patients with acquired immunodeficiency syndrome, *N. Engl. J. Med.* **312**:874–879.

Piette, A. M., Tusseau, F., Vignon, D., Chapman, A., Parrot, G., Leibowitch, J., and Montagnier, L., 1986, Acute neuropathy coincident with seroconversion for anti-LAV/HTLV-III, *Lancet* **1**:852.

Polk, B. F., Fox, R., Brookmeyer, R., Kanchanaraksa, S., Kaslow, R., Visscher, B., Rinaldo, C., and Phair, J., 1987, Predicators of the acquired immunodeficiency syndrome developing in a cohort of seropositive homosexual men, *N. Engl. J. Med.* **316**:61–66.

Popovic, M., Sarngadharan, M. G., Read, E., and Gallo, R. C., 1984, Detection, isolation and continuous production of cytopathic retroviruses (HTLV-III) from patients with AIDS, *Science* **224**:497–500.

Price, R. W., Brew, B., Sidtis, J., Rosenblum, M., Scheck, A. C., and Clearly, P., 1988, The brain in AIDS: Central nervous system HIV-1 infection and AIDS dementia complex, *Science* **239**: 586–592.

Rasheed, S., Norman, G. L., Gill, P. S., Meyer, P. R., Cheng, L., and Levine, A. M., 1986a, Virus-neutralizing activity, serologic heterogeneity, and retrovirus isolation from homosexual men in the Los Angeles area, *Virology* **150**:1–9.

Rasheed, S., Gottlieb, A. A., and Garry, R. F., 1986b, Cell killing by UV-inactivated human immunodeficiency virus, *Virology* **154**:395–400.

Rasheed, S., Shu, S., and Norman, G. L., 1987a, Acquired immune deficiency syndrome: Diagnostic procedures for the antibody and retrovirus, in: *Viral Hepatitis and AIDS* (V. M. Villarejos, ed.), San Jose, Costa Rica LSU-ICMRT, pp. 31–52.

Rasheed, S., Norman, G. L., Shu, S., Gill, P. S., and Levine, A., 1987b, High expression of HIV-p24 antibodies as predictors for the development of AIDS, *RNA Tumor Virus Meeting*, Cold Spring Harbor, p. 149.

Rasheed, S., Su, S., and Larsen, R. A., 1988, Correlation of HIV P24 levels in cerebrospinal fluid (CSF) and encephalitis in HIV-infected patients. *Int. Conf. AIDS*, **2**:365.

Rasheed, S., Yao, K. X., and Zhou, J. T., 1989, Genetic analysis of Burkitt's lymphoma cells from a patient with AIDS, *Int. Conf. AIDS*, p. C-703.

Resnick, L., and Shapshak, P., 1987, Serological characterization of HTLV-III/LAV infection by Western blot and radioimmunoprecipitation assays, *Arch. Pathol. Lab. Med.* **111**:1040–1044.

Resnick, L., DiMarzo-Veronese, F., Shopbach, J., Tourtellotte, W. W., Ho, D. D., Muller, F., Shapshak, P., and Gallo, R. C., 1985, Intra-blood-brain-barrier synthesis of HTLV-III-specific IgG in patients with AIDS or AIDS-related complex, *N. Engl. J. Med.* **313**:1498–1504.

Shaw, G. M., Harper, M. E., Hahn, B. H., Epstein, L. G., Gajdusek, D. C., Price, R. W., Navia, B. A., Petito, C. K., O'Hara, C. J., Groopman, J. E., Cho, E. S., Oleske, J. M., Wong-Staal, F., and Gallo, R. C., 1985, HTLV-III infection in brains of children and adults with AIDS encephalopathy, *Science* **227**:177–182.

Starich, B. R., Hahn, B. H., Shaw, G. M., McNeely, P. D., Modrow, S., Wolf, H., Parks, E. S., Parks, W. P., Josephs, S. F., Gallo, R. C., and Wong-Staal, F., 1986, Identification and characterization of conserved and variable regions in the envelope gene of HTLV-III/LAV, the retrovirus of AIDS, *Cell* **45**:637–648.

Stephens, R. M., Casey, J. W., and Rice, N. R., 1986, Equine infection anemia virus gag and pol genes: Relatedness to visna and AIDS virus, *Science* **231**:589–594.

Terwilliger, E., Sodroski, J. G., Rosen, C. A., and Haseltine, W. A., 1986, Effects of mutations within the 3′ orf open reading frame region of human T-cell lymphotropic virus type III (HTLV-III/LAV) on replication and cytopathogenicity, *J. Virol.* **60**:754–760.

Wiley, C. A., Schrier, R. D., Nelson, G. A., Lampet, P. W., and Oldstone, M. B. A., 1986, Cellular localization of human immunodeficiency virus infection within the brains of acquired immune deficiency syndrome (AIDS) patients, *Proc. Natl. Acad. Sci. USA* **83**:7089–7093.

Wong-Staal, F., Shaw, G. M., Hahn, B. H., Salahudin, S. Z., Popovic, M., Markham, P. D., Redfield, R., and Gallo, R. C., 1985, Genomic diversity of human T-lymphotropic virus type III, *Science* **229**:759–762.

Part II

Virological and Immunological Study of Schizophrenia

Chapter **6**

Prenatal Viral Infection as an Etiological Agent in Adult Schizophrenia

Evidence for Two Models

Christopher E. Barr and Sarnoff A. Mednick

There is a significant body of literature suggesting structural abnormalities in the brains of schizophrenics; these abnormalities appear to be nondegenerative and may be perinatal in origin (Kovelman and Scheibel, 1986; Weinberger, 1987; Bogerts, 1988; Lyon *et al.*, 1989). Though researchers have focused on delivery complications (McNeil, 1988) as the source of these perinatal abnormalities, there are several lines of evidence that indicate schizophrenia may also result from a disturbance of gestation. These include postmortem histopathological studies of the brains of adult schizophrenics and studies showing an association between risk of prenatal viral infection and subsequent increases in the birthrate of schizophrenics.

In this chapter an attempt will be made to assess the kind of brain damage found in schizophrenics, when there is reason to believe it originated prenatally. The evidence for midgestational viral infection as an etiological factor in schizophrenia will be reviewed, in the context of fetal neural development. The ways in which prenatal viral infection might interfere with fetal neural development will be

Christopher E. Barr and Sarnoff A. Mednick • *Department of Psychology, University of Southern California, Los Angeles, California 90089-1111.*

discussed (i.e., by causing defects of neuronal migration or destruction of cells) along with their implications for future research.

PART I: HISTOPATHOLOGICAL AND EPIDEMIOLOGICAL EVIDENCE

Histopathological Studies

In the first half of this century, over 200 articles on the neuropathology of schizophrenia were published, without any pattern of pathological changes characteristic of schizophrenia being generally agreed on (Bogerts, 1988). A number of methodological issues may have contributed to the failure of classical neuropathologists' attempts to find a lesion pathognomonic for schizophrenia: lack of controls, variation in the criteria for schizophrenia and in psychodiagnostic methods (retrospective versus premortem), and use of qualitative rather than quantitative methods. The qualitative approach was noted to be vulnerable to the tendency for idiosyncratic theories to bias the gathering and interpretation of data (Kirch and Weinberger, 1986). By the 1950s, failure to arrive at a characteristic lesion, plus dramatic new biochemical findings, led to a decline in neuropathological studies. More recent CT findings of enlarged ventricles, and apparent cortical atrophy, have led to a revival of interest in neuroanatomical research in schizophrenia.

The more recent histopathological studies have been characterized by the use of quantitative methods, and more rigorous methodology than was generally true of their precursors (Bogerts, 1988; Kirch and Weinberger, 1986). The quantitative approach employs more objective measures and methods, such as: the number, size, or spatial orientation of individual cells, the volume of particular structures, the intensity of glial staining, observers blind to diagnosis, and statistical comparisons with carefully matched controls. Accordingly, the studies reviewed here will be primarily of the quantitative type, though a few relevant qualitative studies will also be mentioned. The discussion is not intended as an exhaustive review, and is limited to a sampling of studies which allow some inferences to be drawn about the stage of development in which the observed aberrations occurred.

McLardy (1974) found that 12 of 30 schizophrenics (with 7 controls) had strikingly thinner bilateral granule cell layers in the hippocampal formation. Zinc content was also reduced by 50% in the granule cell layer. No other brain areas were examined. McLardy concluded that these cell changes were not a result of degeneration but were consistent with developmental arrest.

Jakob and Beckmann (1986) examined 64 schizophrenic brains (with 10 controls). Of the 64, 42 had unusual patterns of temporal sulci and gyri. Of these 42, 20 had cytoarchitectonic abnormalities in the rostral entorhinal region of the parahippocampal gyrus, usually a poorly developed structure in the upper layers with heterotopic displacement of single pre-alpha-cell groups. Other brain regions were not investigated and no evidence of gliosis was found. The authors suggested that the ectopic cells resulted from a disturbance of neuronal migration during the second trimester.

Kovelman and Scheibel have found evidence of pyramidal cell disorientation in the left hippocampus of schizophrenics (Scheibel and Kovelman, 1981; Kovelman and Scheibel, 1984), and that the degree of disorganization was associated with severity of illness but not with advancing age. In the latest study, with ten male, paranoid schizophrenics (and eight age-matched controls), investigators were blind to the diagnostic status of the subjects, neuron misalignment was measured quantitatively, and diagnosis was confirmed premorbidly by several physicians.

Falkai and Bogerts (1986) examined the density of neuronal and glial cells in the hippocampus and found evidence for a decreased number of neurons, in the absence of gliosis, for schizophrenics as compared to controls. A similar finding was obtained for the entorhinal region (Falkai *et al.*, 1988). The results of the two studies were interpreted as due to a developmental hypoplasia rather than a degenerative process.

Benes *et al.* (1986) evaluated neuron and glial cell density, neuron size, and neuron/glial cell ratios of ten schizophrenics (and ten controls) in the prefrontal, anterior cingulate, and primary motor cortex. Neuron densities were found to be significantly lower in layer VI of the prefrontal, layer V of the anterior cingulate, and layer III of the motor cortex. There were no significant differences in the neuron/glial cell ratios between schizophrenics and controls. The density of glial cells was also lower in schizophrenics than controls. In other words, Benes *et al.* found quantitative evidence of reduced numbers of neurons in the absence of gliosis.

In addition, multiple regression techniques were employed to remove the effects of other variables which might account for the differential neuron density such as age, neuroleptic exposure, and perimortem events (hypoxia, duration of postmortem interval before brain fixation, duration of fixation). The difference in neuron densities between the two groups was maintained after these confounds were statistically removed. The authors interpreted these findings as arguing against a process of neuronal degeneration. The findings were, however, consistent with the hypothesis of developmental dysplasia.

Indications of Prenatal Damage

Several different characteristics of these study results might lead us to infer that the observed pathology occurred prenatally, perhaps in the second trimester.

1. Ectopic neurons, cells of a type that should appear in one layer of the cortex but appear in another, e.g., heterotopic pre-alpha cells, have been reported by

Jakob and Beckmann. Neurons migrate to their correct position during fetal neural development (generally in the second trimester) and these results are consistent with a disruption of neuronal migration.

2. Misalignment of neurons, e.g., the disarray of hippocampal pyramidal cells found by Kovelman and Scheibel. After these neurons migrate to their correct final positions, they must also establish the proper spatial orientation with respect to one another. Kovelman and Scheibel (1984) report after reviewing the literature that the finding of "isolated, misplaced, or ectopic neurons indicates that such cells, when they appear, are considered as developmental anomalies."

3. Reductions in neuron density in the absence of gliosis or mineralization. Gliosis is a nonspecific response to cellular damage and may result from hemorrhage, infection, autoimmune response, or other insults. It is believed that the ability of astrocytes to respond with hypertrophy or proliferation begins to appear only during the sixth or seventh month of gestation (Gilles *et al.*, 1983).

Reduced numbers of neurons without an increase in glial cells suggest either a failure of neurons to develop or migrate to the site in question, cell death prior to the third trimester, or a perimortem effect, e.g., hypoxia, in which neuron destruction leads to death before gliosis can develop. Because the latter explanation is also consistent with the observed findings, the lack of gliosis should be considered a weaker indicator of possible developmental disruption. It is important to note, however, that Benes *et al.* took pains to remove the effects of possible specimen preparation and perimortem confounds and found that the difference in neuron densities between schizophrenics and controls was still maintained.

4. Neuronal loss in the absence of mineralization may also suggest a developmental rather than degenerative process, as McLardy (1974) indicated. In this case, mineral deposits are assumed to be a form of cellular debris, rather than being a cause of neuron destruction itself. From this standpoint, reduction in neuron density without mineralization would suggest an aberration in cell migration or mitosis rather than atrophy. Further investigation of this hypothesis is required before it can be given much weight.

In summary, there is a range of indicators of prenatal damage in the preceding studies. Some of these indicators seem fairly reliable, i.e., neuronal ectopia and disarray, while others are more suggestive, i.e., reduced neuron density in the absence of gliosis or mineralization.

As Kirch and Weinberger (1986) report, "Every area of the central nervous system, including the spinal cord, has been identified as showing structural abnormalities in schizophrenia." Yet there has been little consensus as to any lesion or pattern of pathology characteristic of schizophrenia. It is interesting to note, however, that when findings are limited to carefully controlled studies, a more delimited pattern of pathology emerges, implicating prenatal, possibly second-trimester developmental disruption. The findings reviewed above all indicate histological abnormalities in either (1) the hippocampus or parahippocampal gyrus or (2) areas of the frontal cortex, i.e., the prefrontal cortex, the anterior cingulate gyrus, and the primary motor cortex. Weinberger (1987) has hypothesized that a "lesion" in a mesolimbic, mesocortical dopamine "circuit" (specifically, dorsolateral prefrontal cortex) may be responsible for schizophrenic symptomatology. Benes and Bird (1987) note that the cingulate gyrus has extensive connections with the dorsolateral prefrontal cortex and that, as part of Papez's loop, it is interconnected with the hippocampus.

It is tempting to speculate that fetal neurodevelopmental disruption, occurring in the second trimester, impacts specifically on brain structures involved in a mesolimbic, mesocortical "psychosis circuit." However, this line of speculation is premature, given the relatively small number of sites studied in which the possibility of prenatal developmental disruption can be evaluated. It may be that when ectopic cells, neuronal disarray, or neuronal thinning in the absence of gliosis, are evaluated in other sites, we may find widespread evidence of prenatal developmental disruption.

Prenatal Viral Infection and Schizophrenia

The second type of studies suggesting that a disturbance of prenatal development might play an etiological role in schizophrenia are those showing an association between prenatal viral infection, and increased risks of adult schizophrenia in the offspring.

Within the context of an ongoing prospective study of individuals at high-risk for schizophrenia, Machon *et al.* (1983) found that those born in a densely populated urban area (and therefore at increased risk of viral infection), in winter months, and who were at higher genetic risk, showed a markedly higher rate of schizophrenia (23.3%) than others who did not meet these three criteria. Overall the high-risk group had an 8.9% schizophrenia rate, while the risk of schizophrenia in the general population is about 1%.

In a follow-up study of the same population, Machon *et al.* (1987) noted that the increased rate of schizophrenia found in the genetic high-risk, urban, winter-born group appeared to be accounted for by the presence or absence of pregnancy and birth complications (PBCs). Within this group the schizophrenia rate for those with PBCs was 30% but only 9% for those without PBCs, i.e., the average rate for the high risk group. It was speculated that prenatal viral exposure may be responsible for both subtle neurological damage to the fetus and in addition the increase in PBCs. In this case the PBCs are simply a marker for viral infection and the latter factor is the etiological agent. An alternate explanation was that viral infections, or some other seasonally varying factor, caused PBCs, which in turn were responsible for the increase in schizophrenia.

Indirect evidence for the role of viral infection in the etiology of schizophrenia was provided by Mednick *et al.* (1988). In 1957 the residents of Helsinki experienced a severe type A2 influenza epidemic. Those individuals who were in their second trimester of fetal development during this epidemic had a higher risk of being hospitalized for schizophrenia, compared to those born in the same months and same city for the six previous years. The apparent effect was observed in males and females and replicated across several psychiatric hospitals. It would seem that there is a specific prenatal "window of vulnerability" to the effects of influenza on subsequent adult schizophrenia.

Currently unpublished analyses of the Helsinki data indicate that the viral effect may be associated with a subtype of schizophrenia. It was noted that the index group schizophrenics who were in their second trimester during the epidemic were more likely than control group schizophrenics to receive ICD-8 subdiagnoses of Other or Unspecified schizophrenia (53 versus 28%). Second-trimester-exposed index subjects were also more likely to be diagnosed as schizophrenic on their first psychiatric admission (23.5 versus 13.2%) than were controls. Indexes of chronicity such as: age at first admission, number of psychiatric admissions, and number of days hospitalized, were not significantly associated with index schizophrenics for any trimester of exposure.

This pattern of results is difficult to interpret because we do not yet know what kind of symptoms or neurological differences are associated with Other or Unspecified subdiagnoses and a schizophrenia diagnosis on first admission. However, these findings do imply that second-trimester influenza infection is affecting the course of the subsequent schizophrenic illness.

Influenza and Schizophrenia in Denmark

The Helsinki study was limited to a single city, a single epidemic, and employed a relatively small number of schizophrenic subjects. In order to expand on the Helsinki findings, Barr *et al.* (1989) carried out a follow-up study in Denmark. This investigation was designed to replicate the Helsinki study and extend it by: using a different country, extending the period of time covered to 40 years (1911 to 1950), studying an entire national population of hospitalized schizophrenics, and evaluating the effects of all influenza epidemics over 40 years, rather than a single epidemic.

We obtained a record of the number of individuals born per month in Denmark, between January 1, 1911 and December 31, 1950. For the same time period we also obtained the number of these individuals who eventually were diagnosed schizophrenic, the number of influenza cases, reported monthly, and data on the size of the Danish population. The schizophrenic birthrate was expressed as number of births of schizophrenics per month, per thousand live births. Influenza incidence was defined as the number of cases per 1000 population for each month.

Problem: The Winter Concurrence

It would seem that the most obvious way to approach the data is to determine whether the months in which influenza is highly prevalent are followed by an increase in the births of schizophrenics. We already know that those high-influenza months occur most often in the winter, and that there is a tendency for schizophrenics to be born in the winter. There are three types of explanations for this concurrence.

1. It may be that the winter increase of influenza and of schizophrenic births are not causally related. For example, high summer temperatures early in pregnancy may increase schizophrenic births in winter, while winter temperature may increase the risk of influenza. Nonetheless, a correlation would be found between schizophrenia and influenza because of their winter coincidence. In other words, the highest influenza months would be associated with a higher schizophrenic birthrate, simply because both events happen in the winter, though for two different reasons.

The essential feature of this kind of two-factor theory is that the two causes are independent of each other. Accordingly, we assume that an unusually hot summer does not imply an unusually cold winter. Using the example above, an especially hot summer should produce more winter schizophrenic births than normal. However, we would not expect any more or less winter influenza than normal. In short, we would not expect that an unusually high level of influenza (for the time of year) would be followed by an unusually high increase in schizophrenic births, unless there were some kind of relationship between the two variables.

2. The second possible explanation of the winter concurrence is that a single winter-related third factor (e.g., cold temperature, decreased immune response, dietary deficiency) produces both the winter increase of influenza and schizophrenic births. According to this conception, influenza is just a correlate of the real etiological agent, and has no direct causal significance.

3. The final interpretation of the winter concurrence of influenza and schizophrenia rates is that prenatal influenza infection directly increases the risk of adult schizophrenia. The acceptability of this interpretation is increased if the other two hypotheses are rejected.

Analyses

As indicated above, simply correlating monthly influenza and schizophrenic birthrates would only demonstrate what we already know, i.e., that there is a winter concurrence of influenza and schizophrenia. In order to rule out possible two-factor or third-factor explanations, various statistical methods were used to remove the effects of season from monthly influenza and schizophrenic birthrates.

Each of the 480 months of the year was

1. Classified as being average, unusually high, or unusually low in influenza incidence for that time of the year, and
2. Received a deviation score for schizophrenic birthrates, representing the degree to which it exceeded or fell short of the level expected for that time of year.

For example, June 1921 was categorized as a high-influenza month; those born in June 1921 were in their ninth month of gestation in a high-influenza month. The categorization of each monthly influenza rate as high, medium, or low was paired with that month's deviation score for schizophrenic births. An ANOVA compared the schizophrenia deviation score for high- versus medium- versus low-influenza month groups. This ANOVA tested the association between influenza level in the month of birth and schizophrenic birthrate. This type of ANOVA was then repeated for the eighth through first months of gestation.

Results

Figure 1 plots the results of exposure to unusually high, medium, or unusually low levels of influenza, at different points in fetal development, on subsequent schizophrenic birthrate. The three influenza groups were defined as being higher than, lower than, or equal to, the amount expected for that time of year. Schizophrenic birthrate was measured using seasonal deviation scores.

The only significant association occurred in the sixth month of gestation ($p = 0.002$, $F = 6.178$). T-test results show that the schizophrenic birthrate for the medium- and low-influenza groups did not differ from each other. However, the high-influenza month group had a significantly greater schizophrenic birthrate than either of the other two groups. This indicates that influenza infection is only a risk factor for schizophrenia when it occurs in the sixth month of gestation.

Using a similar method we also noted that unusually high levels of influenza, in the summer, are significantly associated with increase in the risk of schizophrenia for those exposed at the end of the second trimester. This combination of results indicates that neither a winter-related third factor, or two-factor theory accounts for sixth-month effect of influenza on adult schizophrenia.

Limitations

This study has several limitations:

1. We do not know how many of the schizophrenic subjects of the study actually experienced a viral infection in their sixth month of gestation.

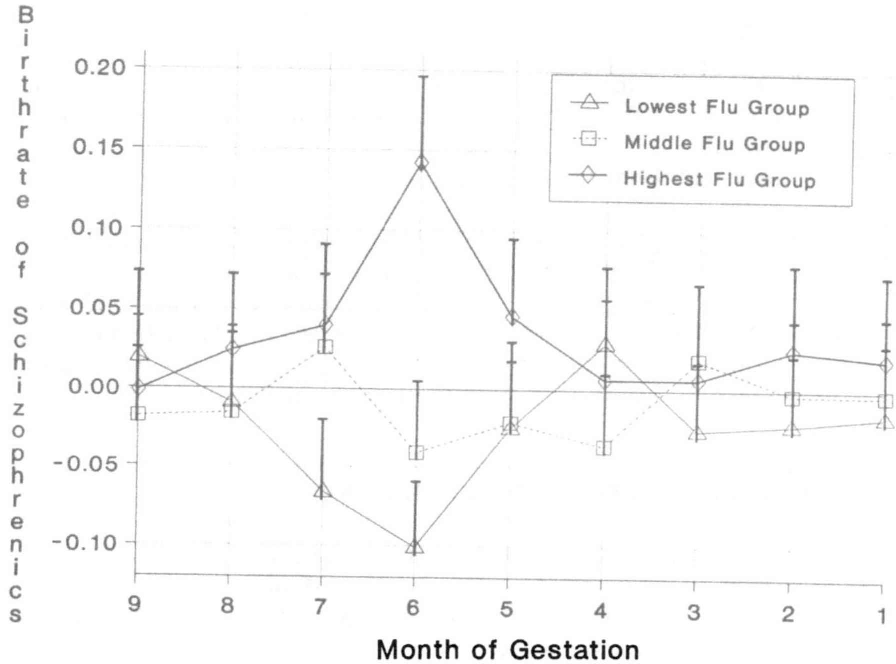

Figure 1. The mean schizophrenia birthrate following three levels of exposure to influenza at each of the 9 months of gestation. The schizophrenia birthrate is expressed as a deviation score, and the three influenza groups are defined using deviation scores.

During peak epidemic periods the number of recorded infection cases was as high as 23% of the population. How many other individuals who were infected subclinically and thus did not seek medical attention is difficult to determine. For a severe Helsinki epidemic the subclinical incidence has been estimated at approximately 30% (Hakosalo and Saxen, 1971).

2. The timing of gestation is based on birth dates, which are ascertained only to the nearest month. We do not know which of the subjects in the sample were born prematurely.
3. The diagnosis of schizophrenia was made according to Danish hospital, rather than research standards.
4. To the extent that the population of schizophrenics contained in our database were resident hospital patients, our sample may be biased toward a more chronic population.

Conclusions

1. Exposure to increased levels of influenza at the end of the second trimester (sixth month) is associated with increased risk of adult schizophrenia.
2. It is unlikely that this association results from a third, winter-related factor.
3. We have replicated a previous finding of an association between high levels of influenza in the second trimester, and subsequent increases in rates of adult schizophrenia. This study suggests that the window of vulnerability is narrower than a trimester, and may be centered on the sixth month of fetal neural development, a period characterized by neuronal migration and especially rapid brain growth.

PART II: PRENATAL DEVELOPMENTAL PROCESSES

The studies of prenatal viral infection suggest that a second-trimester disruption of fetal neural development may increase the risk of eventual adult schizophrenia. A hypothesis which invokes prenatal viral infection as an etiological factor in schizophrenia must address several questions:

1. What ontogenic process might be vulnerable to a viral infection?
2. How, specifically, might a viral infection interfere with those processes?
3. What testable implications are generated by the different ways in which a virus might disrupt fetal development?

Neuronal Migration

Jakob and Beckmann (1986) and Kovelman and Scheibel (1984) have hypothesized that fetal neuronal migration has been disrupted in some of the brains of adult schizophrenics they have examined. Rakic (1972, 1974, 1988a,b) has investigated the process of cortical neuronal migration over the last two decades. The following description of neuronal migration is based mainly on his work.

Developing neurons are produced in the proliferative zone, an area of epithelium near the lateral cerebral ventricle. Within the proliferative zone, precursor or stem cells are organized into columns called proliferative units. Each proliferative unit has an associated glial fiber which leads to the cortical surface. Although the cortex folds and shifts throughout development, the connection between a proliferative unit and its cortical endpoint is maintained by the glial fiber. Each proliferative unit produces a series of young neurons which migrate up the common glial fiber. The different layers of cortex are made up of cells which migrated at different times. Therefore, the cortical layer in which disruption of migration is apparent, gives us a rough indication of the timing of the disturbance.

Neuronal migration begins in the first trimester and has tapered down by the third trimester. However, it may extend as late as "the end of the second half of gestation" according to Rakic (1988a). Because of differential rates of maturation, the stage of migration at one site may be as much as a month ahead or behind that of another area, in the same brain. This adds some further uncertainty to the extent of neuronal migration occurring after midgestation.

As cells migrate up the glial guide, they encounter a number of other cellular processes which logically they might align with, but do not. What accounts for the migrating neuron's ability to follow the glial fiber? It is generally hypothesized that neuronal and glial cell surfaces contain cell adhesion molecules. A number of candidate molecules have been proposed (Rakic, 1988a). If these molecules are lacking or their chemical action interfered with, a migratory deviation or failure may occur.

Implications for Neuropathology

The radial unit hypothesis of fetal neural development has several implications for the kind of structural aberrations found in the brains of schizophrenics. We might expect to see thinning of the cortex, without shrinking of a particular cortical area, if cells are interrupted in migration. Damage that occurs earlier during the formation of the proliferative units, should also reduce the number of ontogenic columns and therefore the surface area of the affected cortical region, without reducing its thickness. The findings of ectopic cells, and reduced neuron densities in the studies reviewed earlier, as well as other findings of thinning of the hippocampal formation, parahippocampal gyrus, and amygdala (Bogerts *et al.*, 1984; Brown *et al.*, 1984), suggest that, at least for some schizophrenics, a disruption of neural migration occurs.

It is possible that viral infection has nothing to do with disturbances of neuronal migration. Evidence exists for a genetic mutation which produces disruption of neuronal migration, with resulting neuropathology, i.e., the reeler mouse (Rakic, 1988a). It may be, therefore, that disruption of neuronal migration is an entirely genetically controlled event. If viral infection plays no role in disruption of neuronal migration, what other developmental processes might be involved?

Neuronal Destruction

Another major feature of second-trimester neurological development is a burst of brain growth which shows its greatest acceleration at week 24.5 (Gilles *et al.*, 1983, p. 317). There in an abrupt increase in cerebral volume, hemispheric surface area, and decrease in the volume of the lateral ventricle (Gilles *et al.*, 1983, pp. 316–317), all occurring around the sixth month. A viral infection at this point may cause the loss of cells important in the etiology of schizophrenia and account for enlarged ventricles and the relatively greater size of sulci, i.e., the apparent "atrophy" of a number of cerebral structures commonly noted in adult schizophrenics. Around this period the ability of astrocytes to proliferate or respond hypertrophically is thought to begin (Gilles *et al.*, 1983, p. 319). Therefore, we might see evidence of gliosis, in schizophrenic brains, resulting from an infection at this time, and such findings have been reported.

Stevens (1982) studied brain sections from 25 schizophrenics and 20 controls and found increased fibrillary gliosis in periventricular structures of the diencephalon, the periaqueductal regions of the mesencephalon, the basal forebrain, the hippocampus, and subependymal regions of the inferior horn of the lateral ventricles. Stevens interpreted her findings as resulting from a previous inflammation, possibly due to a virus. Nieto and Escobar (1972) compared brains of 10 younger schizophrenics (age 29 to 52) to 4 controls. They found greater gliosis in the schizophrenic subjects in the reticular formation, hypothalamus, thalamus, periaqueductal gray matter, and hippocampus. This type reaction does not necessarily represent a prenatal infection, but it is suggestive, in light of the epidemiological evidence from Denmark and Helsinki.

Ependymal Discontinuities

Lyons *et al.* (1989), in discussing the work of Mollgard, reported a "cerebrospinal fluid–brain barrier" (CSF–BB) found only in fetal brains. The CSF–BB includes a protein-tight layer of ependymal cells. Gilles *et al.*, (1983, pp. 113–116) also note that at the end of the second trimester, discontinuities appear in the ependymal lining in three locations: over the hippocampus, in the posterior portions of the lateral ventricles, and on the undersurface of the rostral corpus callosum (i.e., at the surface of the basal ganglia). Mollgard indicated that a virus would have easier to access to the fetal brain at these locations because of gaps in the ependymal layer. Findings implicating neuron loss and disarray in the hippocampus of schizophrenics have been reviewed above. Evidence of gliosis, neuron loss, and reduced volume of basal ganglia structures have been provided by Stevens (1982) and Bogerts *et al.* (1984). Therefore, at least for the hippocampus and basal ganglia, there is evidence that structures near these ependymal gaps may be at risk for insult, in the brains of those who later become schizophrenic.

Hemorrhage

The germinal matrix, a structure of tissue which supports the development of other cells, is rapidly dissolving during the end of the second trimester. Based on data from the NINCDS Collaborative Perinatal Project, Gilles *et al.* (1983, pp.

316–320) reported that the dissolution of the germinal tissue and its capillary bed is associated with an increased risk for periventricular hemorrhage, which in turn may be associated with enlarged ventricles. Both hemorrhage and ventricular enlargement are found in premature infants, which may be related to delivery complications. However, Gilles *et al.* (1983, p. 324) note that stillborn infants have surprisingly similar rates of large macroscopic and microscopic ventricular hemorrhages, suggesting the possibility that factors antecedent to birth may account for a significant portion of intracranial hemorrhages. One such prenatal factor related to hemorrhage is infection. Gilles *et al.* (1983, pp. 204–216) noted that respiratory infection was a significant risk factor for hemorrhage in the germinal matrix, but not elsewhere (e.g., subarachnoid). Intraventricular hemorrhage may account for the enlarged ventricles and periventricular glial scarring noted in the brains of schizophrenics.

In summary then, there is evidence for vulnerability to periventricular hemorrhage because of germinal matrix dissolution, at the end of the second trimester. Also at this time ependymal gaps may make portions of the periventricular area more vulnerable to viral infection. Finally, the epidemiological evidence indicates that the end of the second trimester is a time when viral infection is most likely to produce schizophrenia. It may be that the capillary bed of the germinal matrix, at this vulnerable period, is most likely to hemorrhage due to virally induced tissue destruction. As indicated earlier, respiratory infections, which include influenza, are a risk factor for germinal matrix hemorrhage.

PART III: VIRAL INFECTION AND FETAL DEVELOPMENTAL DISRUPTION

Thus far, discussion of the three areas a prenatal viral theory of schizophrenia should address has been limited to the first; the fetal developmental processes (neuronal migration, and rapid growth at the end of the second trimester) that might be impacted by a viral infection. Accordingly, we shall turn to an examination of some specific mechanisms by which a viral infection might interfere with fetal neural development and the implications these hypotheses have for further research.

Neuronal-Cell Adhesion Molecules

Conrad and Scheibel (1987) have proposed an etiological model of schizophrenia that identifies interruption of neuronal migration into the hippocampus, as the cause of schizophrenia. Neuraminidase-bearing viruses are the specific agent of disruption in this account.

As a migrating neuron enters the primitive hippocampus, it may be required to adhere and detach at precise intervals in order to complete the migratory process.

This is necessary for neurons to: (1) pass other neurons which arrived earlier, (2) separate from the glial guide, (3) form laminations by clustering side by side (not end to end) with proper polar orientation, (4) draw apart from other neurons as the neuropil matures.

Conrad and Scheibel's hypothesis is that neuronal-cell adhesion molecules (N-CAMs) are responsible for the adhesive and uncoupling processes required of migrating neurons. Sialic acid makes up one portion of N-CAMs and is closely related to their cell binding properties. Differing concentrations of two forms of sialic acid (the adult, or A form and the embryonic, or E form) may control the alternation between states of greater or lesser cell adhesion. Influenza viruses (among some others) are known to contain neuraminidase, an enzyme which is capable of converting the E form of sialic acid into its A form. It is thought that the presence of these types of viruses in the fetal brain alters the relative concentrations of sialic acid moieties of N-CAMs, and thereby disrupts the migration and alignment process in the primordial hippocampus. They go on to suggest that one way of reconciling this environmental insult model of schizophrenia with the evidence for a genetic component to the disease, is to posit that what is inherited is actually a compromised immune system. That is, the mothers of schizophrenics are those women who are, on the basis of genetics, most vulnerable to viral infection.

Research Implications

One testable implication of this theory is that schizophrenia is the end product of prenatal infection caused by a limited number of diseases, i.e., neuraminidase-bearing viruses. Therefore, diseases which do not bear this enzyme should not increase the risk of subsequent schizophrenia. We are currently conducting research to evaluate this hypothesis.

A second hypothesis is that the number of schizophrenic offspring in a given period of time should be proportional to the number of women who suffered viral infection during some critical period of gestation, regardless of their genetically determined immunocompetence. Accordingly, an epidemic of influenza should produce a proportionate increase in the birthrate of schizophrenics.

Febrile Hyperthermia

Edwards (1986) has reviewed the evidence for hyperthermia as a teratogen in mammalian species. He has found that the fetal CNS is more susceptible to damage by heat than are other tissues. He notes that a threshold temperature increase of 1.5–2.5°C is sufficient to produce malformations in fetuses of experimental animals. This temperature increase is within the range of those induced by febrile infections (about 103°F in humans). Proliferating cells are especially sensitive to hyperthermia. Mitotic cells exposed to threshold temperature increases, cease mitosis and with sufficient exposure, die. Though cell death is estimated to cause most of the CNS damage, other disturbances are known to occur. These include microvascular leakage leading to hemorrhage and edema. Edwards sees no reason to suppose that humans have an abnormally high threshold to heat damage and reviews findings of miscarriage, microphthalmia, mental retardation, micrencephaly, and other neurological problems, following human fetal exposure to febrile infection. It is clear that fever may interrupt neural development throughout gestation and produce different kinds of damage. According to Rakic's radial unit hypothesis, early hyperthermia could reduce the number of proliferative units, resulting in micrencephaly. A later disruption would reduce the number of cells available for migration, leading to thinner cortical layers in areas still receiving new cells. According to the findings of Gilles *et al.*, we might expect that at the end of the second trimester, when the periventricular area was most vulnerable, fever might produce hemorrhage with corresponding ventricular enlargement and glial scarring.

Research Implications

One clear hypothesis that is derivable from Edwards' work is that if fever is the component of influenza infection responsible for the damage often observed in brains of schizophrenics, then a wide variety of other diseases should raise the risk of adult schizophrenia. Research is currently under way to test this hypothesis.

SUMMARY AND CONCLUSIONS

Two basic models of prenatal influenza infection as an etiological agent in schizophrenia have been discussed; i.e., as a disturbance of neuronal migration, or as a cause of cell death in neurons which have reached their terminal positions. Other viral models of schizophrenia have been proposed in the literature, such as the hypothesis that schizophrenia results from exposure to a slow virus, either before or after birth. We have chosen to restrict this discussion to models which are tied to specific periods of prenatal development.

A variety of avenues by which a viral infection might cause the kind of brain damage observed in schizophrenics have been reviewed. These include interference with N-CAM activity, and destruction of neural cells either directly or indirectly, e.g., by hemorrhage, or fever effects.

It is premature to speculate as to which of these models is correct. The histopathological evidence supports both. There are findings of ectopic or disarrayed neurons, and thinner cortical layers, consistent with a disruption of migration. Alternatively, findings of ventricular enlargement and glial scarring suggest destruction of more mature neurons. Other evidence, indicating that influenza infection is a risk factor for hemorrhage, supports the latter interpretation. Our best evidence for the window of vulnerability to viral infection, points to the sixth month. This estimate remains inexact for a number of reasons and does not clearly distinguish between the two models.

The possibility exists that both types of viral insult are operative in the etiology of schizophrenia. Cannon and Mednick (1990) have hypothesized that schizophrenia results from a two-part process, the first of which is a disruption of neuronal migration, which may be caused by genetic defect, or viral infection, either alone or in combination. The second factor consists of either ventricular enlargement resulting from hemorrhage or anoxia, or a traumatic social environment in childhood. The Cannon–Mednick model indicates that viral infection may be an etiological factor at either or both stages.

In conclusion, we recognize that we have permitted ourselves considerable latitude in the expression of highly speculative, and controversial, interpretations of research in disparate fields. This has, of course, been done to help generate new hypotheses worthy of being tested.

ACKNOWLEDGMENTS The writing of this chapter was supported by a grant from the Scottish Rite Schizophrenia Research Program, and by the National Institute of Mental Health grants 5R01 MH37692 and 5R01 MH37902, and by Research Scientist Award K05-MH00619 (Dr. Mednick).

REFERENCES

Barr, C. E., Mednick, S. A., and Huttunen, M. O., 1989, Prenatal influenza infection as an etiological factor in schizophrenia, Poster presented at the 2nd International Congress on Schizophrenia Research, San Diego.

Benes, F. M., and Bird, E. D., 1987, An analysis of the arrangement of neurons in the cingulate cortex of schizophrenic patients, *Arch. Gen. Psychiatry* **44:**608–616.

Benes, F. M., Davidson, J., and Bird, E. D., 1986, Quantitative cytoarchitectural studies of the cerebral cortex of schizophrenics, *Arch. Gen. Psychiatry* **43:**31–35.

Bogerts, B., 1988, Neuropathological abnormalities and their clinical correlates in schizophrenia, Paper presented at the National Institute of Mental Health conference on Fetal Neural Development and Schizophrenia, Washington, D.C.

Bogerts, B., Meertz, E., and Schonnfeldt-Bausch, R., 1984, Basal ganglia and limbic system pathology in schizophrenia, *Arch. Gen. Psychiatry* **42:**784–791.

Brown, R., Colter, N., Corsellis, J. A. N., Crow, T. J., Frith, C. D., Jagoe, R., Johnstone, E. C., and Marsh, L., 1984, Postmortem evidence of structural brain changes in schizophrenia, *Arch. Gen. Psychiatry* **43:**36–42.

Cannon, T. D., and Mednick, S. A., 1990, Genetic and perinatal determinants of structural brain deficits in schizophrenia, *Arch. Gen. Psychiatry* **46:**883–889.

Conrad, A. J., and Scheibel, A. B., 1987, Schizophrenia and the hippocampus: The embryological hypothesis extended, *Schiz. Bull.* **4:**577–587.

Edwards, M. J., 1986, Hyperthermia as a teratogen: A review of experimental studies and their clinical significance. *Teratogenesis Carcinogenesis Mutagenesis* **6:**563–582.

Falkai, P., and Bogerts, B., 1986, Cell loss in the hippocampus of schizophrenics, *Eur. Arch. Psychiatry Neurol. Sci.* **236:**154–161.

Falkai, P., Bogerts, B., and Rozumek, M., 1988, Limbic pathology in schizophrenia: The entorhinal region—a morphometric study, *Biol. Psychiatry* **24:**515–521.

Gilles, F. H., Leviton, E., and Dooling, E. C., 1983, *The Developing Human Brain*, John Wright, Massachusetts.

Hakosalo, J. K., and Saxen, L., 1971, Influenza epidemic and congenital defects, *Lancet* **2:**1346–1347.

Jakob, H., and Beckmann, H., 1986, Prenatal developmental disturbances in the limbic allocortex in schizophrenics, *J. Neural Transm.* **65:**303–326.

Kirch, D. G., and Weinberger, D. R., 1986, Anatomical neuropathology in schizophrenia: Post-mortem findings, in: *Handbook of Schizophrenia*, Volume 1 (H. A. Nasrallah and D. R. Weinberger, eds.), Elsevier, Amsterdam, pp. 325–348.

Kovelman, J. A., and Scheibel, A. B., 1984, A neurohistological correlate of schizophrenia, *Biol. Psychiatry* **19**(12):1601–1621.

Kovelman, J. A., and Scheibel, A. B., 1986, Biological substrates of schizophrenia, *Acta Neurol. Scand.* **73:**1–32.

Lyon, M., Barr, C. E., Cannon, T. D., Mednick, S. A., and Shore, D., 1989, Fetal neural development and schizophrenia, *Schiz. Bull.* **15**(1):149–161.

Machon, R. A., Mednick, S. A., and Schulsinger, F., 1983, The interaction of seasonality, place of birth, genetic risk and subsequent schizophrenia in a high risk sample, *Br. J. Psychiatry* **143:** 383–388.

Machon, R. A., Mednick, S. A., and Schulsinger, F., 1987, Seasonality, birth complications and schizophrenia in a high risk sample, *Br. J. Psychiatry* **151:**122–124.

McLardy, T., 1974, Hippocampal zinc and structural deficit in brains from chronic alcoholics and some schizophrenics, *J. Orthomol. Psychiatry* **4**(1):32–36.

McNeil, T. F., 1988, Obstetric factors and perinatal injuries, in: *Handbook of Schizophrenia*, Volume 3 (M. T. Tsuang and J. C. Simpson, eds.), Elsevier, Amsterdam, pp. 319–344.

Mednick, S. A., Machon, R. A., Huttunen, M. O., and Bonnet, D., 1988, Adult schizophrenia following prenatal exposure to an influenza epidemic, *Arch. Gen. Psychiatry* **45:**189–192.

Nieto, D., and Escobar, A., 1972, Major psychosis, in: *Pathology of the Nervous System* (J. Minkler, ed.), McGraw–Hill, New York, pp. 2654–2665.

Rakic, P., 1972, Model of cell migration to the superficial layers of fetal monkey neocortex, *J. Comp. Neurol.* **145:**61–84.

Rakic, P., 1974, Neurons in rhesus monkey visual cortex: Systematic relation between time of origin and eventual disposition, *Science* **183:**425–427.

Rakic, P., 1988a, Defects of neuronal migration and the pathogenesis of cortical malformations, *Prog. Brain Res.* **73:**15–37.

Rakic, P., 1988b, Specification of cerebral cortical areas, *Science* **241:**170–176.

Scheibel, A. B., and Kovelman, J. A., 1981, Disorientation of the hippocampal pyramidal cell and its processes in the schizophrenic patient, *Biol. Psychiatry* **16**(1):101–102.

Stevens, J. R., 1982, Neuropathology of schizophrenia, *Arch. Gen. Psychiatry* **39:**1131–1139.

Weinberger, D. R., 1987, Implications of normal brain development for the pathogenesis of schizophrenia, *Arch. Gen. Psychiatry* **44:**660–669.

Chapter 7

An Influenza Epidemic and the Seasonality of Schizophrenic Births

E. Fuller Torrey, Ann E. Bowler, and Robert Rawlings

INTRODUCTION

The occurrence of psychosis following epidemics of influenza was noted as early as 1846 (Rorie, 1901). In the wake of the 1889–1890 influenza pandemic, Althaus (1893) reviewed 34 articles on "psychoses following influenza" which had been published in the preceding 3 years. The deadly influenza pandemic of 1918–1919 was also followed by a spate of articles, including Menninger's (1926) review of 200 postinfluenzal psychoses admitted to a single hospital of which "one-third *looked* like and were labeled dementia praecox." More recently the influenza pandemic of 1957, caused by an influenza A viral strain which was especially neurotropic, produced reports of manic and schizophrenic-like psychoses from at least six countries (Bental, 1958; Lloyd Still, 1958; Prokop, 1958; Soeiro, 1958; Loo *et al.*, 1957; Chistovich, 1959).

If the influenza virus can occasionally cause psychoses in adults, might it also infect the brains of developing fetuses or newborns and, after a latent period of 15 or 20 years, cause similar psychoses? The realization that the influenza virus may cause Parkinson's disease after a latent period of many years lends credibility to

---

E. Fuller Torrey and Ann E. Bowler • *Twin Studies Unit, NIMH Neurosciences Center, St. Elizabeths Hospital, Washington, D.C. 20032.* Robert Rawlings • *Division of Biometry and Epidemiology, National Institute on Alcohol Abuse and Alcoholism, Rockville, Maryland 20857.*

this model (Ravenholt and Foege, 1982). In addition, it might explain the well-defined and consistently replicated 5–15% winter-spring excess of schizophrenic births (Bradbury and Miller, 1985; Boyd *et al.*, 1986).

The possibility that the influenza virus might be acquired early in life and cause schizophrenia-like disease many years later has been suggested by three recent studies. Watson *et al.* (1984), in a study of veterans with schizophrenia in Minnesota, concluded that there were "specific relationships between winter schizophrenic births and the prevalence of both pneumonia and influenza." Torrey *et al.* (1988), in a study of schizophrenic births and reportable viral illnesses in Connecticut between 1920 and 1955 using time series spectral analysis, reported that influenza was significantly related to schizophrenic births ($p < 0.005$) with the strongest correlation occurring at about the time of birth. Finally, Mednick *et al.* (1988), in a study of schizophrenic births and the 1957 influenza epidemic in Finland, found a significant ($p < 0.05$) excess of individuals with schizophrenia who had been in midtrimester fetal development during the 1957 epidemic. The present study is an attempt to replicate the findings of Mednick *et al.* by examining the birth pattern of individuals now diagnosed with schizophrenia to determine whether this birth pattern has any relationship to the 1957 influenza epidemic.

METHODOLOGY

The incidence of influenza cases during the 1957 pandemic peaked in the United States in October of that year with a secondary peak (as measured by influenza-related deaths) occurring in February of 1958 (Langmuir, 1961). The influenza did not occur evenly across states but affected some much more widely than others. Selected for study were the 17 states which, according to 1957 data collected by the Centers for Disease Control, had the highest percentage of counties reporting influenza outbreaks (MMWR, 1957). Data were requested from an additional three states (Louisiana, Utah, Hawaii) because of the unusual pattern of the influenza epidemic in those states. Each of the states was asked to provide the month and year of birth of all individuals now diagnosed with schizophrenia who were receiving mental health services in the state.

Of the 17 states, 10 were able to provide month and year of birth of individuals currently diagnosed with schizophrenia who were born from January 1950 to December 1959 (Table 1). Approximately three-quarters of the schizophrenics were diagnosed using DSM-III criteria and one-quarter using DSM-II. Each of the 10 states provided data without duplication of patients except for Mississippi where a minor degree of duplication was thought to occur. The total number of individuals with schizophrenia in the 10 states born 1950–1959 was 43,778 including 405 born in October 1957, the peak of the influenza epidemic. Data were also obtained from United States vital statistics on all births for the same states for 1950–1959 ($N =$

Table 1. Individuals with Schizophrenia Born 1950–1959 in Ten States

	No. of patients	Source of patients
Connecticut	413	Inpatients as of 2/29/88
Georgia	9,717	Hospital admissions 1976–1987
Iowa	742	Hospital and outpatient admissions 1983–1988
Maine	1,598	Community hospital discharges 1973–1987
Maryland	3,642	Hospital residents 1987 and first admissions 1982–1987
Mississippi	1,775	Hospital admissions 1984–1988, not unduplicated but little overlap because of regional admissions
New York	14,755	Hospital admissions 1982–1987
Ohio	5,739	Hospital admissions 1983–1987
Oregon	180	Inpatients as of 6/28/88
Wisconsin	5,253	Patients who initiated services with state facilities, 1980–1984
Total	43,814	

10,496,686) and the schizophrenic birthrate per 10,000 total births for each month was calculated (Table 2); the average monthly rate was 41.7. A time series analysis was undertaken with the data deseasonalized and trends removed by differencing; the resultant series was examined for any unusual changes after 1957. Chi square tests were used to compare the observed and expected percentage of schizophrenic births and total births; months in which influenza was thought to influence schizophrenic births were compared with the same months for all other years.

Table 2. Schizophrenic Birth Rate per 10,000 Total Births by Month, 1950 to 1959, Ten States

	1950	1951	1952	1953	1954	1955	1956	1957	1958	1959	Totals
Jan.	48.1	43.9	42.2	45.7	47.8	49.4	49.4	47.6	48.6	46.2	46.9
Feb.	41.6	40.7	45.1	40.5	47.9	46.8	45.4	40.2	39.8	41.3	42.9
Mar.	41.8	43.8	35.6	43.5	41.5	41.4	45.2	43.1	39.4	39.2	41.5
Apr.	45.9	33.4	40.7	40.9	43.3	40.6	45.6	40.9	41.6	37.8	41.0
May	41.7	45.1	40.4	41.6	39.3	35.8	40.2	41.4	42.5	38.0	40.6
Jun.	41.6	37.3	38.9	43.5	45.6	43.5	39.8	45.1	36.1	38.5	40.8
Jul.	39.9	37.6	43.9	41.8	45.0	40.9	42.4	41.7	36.3	37.0	40.7
Aug.	36.0	44.0	37.3	41.6	41.3	43.6	42.9	38.9	39.1	37.8	40.1
Sep.	41.8	42.2	39.4	47.1	43.6	41.2	41.4	42.4	39.7	34.1	41.2
Oct.	38.3	41.2	42.0	41.2	42.2	38.4	40.0	41.3	40.4	35.6	40.1
Nov.	44.4	37.4	43.7	45.3	48.1	42.7	41.1	44.4	36.9	37.4	42.1
Dec.	43.4	44.7	45.6	42.4	46.2	44.3	46.7	43.1	36.9	38.4	43.2
Totals	41.9	41.0	41.2	42.9	44.5	42.1	43.4	42.5	39.7	38.4	41.7

RESULTS

Contrary to our hypothesis, there was no significant elevation of the schizophrenic birthrate immediately preceding, during, or after the 1957 influenza epidemic (Table 3). In looking initially at the raw numbers of schizophrenic births there did appear to be an elevation but this was found to be illusory when the schizophrenic births were put in relationship to general births; October 1957 had in fact a greater number of *general* births than all except 3 other months in the 120 months studied.

The most significant finding of the study was the seasonality of schizophrenic births, similar to that which has been observed in previous studies. As Fig. 1 shows, the peak month for schizophrenic births in the ten states for the years 1950–1959 was January with December and February also elevated. The magnitude of the increased schizophrenic birthrate for January alone was 12.4% ($\chi^2 = 59.87$; $p < 0.0001$) and for December–February together it was 5.9% ($\chi^2 = 29.12$; $p < 0.0001$). The difference between the months with the highest rate (January, 1955 and 1956; 49.4 schizophrenic births per 10,000 total births) and the month with the

Table 3. Schizophrenic Births as a Percentage of Total Births in Relation to the 1957 Influenza Epidemic in Ten States

	Birth period	*n*	χ^2 (d.f.=1)	*p* value
	Influenza peak month			
Index	Oct. 1957	405	0.418	<0.52
Control	Oct. 1950–56, 58, 59	98,054		
	Influenza peak 3-month period			
Index	Sept., Oct., Nov. 1957	1,215	1.743	<0.187
Control	Sept., Oct., Nov. 1950–56, 58, 59	285,038		
	Influenza epidemic months			
Index	Sept. 1957–Jan. 1958	2,045	1.694	<0.193
Control	Sept. 1950–56, 58, 59, Jan. 1950–57, 59	466,280		
	First trimester pregnancy months			
Index	April, May, June 1958	1,076	0.361	<0.548
Control	April, May, June 1950–57, 59	268,574		
	Second trimester pregnancy months			
Index	Jan., Feb., Mar. 1958	1,128	0.983	<0.321
Control	Jan., Feb., Mar. 1950–57, 59	264,818		
	Third trimester pregnancy months			
Index	Oct., Nov., Dec. 1957	1,200	0.916	<0.336
Control	Oct., Nov., Dec. 1950–56, 58, 59	279,914		

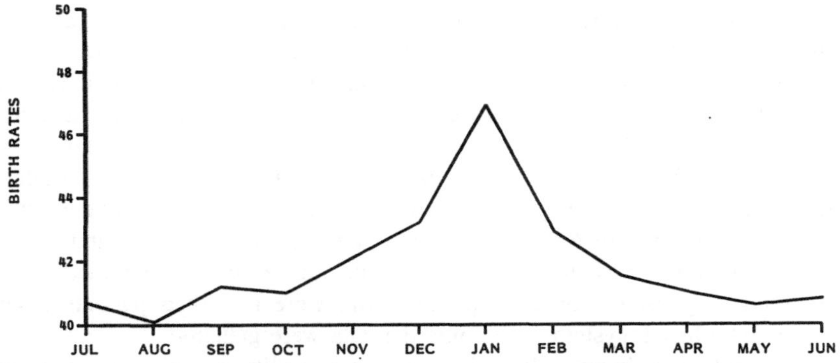

Figure 1. Schizophrenic birthrate by month, 1950–1959, per 10,000 total births, ten states.

lowest rate (April 1951; 33.4) was 48% more schizophrenic births during the high months.

Since New York State data comprised one-third of the total number of schizophrenic births studied, the other nine states were analyzed separately. A January excess of schizophrenic births was also found in these nine states showing a seasonal association between month of birth and births of schizophrenics (χ^2 d.f. = 11; $p < 0.0001$). When the states were divided geographically, the northeastern states (New York, Connecticut, and Maine) and the southeastern states (Georgia and Mississippi) both had a highly significant association between schizophrenic births and birth month ($p < 0.0001$ for both groups of states). The other group of states (Maryland, Ohio, Iowa, and Wisconsin) also had an excess of schizophrenic births in January but it failed to achieve a statistical significance association ($p < 0.077$).

DISCUSSION

The fact is firmly established that influenza infections in adults may occasionally cause a syndrome which is clinically identical to schizophrenia. The results of the present study suggest that if epidemic influenza infects the brain during the perinatal period, it does not produce the symptoms of schizophrenia later in life frequently enough to be detected statistically. As such, the results fail to reinforce previous suggestions that influenza *in utero* or shortly after birth may be etiologically related to schizophrenia, or that epidemics of influenza account for the winter–spring seasonality of schizophrenic births.

There are three important limitations to our conclusions. First, the comparison of schizophrenic births and general births in each state does not take into account the fact that many individuals with schizophrenia may have been born in other states; states do not record place of birth in psychiatric data collection so it is not possible to assess the magnitude of this interstate migration. Second, different strains of the influenza virus may vary geographically in both virulence and neurotropism (Wright *et al.*, 1980), and it is possible that the 1957 virus in Finland where the Mednick *et al.* study was done was different from the strain in the United States. Third, it should be remembered that the data are based not on all individuals with schizophrenia born in those states during those years, but rather on the individuals diagnosed with schizophrenia who were identified patients in the public mental health system at the time the data were gathered.

The present study strongly replicates the seasonality of schizophrenic births reported previously in the United States (Torrey *et al.*, 1977) and in at least ten other northern hemisphere countries (Bradbury and Miller, 1985; Boyd *et al.*, 1986). The number of schizophrenic births in the present study (N = 43,778) was almost as large as the previous United States study (N = 53,584) but utilized completely different patients. The previous study reported a significant peak of schizophrenic births from December to May, most marked in March and April, whereas the present study found a peak of schizophrenic births from December to February. The studies differed in the states included, the years of schizophrenic births (1920–1955 in the previous study; 1950–1959 in the present study); the years of admission for the patients; and the diagnostic criteria (all DSM-II in the previous study; predominantly DSM-III in the present study).

Despite the failure of the present study to link perinatal influenza infections to schizophrenic births, a viral cause for the observed schizophrenic birth seasonality continues to be a reasonable and attractive hypothesis (Torrey, 1987). Upper respiratory viruses are especially interesting possibilities since the upper respiratory tract in infants is less than 2 cm from the medial temporal lobe of the brain which is the area suspected of being involved in schizophrenia. It is known that viruses can migrate along the trigeminal nerve (Weiner and Fleming, 1984), which innervates the upper respiratory tract, to the trigeminal ganglion immediately proximate to the medial temporal cortex. A variety of routes are possible from the trigeminal ganglion to the brain tissue, the most likely being along the course of nerves which run from the ganglion to innervate meninges of the anterior and middle fossae of the brain; this method of viral spread has been proposed to account for the prominent localization of herpes simplex encephalitis in the temporal and orbitofrontal lobes (Davis and Johnson, 1979). In this connection it is of interest to note that some temporal lobe neuropathology in schizophrenia is consistent with the spread of virus from CSF to brain cells rather than hematogenously (Colter *et al.*, 1987). Upper respiratory viral infections in infancy, therefore, should continue to be explored for possible etiological connections to the seasonality of schizophrenic births.

ACKNOWLEDGMENTS We thank the following persons who kindly provided data for this study: Hilary Hamlin, Connecticut Department of Mental Health; Dr. Alan Ziglin, Georgia Division of Mental Health, Mental Retardation and Substance Abuse; Donna Hamano, Hawaii Division of Mental Health; Timothy Carroll, Iowa Division of Mental Health, Mental Retardation and Developmental Disabilities; Dr. Richard Heine, Kentucky Division of Mental Health; Julita Klavens, Maine Department of Mental Health and Mental Retardation; Timothy Santoni, Maryland Department of Health and Mental Hygiene; Dr. Susan Bowen, Mississippi Department of Mental Health; Dr. Shula Minsky, New Jersey Division of Mental Health and Hospitals; Hilda LaSalle, New York State Office of Mental Health; Joseph Wiant, Ohio Department of Mental Health; James Carlson, Oregon Division of Mental Health; Ronald Tremper, Rhode Island Department of Mental Health, Retardation and Hospitals; Dr. Ray Preston, Utah State Hospital; and Deborah Wills, Wisconsin Office of Mental Health.

REFERENCES

Althaus, J., 1893, On psychoses after influenza, *J. Ment. Sci.* **39**:163–176.

Bental, E., 1958, Acute psychosis due to encephalitis following Asian influenza, *Lancet* **2**:18–20.

Boyd, J. H., Pulver, A. E., and Stewart, W., 1986, Season of birth: Schizophrenia and bipolar disorder, *Schiz. Bull.* **12**:173–186.

Bradbury, T. N., and Miller, G. A., 1985, Season of birth in schizophrenia: A review of evidence, methodology, and etiology, *Psychol. Bull.* **98**:569–594.

Chistovich, A. S., 1959, The value of microbiological testing in the diagnosis and therapy of mental diseases, *Nauch. Konferen. Posvyashch.* **20**:113–119.

Colter, N., Battal, S., Crow, T. J., Johnstone, E. C., Brown, R., and Bruton, C., 1987, White matter reduction in the parahippocampal gyrus of patients with schizophrenia [letter], *Arch. Gen. Psychiatry* **44**:1023.

Davis, L. E., and Johnson, R. T., 1979, An explanation for the localization of herpes simplex encephalitis, *Ann. Neurol.* **5**:2–5.

Langmuir, A. D., 1961, Epidemiology of Asian influenza, *Am. Rev. Resp. Dis.* **83**:2–10.

Lloyd Still, R. M., 1958, Psychosis following Asian influenza in Barbados, *Lancet* **2**:20–22.

Loo, M. P., Eloy, G., and Duflot, M. J.-P., 1957, Infections et psychoses, *Ann. Med. Psychol.* **115**: 737–744.

Mednick, S. A., Machon, R. A., Huttunen, M. O., and Bonett, D., 1988, Adult schizophrenia following prenatal exposure to an influenza epidemic, *Arch. Gen. Psychiatry* **45**:189–192.

Menninger, K. A., 1926, Influenza and insanity, *Am. J. Psychiatry* **5**:469–529.

Morbidity and Mortality Weekly Reports (MMWR), 1957, National Office of Vital Statistics, U.S. Public Health Service, Washington, D. C.

Prokop, H., 1958, Psychosen im rahmen der grippeep: demie 1957/58, *Arch. Psychiatr.* (Berlin) **197**:484–500.

Ravenholt, R. T., and Foege, W. H., 1982, 1918 influenza, encephalitis lethargica, Parkinsonism, *Lancet* **2**:860–864.

Rorie, G. A., 1901, Post-influenzal insanity in the Cumberland and Westmoreland asylum, with statistics of sixty-eight cases, *J. Ment. Sci.* **47**:317–326.

Soeiro, L. N., 1958, Pricoses gripais, *J. Med. (Porto)* **37**:757–759.

Torrey, E. F., 1987, Viruses as the possible cause of schizophrenic birth seasonality, in: *Seasonal Effects on Reproduction, Infection and Psychoses* (T. Miura, ed.), SPB Academic Publishing, The Hague.

Torrey, E. F., Torrey, B. B., and Peterson, M. R., 1977, Seasonality of schizophrenic births in the United States, *Arch. Gen. Psychiatry* **34**:1065–1070.

Torrey, E. F., Rawlings, R., and Waldman, I. N., 1988, Schizophrenic births and viral diseases in two states, *Schiz. Res.* **1**:73–77.

Watson, C. G., Kulcala, T., Tilleskjor, C., and Jacobs, L., 1984, Schizophrenic birth seasonality in relation to the incidence of infectious diseases and temperature extremes, *Arch. Gen. Psychiatry* **41**:85–90.

Weiner, L. P., and Fleming, J. O., 1984, Viral infections of the nervous system, *J. Neurosurg.* **61**: 207–224.

Wright, P. F., Thompson, J., and Karzon, D. T., 1980, Differing virulence of H, N, and H3N2 influenza strains, *Am. J. Epidemiol.* **112**:814–819.

Chapter **8**

Virological and Immunological Study of Schizophrenic Patients in Relation to CT Scan Abnormality

Carlo Lorenzo Cazzullo, Emilio Sacchetti, Antonio Vita, Susanna Brambilla, Roberta Mancuso, Carlo Ezio Vaccari, Domenico Caputo, and Pasquale Ferrante

INTRODUCTION

The application of up-to-date biomedical technologies together with the acquisition of homogeneous epidemiological and clinical data coming from different geographical areas seem to indicate that the abnormalities of biological order play an important role in the pathogenetic mechanisms of schizophrenia.

There is now consistent evidence that a high percentage of schizophrenic patients have morphological abnormalities of the brain. This was shown by several pneumoencephalographic observations in the 1960s and by a great number of

---

Carlo Lorenzo Cazzullo, Emilio Sacchetti, Antonio Vita, and Susanna Brambilla • *Institute of Clinical Psychiatry, University of Milan, 20122 Milan, Italy.* Roberta Mancuso, Carlo Ezio Vaccari, Domenico Caputo, and Pasquale Ferrante • *Multiple Sclerosis University Center "Don C. Gnocchi," 20148 Milan, Italy.*

recent tomographic investigations. Particularly, enlargement of the cerebral ventricles and cortical atrophy have been noted (Weinberger *et al.*, 1983; Shelton and Weinberger, 1988). Though nonspecific, these changes would indicate that a neuropathological process has occurred in the brains of a proportion of schizophrenic patients.

In a previous study we found that the mean ventricular brain ratio of schizophrenic patients was significantly higher than that of healthy controls. Furthermore, a quarter of the patients showed pathological enlargement of cerebral ventricles. An even higher proportion of patients also showed signs of cortical atrophy, i.e., enlargement of convexity sulci and of interhemispheric and Sylvian scissures; these anomalies are of outstanding importance if related to the patients' age. Ventricular size is not correlated with the patients' age and duration of illness. In fact, pathological enlargement is found with the same frequency both in chronic schizophrenic patients and in subjects studied during their first psychotic episode (Vita *et al.*, 1988). Finally, ventricular enlargement seems to be a stable measure over time in the individual patient. In fact, patients retested by CT scan after some years (Shelton and Weinberger, 1988; Vita *et al.*, 1988; Reveley *et al.*, 1982; Turner *et al.*, 1986) had ventricular enlargement values overlapping the initial ones.

These results clearly indicate that ventricular enlargement does not seem to be a secondary change due to chronicity or treatment but rather a primary and early anomaly in schizophrenia probably preceding its clinical onset, with possible etiopathogenetic relevance.

Even though the exact origin of ventricular enlargement is still unknown, a body of evidence suggests that environmental determinants may be involved in its etiology. In this regard, several authors observed a greater incidence of ventricular dilatation in patients with no family history of schizophrenia (Reveley *et al.*, 1982; Turner *et al.*, 1986). Our research confirms these findings. In fact, we noted that 33% of the subjects with a negative family history showed ventricular dilatation versus only 15% of those with a positive family history (Sacchetti *et al.*, 1987). These results indicate that ventricular enlargement may identify a group of schizophrenic patients whose pathology is not exclusively dependent on genetic factors and where environmental determinants may play a pathogenetic role.

The etiopathogenesis of the cerebral abnormalities is complex, even though experimental neurology has long pointed out that the changes in the brain parenchyma around the ventricles are primarily correlated with the physiopathology of the blood–brain barrier (BBB), which is always involved in any inflammatory reaction that produces blood circulating antigens. Such antigens meet the BBB as a first filter and trigger a pathology that spreads through the ependyma to the surrounding parenchyma. Thus, various agents able to alter the BBB may be of outstanding importance in the genesis of ventricular dilatation.

Among the exogenous risk factors able to trigger the immunological mechanisms from which parenchymal alterations may ensue, viruses are highly suspected to be involved in the etiopathology of schizophrenia owing to their features and pathogenetic abilities. Therefore, in recent years several studies have been carried out to investigate the relationship between viruses and schizophrenia by isolation techniques, antibody investigations, and by molecular biology approaches for the research of viral nucleic acids in the brain or different biological materials from patients (Crow, 1983; Aulakh *et al.*, 1981).

Partly discordant results were found for antibody response anomalies against some viruses and particularly cytomegalovirus and herpes simplex virus, which can cause latent infections (Torrey *et al.*, 1982; Libikova, 1983).

More recently, the possibility that one or more retroviruses may play a role in the etiology of the disease has been put forward, either referring to an unidentified member of the HTLV family or taking into account a possible action by similar retroviral genomic sequences situated in particular chromosomal areas (Crow, 1987).

In this regard, trying to elucidate immunological and virological aspects which may suggest a viral involvement in the etiology of schizophrenia, we performed an evaluation study of the levels of specific antibodies against some viruses and of some specific immunological parameters. The data have been evaluated on the basis of the presence or lack of ventricular dilatation and/or cortical atrophy in schizophrenic patients and compared with a group of healthy controls.

MATERIALS

Twenty-seven schizophrenic patients (12 with and 15 without ventricular enlargement) and 28 healthy subjects were studied. In Table 1 some epidemiological and clinical parameters of the cases and controls are given.

Table 1. Epidemiological and Clinical Aspects of the Schizophrenic Groups and Healthy Controls

	Patients with increased VBR	Patients with normal VBR	All patients	Healthy controls
Number	12	15	27	28
Male	5	11	16	16
Mean age	33.8 yr	29.6 yr	31.4 yr	30.3 yr
Mean age at onset	22.5 yr*	18.7 yr*	20.5 yr	—
Mean disease duration	12.8 yr†	8.7 yr†	10.5 yr	—
Mean VBR	10.0	3.4	5.8	—
Cortical atrophy	50%	33%	40.7%	—

*,† $p > 0.05$, Student's *t* test.

Controls matched by age and sex have been chosen; for this reason no difference related to these two parameters can be expected between the patients and the controls.

The schizophrenic patients with ventricular enlargement differ, but not significantly, from the group without ventricular enlargement; the mean age of the subjects, the mean age of onset, and the mean duration of the disease are higher in the former group than in the latter.

Fifty percent of the cases with ventricular enlargement and thirty-three percent of those without ventricular enlargement showed cortical atrophy at CT scan examination. Finally, it is important to stress that the patients were included in the study independently of the type of symptoms and of the level of therapy.

VIROLOGICAL STUDIES

In the course of the study, antibodies against several viruses were checked in a sample of serum, collected at the same time and stored in the same way, from each patient and control. Particularly, an enzyme-linked immunosorbent assay (ELISA) prepared in our laboratory (Ferrante *et al.*, 1987) was employed for herpes simplex type 1 and type 2 (HSV-1 and HSV-2), cytomegalovirus (CMV), varicella–zoster (VZV), and measles virus antibodies. CMV-specific IgM was searched by means of a commercially available ELA (enzyme-labeled antigen) test. The antibodies to human immunodeficiency virus type 1 (HIV-1) and to HTLV-1 were checked using two commercially available ELISA. Moreover, a Western immunoblot containing purified virus from H9III and MT2 cell lines as antigen and, in the case of HTLV-1 virus, an indirect immunofluorescence assay (IFA) with MT2 and C10MJ2 cells were used.

The results regarding the conventional viruses are reported in Table 2 for each group of subjects as percentage of positivity, mean optical density (OD), and standard deviation of the OD.

No statistically significant differences were observed between the schizophrenic patients and the controls with regard to either the frequencies of positivity or the OD values in the cases of HSV-1, HSV-2, and CMV. Moreover, none of the tested sera showed specific CMV IgM. On the contrary, we observed that the measles antibody levels were significantly higher in the schizophrenic patients than in the healthy controls.

Among the cases, those with normal VBR had higher measles antibody levels than those with ventricular enlargement and, in a significant way, higher than the healthy controls. Taking into account the patients with cortical atrophy, the results showed the same patterns with no difference in the case of the Herpesviridae and still increased measles antibodies in the group without cortical atrophy. A brief summary of the results of HIV-1 and HTLV-1 antibody testing is given in Table 3.

Table 2. Viral Antibody Patterns in the Schizophrenic Patients and Controls

	Patients with increased VBR			Patients with normal VBR			All patients			Healthy controls		
	Positive	Mean OD	S.D.	Positive	Mean OD	S.D.	Positive	Mean OD	S.D.	Positive	Mean OD	S.D.
Herpes simplex type 1	83.3%	1.314	0.755	75.7%	1.321	0.860	77.7%	1.318	0.825	78.5%	1.242	0.872
Herpes simplex type 2	75%	0.296	0.178	75.7%	0.387	0.261	74.0%	0.366	0.212	75.0%	0.306	0.226
Cytomegalovirus IgG	75%	0.441	0.357	40%	0.426	0.339	55.5%	0.431	0.348	89%	0.587	0.288
Cytomegalovirus IgM	0	—	—	0	—	—	0	—	—	0	—	—
Measles	100%	0.555	0.279	100%	0.565	0.151	100%	0.560	0.212	96.4%	0.427	0.222

Mean antibody levels

All patients versus controls	$p = 0.027$
Patients with increased VBR versus controls	$p = 0.14$
Patients with normal VBR versus controls	$p = 0.037$
Patients with increased versus normal VBR	$p = 0.90$

Table 3. Summary of the Results on Retrovirus Antibody Presence in the Studied Groups

	Patients with increased VBR (n = 12)	Patients with normal VBR (n = 15)	Healthy subjects (n = 28)
HIV-1 ELISA	0	1	0
HIV-1 WB	0	1	0
HTLV-1 ELISA	0	0	0
HTLV-1 IFA	0	0	0
HTLV-1 WB	0	2	0

Only one schizophrenic patient was positive when tested by ELISA for HIV antibodies and this positivity was also confirmed by Western immunoblotting (WB). This case was a young drug addict who developed schizophrenia in 1979, at least 2 years before the spread of HIV infection in Italy. When examined by CT scan, he showed neither ventricular enlargement nor cortical atrophy.

The data concerning HTLV-1 antibodies need a short comment. Although neither patients nor controls were positive when tested by ELISA or IFA, we decided to check them again by looking for the presence of a selected reactivity against one or more viral proteins. As shown in Table 3, two schizophrenic patients were referred as positive for HTLV-1; however, the antibody response observed in their sera was clear but restricted to only one viral protein, the 63,000-dalton glycoprotein of the viral envelope.

IMMUNOLOGICAL STUDIES

In the same group of patients we conducted laboratory investigations on the serum levels of some immunological parameters. Table 4 shows the observed levels of IgG, IgM, IgA and of the C3 and C4 fractions of complement. All of the tests were performed by means of a nephelometric method employing the Beckman ICS apparatus.

With regard to the immunoglobulin levels, no statistically significant differences were observed between the schizophrenics and the controls or between the patients with and without ventricular enlargement.

On the contrary, the levels of C3 and C4 were significantly higher in the patients than in the controls. Moreover, the levels were significantly higher in the patients with ventricular enlargement than in the controls while the cases without ventricular enlargement did not differ from the healthy subjects.

It is interesting to stress that, even though not significant, the difference

Table 4. Immunological Data Obtained on the Sera of Schizophrenic Patients and Controls

	Patients with increased VBR		Patients with normal VBR		All patients		Healthy controls	
	Mean value	S.D.	Mean value	S.D.	Mean value	S.D.	Mean value	S.D.
IgG (mg/dl)	1189	338	1241	313	1218	319.46	1275	267
IgM (mg/dl)	132	39	136	72	134.53	58.75	157	93
IgA (mg/dl)	260	236	197	72	225	166	219	72
C3 (mg/dl)	134	22	118	21	125	23	106	23
C4 (mg/dl)	30.1	7.01	24.8	9.0	27	8.5	22.6	6.6

All patients versus controls	C3: $p = 0.0039$	C4: $p = 0.03$
Patients with increased VBR versus controls	C3: $p = 0.0021$	C4: $p = 0.0041$
Patients with normal VBR versus controls	C3: $p = 0.11$	C4: $p = 0.37$
Patients with increased versus normal VBR	C3: $p = 0.70$	C4: $p = 0.10$

between cases with ventricular enlargement and cases without this alteration is greater than that observed between cases without ventricular enlargement and healthy subjects.

In Table 5 the same immunological markers are evaluated in schizophrenic patients according to the presence or absence of cortical atrophy. Also in this case the patients showed a significant increase of C3 and C4 while no difference was observed for the three studied immunoglobulin classes. The highest C3 and C4 levels were seen in the patients with cortical atrophy while the patients without this abnormality did not differ from the controls as observed in Table 4 when ventricular enlargement was considered.

DISCUSSION

The virological investigations that we carried out failed to detect significant differences between schizophrenics and controls and, among the patients, between the group with radiological alterations and the group without them as regards antibodies against HSV and CMV. This finding, which disagrees with other authors' findings (Torrey *et al.*, 1982; Libikova, 1983), needs to be verified on wider groups using more sophisticated virological methods.

As to antimeasles antibodies, which proved to be higher in the unaltered patients than in the controls, in our opinion they may represent specific evidence of immunological reactivity because this observation is common to several diseases, with immunological disorders.

Table 5. Immunological Data Obtained on the Sera of Schizophrenic Patients and Controls in Relation to Cortical Atrophy

	Patients with cortical atrophy		Patients without cortical atrophy		All patients		Healthy controls	
	Mean value	S.D.	Mean value	S.D.	Mean value	S.D.	Mean value	S.D.
IgG (mg/dl)	1168	236	1287	305	1218	319.46	1275	267
IgM (mg/dl)	137	52.3	134.4	70.8	134.53	58.75	157	93
IgA (mg/dl)	196	59.6	230.4	79.5	225	166	219	72
C3 (mg/dl)	131.5	27	118.1	20.3	125	23	106	23
C4 (mg/dl)	29.1	9.11	24.7	8.5	27	8.5	22.6	6.6

All patients versus controls	C3: $p = 0.0039$	C4: $p = 0.03$
Patients with increased VBR versus controls	C3: $p = 0.0091$	C4: $p = 0.02$
Patients with normal VBR versus controls	C3: $p = 0.11$	C4: $p = 0.38$
Patients with increased versus normal VBR	C3: $p = 0.18$	C4: $p = 0.23$

The finding of an antibody response against a single HTLV-1 protein in two cases is too limited, although we previously observed only one positive subject out of 272 healthy Italian men using the same methods (Ferrante *et al.*, 1989).

The most interesting result is without doubt the increased C3 and C4 levels which were higher in the patients with ventricular dilatation or cortical atrophy than in the unaltered patients and the controls. Although, these results were obtained with a fairly small group of patients, yet our observation brings to light an association between radiological alterations in schizophrenia and the presence of a marker of immunological activity (Muller-Eberhard, 1975; Whicher, 1978).

CONCLUSIONS

Our data as a whole clearly indicate that it is possible to find immunological markers related to cortical atrophy and/or ventricular dilatations; these alterations have been found to be frequent in schizophrenia so that the neural substrate proves to be of outstanding importance both for therapeutic approaches and for the evaluation of immunological functions.

The increased C3 and C4 levels in biologically altered subjects is a generic marker of immunological activation and might be considered, with all due cautions, to support the hypothesis of the involvement of an exogenous factor with antigenic properties in the pathogenesis of some schizophrenia cases.

REFERENCES

Aulakh, G. S., Kleinman, J. E., Aulakh, H. S., Albrecht, P., Torrey, E. F., and Wyatt, R. J., 1981, Search for cytomegalovirus in schizophrenic brain tissue, *Proc. Soc. Exp. Biol. Med.* **167**:172–174.

Crow, T. J., 1983, Is schizophrenia an infectious disease? *Lancet* **1**:173–175.

Crow, T. J., 1987, The retrovirus/transposon hypothesis of schizophrenia, in: *Etiopathogenetic Hypothesis of Schizophrenia. The Impact of Epidemiological, Biochemical and Neuromorphological Studies* (C. L. Cazzullo, G. Invernizzi, E. Sacchetti, and A. Vita, eds.), MTP Press, 49–55.

Ferrante, P., Achilli, G., Gerna, G., and Bergamini, F., 1987, Subacute sclerosing panencephalitis: Detection of measles antibody in serum and CSF by enzyme linked immunosorbent assay, complement fixation and hemagglutination inhibition, *Microbiologica* **10**:111–118.

Ferrante, P., Mancuso, R., Finazzi, R., Memoli, M., Lori, F., Cattaneo, E., and Achilli, G., 1989, HTLV-1 antibody prevalence in Italian drug addicts, homosexual males and not at risk subjects, in: *Abstracts of the 89th Annual Meeting of ASM*. New Orleans, Abstract T20, p. 382.

Libikova, H., 1983, Schizophrenia and viruses: Principles of etiologic studies, *Adv. Biol. Psychiatry* **12**:20–51.

Muller-Eberhard, H. J., 1975, Complement, *Ann. Rev. Biochem.* **44**:697–705.

Reveley, A. M., Reveley, M. A., Clifford, C. A., and Murray, R. M., 1982, Cerebral ventricular size in twins discordant for schizophrenia, *Lancet* **1**:540.

Sacchetti, E., Vita, A., Calzeroni, A., Invernizzi, G., and Cazzullo, C. L., 1987, Neuromorphological correlates of schizophrenic disorders: Focus on cerebral ventricular enlargement, in: *Etiopathogenetic Hypothesis of Schizophrenia. The Impact of Epidemiological, Biochemical and Neuromorphological Studies* (C. L. Cazzullo, G. Invernizzi, E. Sacchetti, and A. Vita, eds.), MTP Press, Lancaster, pp. 67–91.

Shelton, R. C., and Weinberger, D. R., 1988, X-ray computerized tomographic studies in schizophrenia, in: *Neurology of Schizophrenia* (H. A. Nasrallah and D. R. Weinberger, eds.), Elsevier. Amsterdam, pp. 207–250.

Torrey, E. F., Yolken, R. H., and Winfrey, C. J., 1982, Cytomegalovirus antibody in cerebrospinal fluid of schizophrenic patients detected by enzyme immunoassay, *Science* **216**:892–894.

Turner, S. W., Toone, B. K., and Brett-Jones, J. R., 1986, Computerized tomographic scan changes in early schizophrenia: Preliminary findings, *Psychol. Med.* **16**:219–225.

Vita, A., Sacchetti, E., Calzeroni, A., and Cazzullo, C. L., 1988, Cortical atrophy in schizophrenia: Prevalence and associated features, *Schiz. Res.* **1**:329–337.

Weinberger, D. R., Wagner, R. L., and Wyatt, R. J., 1983, Neuropathological studies of schizophrenia: A selective review, *Schiz. Bull.* **9**:193–212.

Whicher, J. T., 1978, The value of complement assays in clinical chemistry, *Clin. Chem.* **24**(1):7.

Chapter 9

Viral Persistence and Immune Impairment in Schizophrenia

O. A. Vasiljeva, V. Y. Semke, T. P. Vetlugina, A. I. Zhankov, M. M. Garayev, I. U. Karas, G. V. Logvinovich, N. N. Naidyonova, and T. I. Nevidimova

INTRODUCTION

Investigations of viral persistence and immune system states in mental diseases have been summarized in two recent books (Morozov, 1983; Kurstak *et al.*, 1987). The latter contains data on antibody levels to tick-borne encephalitis, herpes, measles viruses, and other indicators of humoral immunity in schizophrenic patients and healthy individuals living in West Siberia and the Far East. Data obtained during a long-term systematic study on viral persistence, humoral and cell immunity, and interferon in schizophrenics and healthy donors from the above-mentioned regions are given in this chapter.

O. A. Vasiljeva, T. P. Vetlugina, A. I. Zhankov, I. U. Karas, N. N. Naidyonova, and T. I. Nevidimova • *Immunobiology Laboratory of the Mental Health Research Institute, Tomsk Scientific Center of the USSR Academy of Medical Sciences, 634014 Tomsk-14, USSR.* M. M. Garayev • *Biotechnology Laboratory of the Ivanovsky Virology Institute, USSR Academy of Medical Sciences, 123098, Moscow, USSR.* V. Y. Semke and G. V. Logvinovich • *Clinics of the Mental Health Research Institute, Tomsk Scientific Center of the USSR Academy of Medical Sciences, 634014 Tomsk-14, USSR.*

MATERIALS AND METHODS

Specimen Selection

Patients with different schizophrenia forms were studied. Blood serum and CSF samples (over 500) from schizophrenic patients and 660 serum samples from the controls (somatically and mentally healthy volunteers, patients with tick-borne encephalitis and recurrent cutaneous herpes) were investigated. There was a 3-week drug-free period prior to the investigation. Some patients were studied three times: (1) before therapy at the time of hospitalization; (2) 2–3 weeks after hospitalization with neuroleptic (chlorpromazine, chlorprothixenum, haloperidol, triftazinum, majeptil) and electroconvulsive therapy; (3) before discharge.

Virus and Cell Cultures

Herpes simplex virus type 1 strain L_2 (HSV-1) grown in the rabbit kidney cell culture (RK-13) and in the African green monkey kidney cells (Vero) was used. Confluent cell monolayers were inoculated at a multiplicity of infection of 0.1–1 PFU/cell. After the cytopathic effect reached the desired value, the cells were removed, centrifuged, and used for electrophoresis or molecular hybridization. The method of explantation (Pogodina *et al.*, 1981) in virus isolation from schizophrenic materials was used. Primary chick embryo cells and human embryo fibroblasts as well as BHK-12 cell culture, mouse ependymoblastoma of immature type 5, rat Gasserian ganglion neurinoma, BALB/c mouse thymocytes, and rat brain cortex organic culture were employed to study the serum cytotoxic activity of schizophrenics.

Laboratory Animals

Virus isolation from patient blood and CSF was carried out in BALB/c suckling and white suckling mice. Brains from the white suckling mice, intracerebrally inoculated with HSV-1 and uninfected ones were used for molecular hybridization.

Officinal Antigen Preparations

For the lymphocyte stimulation test (LST), antigens of dialyzed preparations of the tick-borne encephalitis vaccine (Institute of Poliomyelitis and Viral Encephalitis, USSR AMS) and the herpetic vaccine (Odessa Bacpreparation Enterprise), phytohemagglutinin (PHA; Difco, Serva) were used.

Serology

Serum and CSF antibodies against influenza A and B, vaccinia viruses, adenovirus type 6, HSV-1, tick-borne encephalitis virus (TBEV), and HIV were detected by neutralization test, complement fixing (CF), hemagglutination inhibition (HI), passive hemagglutination inhibition (PHI) tests, and ELISA.

Analysis of Immunoglobulins, Immune Complexes, T and B Lymphocytes. Phagocytosis

The serum immunoglobulin concentrations were determined using the method of Mancini *et al.* (1964). Immune complexes (IC) were assayed by precipitation with polyethylene glycol-6000 (Serva) as described elsewhere (Haskova *et al.*, 1978). T and B cells were determined according to the lymphocytes' ability to form rosettes with sheep and mouse erythrocytes, respectively; theophylline-sensitive and theophylline-resistant lymphocytes were analyzed by the rosette-formation test after preliminary incubation with 0.01 M theophylline solution at 37°C for 1 hr (Novikov and Novikova, 1979). The capacity of leukocytes to pick up IC was estimated by the method of Vinogradova *et al.* (1986). The standard serum (human serum of known IC concentration) was added at an equal volume to the leukocyte suspension containing 6×10^6 cells/ml and incubated at 37°C. The phagocytic capacity was evaluated by the IC level decrease in serum following 30, 60, or 120 min incubation and expressed in "percent," the initial level being 100%. The effect of levamisolum (500 mg/ml) on phagocytosis was evaluated after the leukocyte suspension had been incubated with the medicine for 1 hr at 37°C.

Determination of Lymphocyte Interferon (IFN)-Synthesizing Ability

10^6 lymphocytes in 1 ml were tested. Newcastle disease virus (10 CPU/lymphocyte) was used as α-IFN inducer (18–20 hr at 37°C), and PHA was used to induce γ-IFN (72 hr at 37° C). IFN titers were determined by the inhibition of vesicular stomatitis virus production in human embryo fibroblast cell culture. The results were read 1–2 days after.

Lymphocyte Stimulation Test with PHA and Viral Antigens

Heparinized blood lymphocytes were isolated by centrifugation in Ficoll Verographin density gradient, with 10^5 cells/150 μl working concentration. Then PHA or officinal antigen preparations of TBEV and HSV were added and incubated in 5% CO_2 at 37°C for 144 hr; 1 Ci/sample of [^{3}H]thymidine was added 18 hr before the end of culturing. The extent of antigen- and PHA-induced lymphocyte proliferation was shown by the stimulation index (SI). For example, SI_{PHA} = cpm PHA-stimulated ^3H incorporation/cpm unstimulated ^3H incorporation.

Electrophoresis and Immunoblotting

Infected and uninfected RK-13 cells were dissolved in the electrophoresis buffer containing 0.0625 M Tris-HCl pH 6.8, 2% SDS, 5% 2-mercaptoethanol, 5 mM EDTA, 10% glycerin, and 0.001% bromphenol blue. The electrophoretic separation of proteins was made in polyacrylamide gel slabs (Studier, 1973); polyacrylamide concentration was 6% in the separating gel and 3% in the concentrating gel at 100–150 V for 4–6 hr with 0.1% SDS using the discontinuous buffer system (Laemmli, 1970). The following proteins were used as molecular weight markers: phosphorylase *b* 94k, bovine serum albumin 67k, ovalbumin 43k, carbonic anhydrase 30k, trypsin inhibitor 20.1k, lactalbumin 14.4k. After electrophoresis the gels were placed in a buffer consisting of 0.025 M Tris (hydroxymethyl) aminomethane, 0.193 M glycine, 20% isopropanol for half an hour; then the proteins were transferred on nitrocellulose membranes in the same buffer for 2–3 hr at 0.4 A (Tsang *et al.*, 1983). The position of protein markers after the transfer was determined using Ponceau S. Then the membranes were cut so that each strip contained proteins from both HSV-1-infected and uninfected RK cells. The strips were processed with schizophrenic sera (18 patients) in the dilution 1:100–1:200 for 2 hr at 37°C and overnight at 4°C, intensely washed with TBS (0.1 M Tris-HCl pH 8.0, 0.15 MNaCl), and exposed for 2 hr at 37°C with peroxidase-labeled antibodies against human IgG. The unbound antibodies were washed with TBS; the strips were treated with a mixture of H_2O_2 and diaminobenzidine to detect the virus-specific proteins. The molecular weights of the virus-specific proteins were determined (Dunker and Rueckert, 1969).

Molecular Hybridization

Total heparinized blood from patients, homogenates of HSV-1-infected and uninfected cell cultures, and mouse brain were treated with proteinase K (200 μg/ml) for 2 hr at 37°C in 0.2 M Tris-HCl pH 8.0, 0.3 M NaCl, 25 mM EDTA, 2% SDS. The general pool of nucleic acids was extracted with phenol–chloroform, precipitated with ethanol at −40°C, pelleted and dissolved in distilled water. The quality of the extracted DNA was tested by 1% NA agarose electrophoresis. DNA of the studied samples was dotted on the nitrocellulose membrane treated with 0.1 N NaOH, neutralized, and dried at room temperature for 2 hr. Prehybridization and hybridization were performed for 24 hr at 64°C in buffer containing Denhart solution 5×, SSPE 5×, 0.1% SDS (Maniatis *et al.*, 1982). The samples were hybridized with [^{32}P]-DNA plasmide pBR322 containing *Eco*RI fragments J, K, and D of HSV-1 strain F genome.

Schizophrenic Serum and CSF Cytotoxic Activity. Analysis of Antithymic and Neurotoxic Activities of Blood Serum from Schizophrenic Patients

The nonspecific cytotoxic activity was estimated in primary chick embryo cells, human embryo fibroblasts, and continuous cell lines of BHK-12, human diploid cells, ependymoblastoma of immature type 5, and a rat Gasserian ganglion neurinoma. In the chick embryo cell culture, the evaluation was made according to the extent of cell monolayer degeneration in the system of four pluses following 30-min contact with negative serum (Vartanian, 1968). The toxic factor titer was estimated. The reversibility of the cell system was determined according to the ability of cells to regenerate 2 days after the culture medium had been changed for a fresh one in samples with serum dilution producing the least but easily determined cytotoxic effect (1.2+). Inactivated sera were investigated with guinea pig complement to evaluate the cytolytic effect in the continuous cell lines (Karmysheva and Ivannikova, 1984).

The specific serum cytotoxic activity was determined in relation to nervous and thymic tissues. The antithymic activity was estimated using the cytotoxic test (Luria and Domashneva, 1973). The results were given as a cytotoxic index (CTI): CTR = $(A - B)/(100 - B)$, where A is the mean percentage of dead thymic cells in the suspension incubated with serum and complement; B is the same, incubated with culture medium. The serum antithymic activity is negative with CTI being 0.00–0.12; positive, 0.13–0.24, superpositive, $\geqslant 0.25$. The serum neurotoxic activity was measured by radiometry using [^{3}H]cholesterine (Perevozchikova and Nazarov, 1980). Organ cultures of the rat brain cortex were incubated by the standard method (Bornstein, 1963). The neurotoxic activity (NTA) was expressed as a percentage of [^{3}H]cholesterine incorporation of the rat brain culture incubated with sera from schizophrenics and healthy donors: NTA = [1 − cpm (schizophrenic serum)/cpm (donors)] × 100. The test is negative if NTA is 0–6%; positive, 7–15%; superpositive, > 15%.

RESULTS AND DISCUSSION

Attempts to Isolate Viruses from Schizophrenic Blood and CSF

Attempts to isolate TBEV were made with blood and CSF from four and seven patients, respectively, with paranoid schizophrenia of continuous and recurrent types of course. It should be noted that patients lived in active TBE foci; therefore, three patients had acute TBE in their histories. The expected persisting TBEV in the studied biological fluids was accumulated by serial passages in suckling mice. Then by the method of explantation of organs from the animals inoculated with

CSF, the virus was detected in two patients with malignant continuous paranoid schizophrenia. The hemagglutination test of 7-, 10-, and 15-day samples of the explant fluids showed the hemagglutinating antigen in titers from 1:2 to 1:32. The antigen for the CF assay prepared from newborn white mouse brain with a typical neuroinfection picture on the 10th day had a 1:256 titer with hyperimmune serum against TBEV, the matching control being negative. The organ prints of the newborn mice fallen ill 6–13 days after inoculation were studied by fluorescent antibodies to TBEV and Venezuelan encephalomyelitis virus. Fluorescent cells were found in all preparations, when anti-TBEV antibodies were used. Most of them were seen on day 9 from the disease onset with negative prints when the uninfected brain and antiserum against Venezuelan encephalomyelitis virus were employed. The histological investigation of the infected brain revealed a chronic inflammatory degenerative process.

Thus, the viruses studied according to their antigenic properties belong to the TBE complex.

The Search for HB_s Antigen and HB_e Antigen in Schizophrenic Sera

The surface HB_s antigen was detected in 15% of schizophrenics studied; HB_e antigen, in one female patient only. According to the anamnesis, these patients with serum hepatitis B virus antigens have never had hepatitis. Similar data were obtained by others (Libikova *et al.*, 1981). They showed HB_s antigen in schizophrenics with a long duration of illness, which suggests that persistent hepatitis B virus plays a certain part in the manifestation of the most severe forms of schizophrenia.

HSV-1 DNA Search in Schizophrenic Patient Blood by Molecular Hybridization Technique

Figure 1 shows an autoradiogram of molecular hybridization of DNA samples from schizophrenic blood. Positive signals showed that considerable amounts of HSV-1 DNA were detected in specimens, which indicated the productive herpesvirus infection. HSV is a neurotropic (Greenwood, 1987) and lymphotropic (Tedder *et al.*, 1987; Downing *et al.*, 1987) virus. Thus, persistent herpesvirus infection may occur on both sides of the blood–brain barrier with a complex relationship. The direct study of an infectious process in the central nervous system is limited, while an indirect assessment of the process may be given by estimation of herpesvirus infection in blood cells.

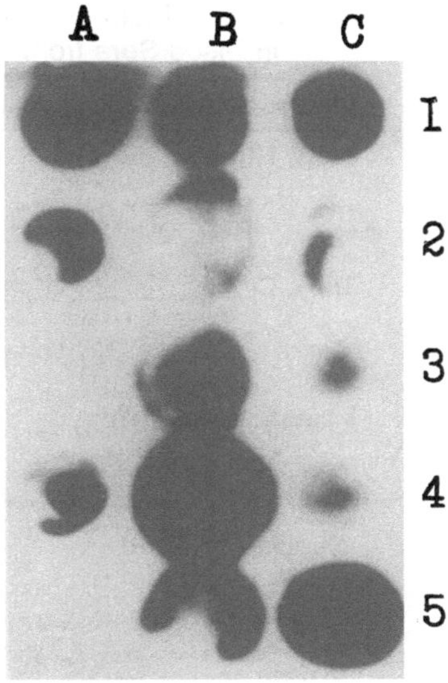

Figure 1. Hybridization of the cloned in pBR322 DNA *Eco*RI J, K, and D fragments to DNA from the studied specimens. A (1), pBR322 DNA (J, K, and D *Eco*RI fragments of HSV-1 DNA); A (2), HSV-infected RK-13 cell DNA; A (3), uninfected RK-13 cell DNA; A (4), HSV-infected mouse brain DNA; A (5), uninfected mouse brain DNA; B and C, total blood DNA of schizophrenic patients.

Viral Antibodies in Acute Schizophrenia and in Healthy Donors

Table 1 shows the distribution of antibody titers to a number of neurotropic and capable-of-persistence viruses.

TBEV. Antibody titers in CF assay in acute schizophrenia were significantly higher than in healthy subjects; high titers were detected only in patients (1:16). It should be noted that patients under 35 had an elevation of mean CF antibody titers and a decrease of antihemagglutinating antibodies to TBEV, but the matching controls have nothing in common. The duration of illness may be the source of difference. The study of 32 CSF samples from acute schizophrenics showed TBEV antibodies in 10 patients. Unlike the present data, the report (Libikova *et al.*, 1977) did not show statistically significant differences between antibody titers in schizophrenics and healthy donors living in TBE foci. The reported antibody titer elevation is in agreement with findings that TBEV persistence is maintained in the presence of high specific antibody titers (Pogodina *et al.*, 1986).

Influenza A and B viruses. Table 1 shows that a high level of anti-influenza immunity in acute schizophrenic patients and healthy subjects was found. We failed to show the antibody titer dependence on schizophrenia progrediency, type, and duration.

Table 1. Distribution of Antibody Titers to Various Viruses in Blood Sera from Schizophrenics and Healthy Donors

Virus serological tests	Antibody (AB) titer	% in patients	% in donors
TBEV, HI	No AB	91	97
	1:10	6	2
	1:20	2	1
	1:40	1	0
TBEV, CF	No AB	55	80
	1:4	33	11
	1:8	7	3
	1:16	5	—
Influenza B virus, HI	No AB	5	9
	1:10–1:40	59	55
	1:80–1:160	34	31
	Over 1:160	2	5
Influenza A virus, HI	No AB	5	5
	1:10–1:40	66	53
	1:80–1:160	20	36
	Over 1:160	9	6
HSV, HI	No AB	2	13
	1:10–1:40	48	32
	1:80–1:160	38	42
	Over 1:160	12	13
Vaccinia virus, HI	No AB	62	85
	1:5	25	9
	1:10	10	4
	1:20	3	2
Adenovirus type 6, CF	No AB	2	1
	1:4	31	44
	1:8	29	33
	1:16–1:32	38	22

HSV. There were no significant differences in titers of HSV antibodies in patients and healthy subjects (Table 1); CSF antibodies were found in one patient only.

Vaccinia virus. Detectable antibody elevation was noted in acute schizophrenic patients (Table 1); two patients had CSF antibodies, indicating a possible persistence of virus in patients studied.

Adenovirus type 6. The number of patients with antibody titers of 1:16–1:32 (Table 1) was found to increase; two patients had CSF antibodies.

HIV. Preliminary investigations of the presence of HIV antibodies in several patients were carried out. Pseudopositive responses were found in 1.2% of cases, but repeat analysis showed negative results. Further investigations of antibodies to HIV in such patients are necessary to study the effect of the infection on the course of mental disease.

Relationship of Clinical Parameters of Schizophrenia with Serum TBEV and HSV Antibody Titers

Data are given in Table 2. A relationship between antibody titers to TBEV and the type of schizophrenia was not found. On the contrary, during improvement a considerable elevation of antibody titers to TBEV in patients with schizophrenia of continuous form and a certain reduction of titers in patients with attack-like schizophrenia were seen. The following are the findings on HSV antibodies: (1) there are no significant differences between titers in patients with various types of course (in the acute phase) and in healthy subjects; (2) the clinical improvement in attack-like schizophrenia is followed by a considerable elevation of antibody titer and in continuous-progredient schizophrenia, by its reduction. The above findings probably reflect the difference in the immunoreactivity of patients with all mentioned types of schizophrenia to the natural focal TBEV and ubiquitous HSV.

Antibody Synthesis to Individual HSV-Specific Proteins

In most schizophrenic patients studied, IgG was found to be synthesized against p125, p120, p115, p110, p107, p99, p93, p89, p85, p80, p66, p60, p56, p50, p46, p36, p33, p28 proteins (Fig. 2). The presence of antibodies to such a wide range of HSV-specific proteins permits discussion of the acute herpesvirus infection in patients. Serum samples obtained at admission, 2–2½ weeks after hospitalization, and 4–6 after hospitalization (sometimes with improvement) failed to show evident changes in the antibody range. This phenomenon needs further investigation. The description of about 50 HSV-1 specific proteins with their antigenicity (Honess and Roizman, 1973) was used for the synthesis analysis of antibodies against individual proteins of this virus in a person during primary and recurrent herpetic infection. Formation of antibody to more than 30 HSV proteins with molecular weights of 212 to 30k was detected (Gilman *et al.*, 1981; Ashley *et al.*, 1988). These findings partly agree with our findings, but the latter

Table 2. Mean Geometric Titer of Antibodies to TBEV and HSV-1 in Schizophrenics with Different Types of Course at an Acute Phase and Remission (CF Assay)

	General pool of patients		Continuous-progredient, paranoid		Attack-like progredient, paranoid		Healthy donors
	Acute	Remission	Acute	Remission	Acute	Remission	
TBEV	1.78	2.29	1.76	2.83	2.70	1.90	1.21
HSV	52.6	63.5	49.5	44.9	38.4	65.3	40.5

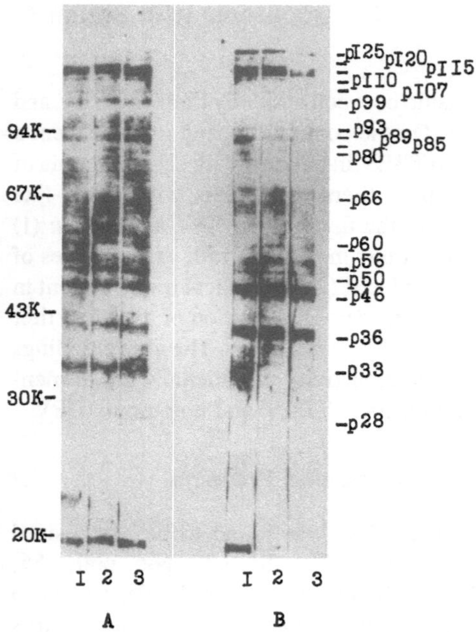

Figure 2. Reactivity of schizophrenic sera in Western blot with HSV-specific proteins synthesized in Vero cells. (A) Reactivity of serum of patient 1 at admission (1); 3–4 weeks after neuroleptic therapy (2); 6 weeks after hospitalization at discharge. (B) Patient 2.

were derived from patients without any clinical signs of herpes at the time of sampling.

The HSV-1 genome (70 genes) complexity and various functions of the virus-specific proteins in the expression of its genetic information (McGeoch *et al.*, 1988) as well as the prognostic character of the antibody synthesis to a series of viral proteins (Kohl, 1985) serve as the basis for further investigation of the antibody synthesis using immunoblotting, a technique which is more informative in this respect than serological tests.

Schizophrenic Blood Lymphocyte Stimulation with Viral Antigens

Table 3 gives data on lymphocyte stimulation and antibody synthesis in schizophrenic patients treated with neuroleptic drugs. A sharp elevation of SI_{HSV} (in comparison with donors) is seen before treatment, but during neuroleptic therapy SI reduces and HSV antibody titers elevate simultaneously. PHA analysis shows that in a number of patients it is lower than in healthy subjects. This is characteristic of patients with viral infections (Semyonov *et al.*, 1982).

Table 3 shows that SI_{HSV} and HSV antibody titers in donors do not depend on age. On the contrary, SI_{HSV} in patients under 35 is reduced during therapy to nearly

Table 3. Antiherpetic Immunity in Schizophrenics and Healthy Donors of Different Groups

Groups	Parameters	Schizophrenic patients: Before treatment	Schizophrenic patients: During treatment	Donors
Pool	SI_{HSV}	2.07 ± 0.37	1.03 ± 0.11	0.59 ± 0.05
	AB titer	98.1 ± 14.0	194.5 ± 33.0	78.6 ± 12.8
Under 35	SI_{HSV}	1.9 ± 0.22	0.91 ± 0.1	0.58 ± 0.07
	AB titer	61.6 ± 10.0	263.7 ± 52.0	81.0 ± 13.0
Over 35	SI_{HSV}	2.31 ± 0.65	1.16 ± 0.19	0.60 ± 0.12
	AB titer	167.2 ± 42.0	129.4 ± 16.0	74.0 ± 16.0

control values with a sharp elevation of antibody titers. In patients over 35, antibody titers are reduced after SI_{HSV} change. This is probably due to the fact that in older patients lymphocyte HSV-sensibilization increases on the one hand, and the ability to quickly respond to viral infections by an intensive antibody synthesis decreases, on the other. The detection of HSV antibody titers in patients resistant to psychopharmacotherapy revealed that the mean SI_{HSV} was 3.84 ± 1.84 before treatment, and then dropped to 1.45 ± 0.34. It should be noted that in some patients it increased. Antibody titer was 40–60 and remained constant. On the other hand, the initially low SI_{HSV} or its decrease to nearly control values during therapy was associated in a number of cases with a reduction of psychopathological symptomatology.

SI_{TBEV} and anti-TBEV hemagglutinin antibodies in schizophrenics are higher than in intact donors, but lower than in patients with acute TBE and in vaccinated subjects. As a rule during pharmacotherapy, parameters under study remain constant, while SI_{TBEV} in TBE patients tends to reduce during recovery.

IFN-genic Lymphocyte Ability in Patients Receiving Psychopharmacological Drugs

To study the effect of psychopharmacotherapy on IFN-genic lymphocyte ability, patients were divided into several groups depending on the initial lymphocyte potency to synthesize α- and γ-IFNs induced by Newcastle disease virus and PHA, respectively. (1) Patients with α-IFN production ≥ 64 U/ml (mean 65 ± 6 U/ml in donors). Prior to their treatment, such patients had mean values of 100 ± 13 U/ml which dropped during therapy up to 34 ± 10 U/ml. (2) Patients with low α-IFN production (0–32 U/ml) detected at the first analysis. Mean values (19 ± 2 U/ml) increased up to 38 ± 7 U/ml during therapy. (3) Patients with γ-IFN production ≥ 32 U/ml (mean 28 ± 4 U/ml in donors). Their mean value (57 ± 7

U/ml) dropped during therapy up to 38 ± 8 U/ml. (4) Patients with low γ-IFN production (0–16 U/ml) detected during the first investigation. Mean 4.7 ± 1.1 U/ml rose up to 29.2 ± 4.0 U/ml during therapy.

In general, among patients with acute schizophrenia the percentage of those with high productivity of both α- and γ-IFNs (64–128 and 32–128 U/ml, respectively) is low; patients with either low synthetic activity of α- and γ-IFNs, or low α- and high γ-IFN's prevail.

Three to four weeks following psychotropic therapy the number of patients with relatively low (36 ± 5 U/ml) α-IFN production and relatively high (30 ± 4 U/ml) γ-IFN production (in donors 65 and 28 U/ml, respectively) increases.

Cytotoxic Properties of Schizophrenic Serum

The cytotoxic activity of blood serum of schizophrenic patients is higher than that of donors against chick embryo cells. BALB/c murine thymocytes, and rat brain cortex ($p < 0.001$). According to the antithymic activity, blood serum of schizophrenic patients is significantly different from that of patients with borderline disorders (0.21 ± 0.02 and 0.5 ± 0.03, respectively). Serum neurotoxic and fibroblastotoxic activities of schizophrenics are negligibly higher than those of donors. The cell degeneration in schizophrenia is irreversible in 79%; the cell monolayer regeneration with the culture medium being changed occurs in 51% of cases with borderline disorders.

Several clinical parameters of schizophrenia influence the serum cytotoxic activity. (1) The neurotoxic activity of blood sera from malignant schizophrenics with manifested productive disorders is maximal (33.8 ± 5.43). The antithymic and fibroblastotoxic activities of schizophrenic sera were found to be independent of the type of course and progrediency of the process. (2) The neurotoxic and fibroblastotoxic activities of schizophrenic sera are significantly higher during the manifested illness (duration of illness less than a year) and in patients with a 10-year illness duration. The antithymic activity was maximal at the time of a more pronounced clinical picture of illness (1–5 years). (3) The antithymic activity levels dropped during pharmacotherapy. Mean values of the neurotoxic and fibroblastotoxic activities changed insignificantly. Cytotoxic parameters were considerably decreased by electroconvulsive therapy rather than by neuroleptic drugs.

Serum cytotoxic activity is not a parameter peculiar to schizophrenic serum only. It is seen in a number of cases. Association of the fibroblastotoxic and neurotoxic activities with a toxicity factor titer was found.

Immunoglobulins, Immune Complexes, T and B Lymphocytes. Phagocytosis

A series of immunological parameters in patients and healthy subjects varies widely (Table 4). Mean values of IgG, IgM, and IgA in patients are higher than in

Table 4. Parameters of the Immune System in Peripheral Blood from Schizophrenics and Healthy Donors

Parameters	Schizophrenics	Healthy donors	p
IC cond. units*	120.6 ± 4.26 (5–460)	103.8 ± 3.86 (35–228)	< 0.01
IgM, mg/ml	1.59 ± 0.11 (0.40–5.4)	1.29 ± 0.09 (0.44–3.0)	< 0.05
IgG, mg/ml	13.3 ± 0.40 (7.4–25.5)	13.6 ± 0.48 (7.4–20.0)	> 0.05
IgA, mg/ml	3.09 ± 0.16 (1.08–5.7)	2.62 ± 0.15 (0.96–5.2)	< 0.05
T lymphocytes, thousand/μl	1.23 ± 0.07 (0.66–1.83)	1.44 ± 0.08 (0.71–2.56)	< 0.05
T lymphocytes, %	71.8 ± 1.77 (35–89)	74.6 ± 2.21 (48–99)	> 0.05
T lymphocytes, theophylline-resistant, %	49.6 ± 2.31 (16–86)	45.8 ± 2.19 (22–78)	> 0.05
T lymphocytes, theophylline-sensitive, %	22.6 ± 1.87 (0–54)	29.7 ± 2.39 (10–56)	< 0.05
B lymphocytes, %	10.2 ± 0.93 (0–23)	13.2 ± 0.98 (4–22)	< 0.05
Phagocytosis, %	79.8 ± 1.64 (45–94)	82.0 ± 1.44 (67–95)	< 0.05

*IC is determined by the extent of optical density multiplied by 1,000 and is expressed in conditional units.

donors. Decrease of the absolute number of T lymphocytes, the relative number of B lymphocytes, and theophylline-sensitive T lymphocytes is noted. Analysis of the relationship between parameters and clinical characteristics of the disease shows that in patients with paranoid, hallucinating–paranoid, and paraphrenic syndromes, IgG, the total concentration of serum immunoglobulins, and IC are higher than in patients with neurosis-like, psychopathy-like, and subdepressive syndromes. These parameters of humoral immunity might reflect the severity of psychopathological disorders.

High IC levels may result from the intensive antibody production (autoantibodies), disturbance of IC elimination due to deficiency of the T-cell system, the change of phagocytic cell function. The capacity of leukocytes to pick up serum IC *in vitro* is lower in schizophrenic patients than in healthy donors. Thus, following 30, 60, and 120 min incubation, serum leukocytes from healthy individuals engulfed 25.8 ± 2.17, 35.8 ± 2.27, and 46.6 ± 1.48% of IC, respectively, while patient leukocytes captured 15.3 ± 2.09, 24.8 ± 1.92, and 33.0 ± 1.96% of IC, respectively ($p < 0.001$ at all points).

Levamizolum produced different effects on phagocytosis in patients and donors. After 1 hr incubation with levamizolum, the leukocyte activity of healthy donors either did not change as compared to control samples (incubation with saline) or slightly increased, while that of patients elevated significantly (42.7 ± 2.45% for patients, 34.6 ± 1.76% for donors). The decreased ability of patient leukocytes to engulf IC might be associated with both a primary impairment of phagocytes and possible inhibition of their receptors with different ligands (Erban and Richtova, 1986).

CONCLUSIONS

The results of biological investigations of patients during different periods of clinical manifestations of schizophrenia have been presented. Such parameters as the viral antibody levels, the index of lymphocyte stimulation with viral antigens, the ability of lymphocytes to produce α- and γ-interferons have been shown to change during pharmacotherapy. Further investigations of these characteristics combined with study of the molecular biology of viral persistence may be useful for understanding the mechanism of homeostatic disturbance in schizophrenic patients and the formation of resistivity to pharmacotherapy.

ACKNOWLEDGMENTS The authors thank O. A. Nikiforova, V. K. Savenko, and M. V. Mishenyov from the Immunobiology Laboratory, Drs. V. F. Lebedeva and A. G. Pereveznyuk from the Clinics of the Mental Health Research Institute, Tomsk Scientific Center of the USSR Academy of Medical Sciences, for technical assistance.

REFERENCES

Ashley, R., Mack, K., Critchlow, C., Shurtleff, U., and Corey, L., 1988, Differential effect of systemic acyclovir treatment of genital HSV-2 infections on antibody responses to individual HSV-2 proteins, *J. Med. Virol.* **24**:309–320.

Bornstein, D. V., 1963, A tissue culture approach to demyelinative disorders, *Natl. Cancer Inst. Monogr.* **11**:197–214.

Downing, R. G., Sewankambo, N., Serwadda, D., Honess, R., Crawford, D., Jarrett, R., and Griffin, B. E., 1987, Isolation of human lymphotropic herpesviruses from Uganda, *Lancet* **2**:390.

Dunker, A. K., and Rueckert, R. R., 1969, Observation on molecular weight determination on PAAG, *J. Biol. Chem.* **244**:5074–5080.

Erban, L., and Richtova, E., 1986, Morphologic changes of leucocy .es in schizophrenic psychosis, *Act. Nerv. Super.* **28**:25–26.

Gilman, S. C., Docherty, J. J., and Rawls, W. E., 1981, Antibody responses in humans to individual proteins of herpes simplex viruses, *Infect. Immun.* **34**:880–887.

Greenwood, R., 1987, Residual mental disorders after herpesvirus infections, in: *Viruses, Immunity, and Mental Disorders* (E. Kurstak, Z. J. Lipowski, and P. V. Morozov, eds.), Plenum Medical, New York, pp. 65–80.

Haskova, V., Kaslik, J., Riha, I., Matl, I., and Rovensky, J., 1978, Simple method of circulating immune complex detection in human sera by polyethylene glycol precipitation. *Z. Immunol. Forsch.* **154**:339–406.

Honess, R. W., and Roizman, B., 1973, Proteins specified by herpes simplex virus. XI. Identification and relative molar rates of synthesis of structural and nonstructural herpes virus polypeptides in the infected cell, *J. Virol.* **12:**1347–1365.

Karmysheva, V. Y., and Ivannikova, G. A., 1984, *Methodial Recommendations on Virus Identification by Cytolytic Effect*, Moscow.

Kohl, S., 1985, Herpes simplex virus immunology: Problems, progress, and promises, *J. Infect. Dis.* **152:**435–440.

Kurstak, E., Lipowski, Z. J., and Morozov, P. V. (eds.), 1987, *Viruses, Immunity, and Mental Disorders*, Plenum Press, New York.

Laemmli, U. K., 1970, Cleavage of structural proteins during the assembly of the head of bacteriophage T4, *Nature* **227:**680–685.

Libikova, H., Stancek, D., Wiedermann, V., Hasto, J., and Breier, S., 1977, Psychopharmacia and electroconvulsive therapy in relation to viral antibodies and infection. Experimental and clinical study, *Arch. Immunol. Ther. Exp.* **25:**641–649.

Libikova, H., Pogady, J., Stancek, D., and Mucha, V., 1981, Hepatitis B and herpes viral components in the cerebrospinal fluid of chronic schizophrenic and senile demented patients, *Acta Virol.* **25:** 182–190.

Luria, E. A., and Domashneva, M. V., 1973, Antithymocyte antibodies in blood serum from schizophrenic patients, *Konsakov J. Neurol. Psychiatry* **12:**1873–1877.

McGeoch, D. J., Dalrymple, A., Davison, A. J., Dolan, A., Frame, U. C., McNab, P., Perry, L. J., and Scott, E., 1988, The complete DNA sequence of the long unique region in the genome of herpes simplex virus type 1, *J. Gen. Virol.* **69:**1531–1574.

Mancini, G., Vaerman, J. P., Carbanora, A. O., and Heremans, J. F., 1964, A single radial-diffusion method for the immunological quantitation of proteins, in: *Proteins of the Biological Fluids* (H. Pelters, Ed.), Elsevier, Amsterdam, pp. 370–373.

Maniatis, T., Fritsch, E. F., and Sambrook, J., 1982, *Molecular Cloning: A Laboratory Manual*, Cold Spring Harbor Laboratory, Cold Spring Harbor, N.Y.

Morozov, P. V. (ed.), 1983, *Advances in Biological Psychiatry*, Volume 12, Karger, Basel.

Novikov, D. K., and Novikova, V. I., 1979, *Cellular Methods of Immunodiagnostics*, Beloruss, Minsk.

Perevozchikova, M. F., and Nazarov, P. G., 1980, Diagnostics of demyelinized diseases of the nervous system based on blood serum effect on nervous tissue culture, in: *Theoretical Grounds of Pathological States*, Nauka, Leningrad, pp. 113–115.

Pogodina, V. V., Levina, L. F., Fokina, G. I., Koreshkova, G. B., Malenko, G. V., Bochkova, N. G., and Rzhakhova, O. E., 1981, Persistence of tick-borne encephalitis virus in infected monkeys. III. Phenotypes of persisting virus, *Acta Virol.* **25:**352–360.

Pogodina, V. V., Frolova, M. P., and Erman, B. A., 1986, *Chronic Tick-borne Encephalitis: Etiology, Immunology*, Nauka, Novosibirsk.

Semyonov, B. F., Kaulen, D. R., and Balandin, I. G., 1982, *Cellular and Molecular Grounds of Antiviral Immunity*, Moscow.

Studier, F. W., 1973, Analysis of bacteriophage T7 early RNA and proteins on slab gels, *J. Mol. Biol.* **79:**237–248.

Tedder, R. S., Briggs, U., Cameron, C. H., Honess, R., Robertson, D., and Whittle, H., 1987, A novel lymphotropic herpesvirus, *Lancet* **2:**390–392.

Tsang, V. G. W., Peralta, J. U., and Simons, A. R., 1983, Enzyme-linked immunoelectrotransfer blot techniques (EITB) for studying the specificities of antigens and antibodies separated by gel electrophoresis, *Methods Enzymol.* **92:**377–391.

Vartanian, M. E., 1968, *Clinico-Biological and Hereditary Laws of Schizophrenia Process*, Moscow.

Vinogradova, T. V., Kapelko, M. A., Veltischev, Y. E., and Stekani, D. V., 1986, Relationship between the level of circulating immune complexes and the phagocytic system function, *Immunology* **5:**63–66.

Chapter 10

Molecular Genetic Studies of Human Cytomegalovirus in Schizophrenia

Hans W. Moises, Rüdiger Rüger, Gavin P. Reynolds, and Bernhard Fleckenstein

INTRODUCTION

Viruses—especially human cytomegalovirus (HCMV)—have been suspected to play a role in the etiology of schizophrenia (Torrey and Peterson, 1973; Torrey *et al.*, 1982, 1983; Crow, 1983). Searching for traces of HCMV infections, serum, blood, CSF, and postmortem brain tissues have been investigated.

Elevated levels of HCMV antibodies were described in serum of schizophrenic patients by Gotlieb-Stematsky *et al.* (1981). Others were unable to replicate these results (Torrey and Peterson, 1973; Lacke *et al.*, 1974; Schindler *et al.*, 1986). Some studies indicated that CSF contained elevated antibody levels against HCMV (Albrecht *et al.*, 1980; Torrey *et al.*, 1982; Kaufmann *et al.*, 1983). Again, others could not confirm these findings (Gotlieb-Stematsky *et al.*, 1981; Rimón, 1985; Shrikhande *et al.*, 1985).

Hans W. Moises • *Department of Genetics, Stanford University School of Medicine, Stanford, California 94305.* Rüdiger Rüger and Bernhard Fleckenstein • *Institute of Clinical Virology, University of Erlangen–Nuremberg, Erlangen, Federal Republic of Germany.* Gavin P. Reynolds • *Department of Pathology, University of Nottingham Medical School, Nottingham, United Kingdom.* Present address of H.W.M.: *Department of Psychiatry, Kiel University Hospital, D-2300 Kiel-1, Federal Republic of Germany.* Present address of R.R.: *Boehringer Mannheim, Department of Genetics, Penzberg, Federal Republic of Germany.*

The search for HCMV in brain autopsy materials from schizophrenic patients has been unsuccessful (Aulakh *et al.*, 1981; Stevens *et al.*, 1984; Taylor *et al.*, 1985; Taylor and Crow, 1986).

The aim of our studies was to use highly sensitive Southern blot hybridization techniques in a search for HCMV DNA in postmortem brain tissue of schizophrenic patients. By employing a series of viral DNA fragments without virus–human DNA homologies cloned in plasmid and cosmid vectors, this method allowed the detection of 0.1 to 0.5 single-copy gene equivalent per cell.

MATERIAL AND METHODS

Brain tissue from seven undisputed schizophrenics, five persons with schizophrenia-like psychoses, three patients with Huntington's chorea, and nine mentally normal individuals (Table 1) was obtained under standard conditions soon after death, collected in the Cambridge Brain Bank Laboratory, and kept frozen at −70°C until isolation of the DNA. About 250 mg of mixed temporal cortex tissue, mainly from Brodmann area 38 temporal pole, was processed and DNA prepared as described by Saldanha *et al.* (1984). Previous experiments had shown that five regions of the HCMV genome contain DNA sequences that hybridize with intermediate repetitive DNA of normal human cells (Rüger *et al.*, 1984). A pool of cosmid and plasmid clones (pCM3-5018, pGHS2-4, pRR3-7) without virus–cell homologies (Rüger and Fleckenstein, 1985) was used as radioactive labeled probes.

^{32}P-labeled HCMV probes (>600 Ci/mmole) (New England Nuclear) were prepared by the nick-repair method (Rigby *et al.*, 1977). Cellular DNA was digested with *Eco*RI and the restriction fragments separated on 0.8% agarose gels. To achieve an optimal transfer, the cellular DNA was fragmented by exposure to UV light and treatment with 0.3 N HCl. After alkali denaturation, the cellular DNA fragments were transferred to nitrocellulose filters in 20×SSC (SSC = 0.15 M NaCl, 0.015 M sodium citrate) by Southern blotting (Southern, 1975). The filters were dried at 80°C for 4 hr. They were preincubated twice with 10×SSC and 5×SSC, respectively. Overnight incubation of the filters with nick-repair labeled HCMV-DNA and washing were carried out as described earlier (Rüger *et al.*, 1984). The hybridization temperatures were chosen 18.0–21.5°C below average T_m of HCMV DNA (Ebeling *et al.*, 1983; Rüger and Fleckenstein, 1985). These conditions allow detection of 0.1 to 0.5 single-copy gene equivalent per cell. Experiments were performed blindly with regard to clinical diagnoses.

RESULTS

The results of a Southern blot experiment are shown in Fig. 1 with DNA from six brains of schizophrenic patients and seven samples of the various other groups.

Table 1. Postmortem Temporal Cortex Samples Used in Hybridization Studies

	Age	Sex	Postmortem delay	Cause of death
Schizophrenia				
1	63	M	26	Coronary atherosclerosis
				Acute pyelitis
2	23	M	64	Asphyxia (hanging)
3	27	F	28	Drowning
4	53	M	34	Congestive heart failure
5	62	F	35	Bronchopneumonia
				Cancer of esophagus
6	56	F	23	Cardiac arrest
				Myocardial infarction
7	65	F	78	Myocardial fibrosis
8	62	F	26	Probable gram-negative bacteremia
9	80	M	54	Bronchopneumonia
10	77	F	43	Pelvic tumor
				Pulmonary embolism
11	56	M	NK[a]	Myocardial infarction
12	23	F	48	Overdose
Huntington's chorea				
1	46	M	36	Bronchial asthma
				Coronary atherosclerosis
2	25	M	NK	Bronchopneumonia
3	42	F	23	Bronchopneumonia, sarcoidosis
Controls				
1	65	M	19	Lobar pneumonia
2	42	M	46	Acute heart failure
3	38	M	13	Coronary thrombosis
4	81	M	63	Not known
5	75	M	46	Not known
6	60	M	51	Acute ventricular dysrhythmia
7	60	F	36	Inhalation of feculent vomit
8	59	M	50	Acute left ventricular failure
9	60	M	71	Acute heart failure
				Coronary atherosclerosis

[a]NK, not known.

A clear hybridization signal was detected with DNA from the temporal cortex of a young man with the full picture of schizophrenia; he died at age 23 by suicide (hanging). It is notable that this patient was first hospitalized at 20 with an acute psychotic disturbance which was difficult to control with neuroleptic treatment. The intensity of the autoradiogram suggested approximately one genome copy per average diploid brain cell. The restriction pattern was distinct from DNA of the HCMV laboratory strain Ad169, and appreciable genetic complexity of hybridizing viral DNA fragments was lower than the molecular weight of DNA probes,

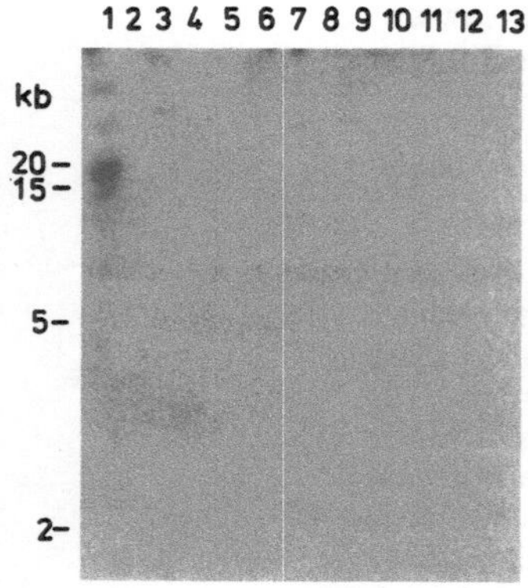

Figure 1. Southern blot hybridization of *Eco*RI-cleaved DNA from the brains of several patients with cloned ^{32}P-labeled HCMV DNA fragments. Lanes 1–6: DNA from schizophrenic patients; lanes 7–9: DNA from normal individuals; lanes 10–13: DNA from Huntington's chorea patients.

indicating substantial sequence divergence. The brain DNA sample did not hybridize with the pure prokaryotic vector. None of the other brain DNA specimens did appreciably hybridize with cloned HCMV DNA.

DISCUSSION

HCMV DNA was found in the temporal lobe of a young schizophrenic patient. This finding could be the result of (1) chance, (2) activation of latent virus infection by immunosuppression, or (3) a causal relationship between viral infection and schizophrenic psychosis.

1. Chance could play a role in the detection of HCMV DNA in the brains of patients and controls. In line with this interpretation would be the fact that Taylor and Crow (1986) found HCMV sequences in the brain of a control case. However, their finding might also be explained by immunosuppression since their control case had received immunosuppressive therapy as treatment for rheumatoid arthritis.

2. Furthermore, minor immunosuppression with increasing age or neuroleptic therapies could contribute to virus reactivation and should be considered as a possible explanation. Considering the young age of the patient and the fact that most schizophrenic patients were treated with neuroleptics, these factors were unlikely to contribute in the present case. Unfortunately, reactivation by other forms of immunosuppression or coinciding primary infection cannot be ruled out.

3. Finally, the suicide of the patient might indicate that he was suffering from an acute psychotic episode which could have been caused by an activation of HCMV in the temporal cortex.

In regard to the literature, neurotropic viruses had been found occasionally in the temporal lobe of patients with endogenous psychoses (Taylor *et al.*, 1985;

Gannicliffe, *et al.*, 1985). Adenoviruses have been found in an elderly schizophrenic (Lord *et al.*, 1975) and DNA of herpes simplex viruses in a depressive woman (Gannicliffe *et al.*, 1985). Furthermore, herpes simplex DNA sequences were detected by molecular hybridization in temporal lobe tissues from five of six patients with severe epilepsy (Gannicliffe *et al.*, 1985). This finding might be relevant for schizophrenia, since a left temporal lobe dysfunction has been long suspected in schizophrenia (Flor-Henry, 1969) and psychoses in temporal lobe epilepsy are sometimes clinically indistinguishable from schizophrenic psychoses (Trimble and Perez, 1982).

Positive brain tissue can be easily missed in analyses of small amounts of brain specimens because of the focal nature of CNS infections from herpes simplex and other viruses (Fraser *et al.*, 1981; Haase *et al.*, 1984). This might explain previous negative results of searches for viruses in schizophrenic brain tissue. *In situ* hybridization of larger parts of the brain may overcome these shortcomings.

CONCLUSION

The demonstration of HCMV DNA in the temporal cortex of a young schizophrenic male indicates the possibility that viral infection of the brain may in some individuals be a contributing factor to the development of a schizophrenic psychosis. However, in the great majority of schizophrenic psychoses there is no indication that infection of the CNS with HCMV has caused the disease. Further studies using the polymerase chain reaction (PCR) will be useful to search for HCMV-sequences in brain tissues at higher sensitivity.

ACKNOWLEDGMENTS This chapter was adapted from an article published in *European Archives of Psychiatry and Neurological Sciences* (1988, **238**:110–113). We thank Professor E. Paykel and Dr. C. M. Wischik from the Cambridge Brain Bank Laboratory for generously providing the brain tissue. H.W.M. was supported by a research grant from the Deutsche Forschungsgemeinschaft MO 429.

REFERENCES

Albrecht, P., Torrey, E. F., Boone, E., Hicks, J. T., and Daniel, N., 1980, Raised cytomegalovirus-antibody level in cerebrospinal fluid of schizophrenic patients, *Lancet* **2**:769–772.

Aulakh, G. S., Kleinman, J. E., Aulakh, H. S., Albrecht, P., Torrey, E. F., and Wyatt, R. J., 1981, Search for cytomegalovirus in schizophrenic brain tissue, *Proc. Soc. Exp. Biol. Med.* **167**:172–174.

Crow, T. J., 1983, Is schizophrenia an infectious disease? *Lancet* **1**:173–175.

Ebeling, A., Keil, G., Nowak, B., Fleckenstein, B., Berthelot, N., and Sheldrick, P., 1983, Genome structure and virion polypeptides of the primate herpesvirus Herpesvirus aotus types 1 and 3: Comparison with human cytomegalovirus, *J. Virol.* **45**:715–726.

Flor-Henry, P., 1969, Psychosis and temporal lobe epilepsy, *Epilepsia* **10**:363–395.

Fraser, N. W., Lawrence, W. C., Wroblewska, Z., Gilden, D. H., and Koprowski, H., 1981, Herpes simplex type 1 DNA in human brain tissue, *Proc. Natl. Acad. Sci. USA* **78**:6461–6465.

Gannicliffe, A., Saldanha, J. A., Itzhaki, R. F., and Sutton, R. N. P., 1985, Herpes simplex viral DNA in temporal lobe epilepsy, *Lancet* **1**:214–215.

Gotlieb-Stematsky, T., Zonis, J., Arlazoroff, A., Mozes, T., Sigal, M., and Szekely, A. G., 1981, Antibodies to Epstein–Barr virus, herpes simplex type 1, cytomegalovirus and measles virus in psychiatric patients, *Arch. Virol.* **67**:333–339.

Haase, A. T., Stowring, L., Ventura, P., Burks, J., Ebers, G., Tourtellotte, W., and Warren, K., 1984, Detection by hybridization of viral infection of the human central nervous system, *Ann. N.Y. Acad. Sci.* **436**:103–108.

Kaufmann, C. A., Weinberger, D. R., Yolken, R. H., Torrey, E. F., and Pofkin, S. G., 1983, Viruses and schizophrenia, *Lancet* **2**:1136–1137.

Lacke, E., Norby, R., and Ross, B. E., 1974, A serological study on mental ill patients. With particular reference to the prevalence of herpes virus infections, *Br. J. Psychiatry* **124**:273–279.

Lord, A., Sutton, R. N. P., and Corsellis, J. A. N., 1975, Recovery of adenovirus type 7 from human brain cell cultures, *J. Neurol. Neurosurg. Psychiatry* **38**:710–712.

Rigby, P. W., Dieckmann, M., Rhodes, C., and Berg, P., 1977, Labelling deoxyribonucleic acid to high specific activity in vitro by nick translation with DNA polymerase I, *J. Mol. Biol.* **113**:237–251.

Rimón, R. H., 1985, Serum and cerebrospinal antibodies to cytomegalovirus in schizophrenia, in: *Biological Psychiatry 1985* (C. Shagass, R. C. Josiassen, W. H. Bridger, K. J. Weiss, D. Stoff, and G. M. Simpson, eds.), Elsevier, Amsterdam, pp. 1077–1079.

Rüger, R., and Fleckenstein, B., 1985, Cytomegalovirus DNA in colorectal carcinoma tissues, *Klin. Wochenschr.* **63**:405–408.

Rüger, R., Bornkamm, G. W., and Fleckenstein, B., 1984, Human cytomegalovirus DNA sequences with homologies to the cellular genome, *J. Gen. Virol.* **65**:1351–1364.

Saldanha, J., Gannicliffe, A., and Itzhaki, R. F., 1984, An improved method for preparing DNA from human brain, *J. Neurosci. Methods* **11**:275–279.

Schindler, L., Leroux, M., Beck, J., Moises, H. W., and Kirchner, H., 1986, Studies of cellular immunity, of serum interferon titers, and of natural killer cell activity in schizophrenic patients, *Acta Psychiatr. Scand.* **73**:651–657.

Shrikhande, S., Hirsch, S. R., Cleman, J. C., Reveley, M. A., and Dayton, R., 1985, Cytomegalovirus and schizophrenia. A test of a viral hypothesis, *Br. J. Psychiatry* **146**:503–506.

Southern, E. M., 1975, Detection of specific sequences among DNA fragments separated by gel electrophoresis, *J. Mol. Biol.* **98**:503–517.

Stevens, J. R., Langloss, J. M., Albrecht, P., Volken, R., and Wang, Y. N., 1984, A search for cytomegalovirus and herpes viral antigen in brains of schizophrenic patients, *Arch. Gen. Psychiatry* **41**:795–801.

Taylor, G. R., and Crow, T. J., 1986, Viruses in human brains: A search for cytomegalovirus and herpes virus 1 DNA in necropsy tissue from normal and neuropsychiatric cases, *Psychol. Med.* **16**:289–295.

Taylor, G. R., Crow, T. J., Higgins, T., and Reynolds, G. P., 1985, Search for cytomegalovirus in postmortem brain tissue from patients with Huntington's chorea and other psychiatric disease by molecular hybridization using cloned DNA, *J. Neuropathol. Exp. Neurol.* **44**:176–184.

Torrey, E. F., and Peterson, M. R., 1973, Slow and latent viruses in schizophrenia, *Lancet* **2**:22–24.

Torrey, E. F., Yolken, R. H., and Winfrey, C. J., 1982, Cytomegalovirus antibody in CSF of schizophrenic patients detected by enzyme immunoassay, *Science* **216**:892–894.

Torrey, E. F., Yolken, R. H., and Albrecht, P., 1983, Cytomegalovirus, a possible etiological agent in schizophrenia, *Adv. Biol. Psychiatry* **12**:150–160.

Trimble, M. R., and Perez, M. M., 1982, The phenomenology of the chronic psychoses of epilepsy, *Adv. Biol. Psychiatry* **8**:98–105.

Chapter **11**

New Experimental Approaches Examining a Viral Etiology of Schizophrenia

Anita Feenstra, Darrell G. Kirch, Mark A. Coggiano, and Richard Jed Wyatt

INTRODUCTION

Viral infections have been suggested as a possible cause of several chronic disorders of the CNS, including multiple sclerosis (Cook and Dowling, 1980; Koprowski *et al.*, 1985; Reddy *et al.*, 1989; Greenberg *et al.*, 1989), Parkinson's disease (Ravenholt and Foege, 1982), Alzheimer's disease (Terry and Davies, 1980), and schizophrenia (Torrey and Peterson, 1976; Tyrrell *et al.*, 1979; Crow, 1983; Wyatt and DeLisi, 1984). Evidence to support a viral etiology of schizophrenia has been based mainly on epidemiological data. These include a season-of-birth effect, where there is an excess of late winter and early spring births (Torrey

Anita Feenstra, Darrell G. Kirch, Mark A. Coggiano, and Richard Jed Wyatt • *Neuropsychiatry Branch, Intramural Research Program, National Institute of Mental Health, Washington, D.C. 20032.* Present address of A.F.: *Zentrum für Molekulare Biologie Heidelberg, D-6900 Heidelberg, Federal Republic of Germany.*

et al., 1977), and a high prevalence of the disease in some geographic areas (Torrey, 1987). Laboratory attempts to more directly substantiate a viral etiology in schizophrenia have focused on alterations in humoral and cell-mediated immunity (Vartanian *et al.*, 1987; DeLisi *et al.*, 1982; Coffey *et al.*, 1983; Kirch *et al.*, 1985; Roos *et al.*, 1985; DeLisi, 1986; Ganguli *et al.*, 1987), which could reflect a challenge by an infectious agent, and on efforts to identify antibodies to specific viruses in blood (DeLisi and Sarin, 1985; King *et al.*, 1985; Robert-Guroff *et al.*, 1985; Torrey and Kaufmann, 1986), CSF (Torrey *et al.*, 1982; Kaufmann *et al.*, 1983), or post-mortem brain material (Stevens *et al.*, 1983). These approaches have led to mixed results with no evidence for a specific virus.

Crow (1984) introduced the concept that retroviruses might be a contributing factor in schizophrenia, thereby combining the viral hypothesis with the apparent genetic component of the disorder. Insofar as retroviruses are RNA viruses with the ability to become integrated into the host cell genome, genetic transmission could be accounted for by germline integration resulting from infection. Alternatively, the patient might be genetically predisposed to a retroviral infection. As human retroviruses have become associated with neuropsychiatric syndromes, interest in a role for retroviruses in the etiology of schizophrenia has increased. The human T-cell lymphotropic virus, HTLV-I, has been associated with a progressive myelopathy, tropical spastic paraparesis (Gessain *et al.*, 1985; Vernant *et al.*, 1987; Osame *et al.*, 1987). HTLV-I infection has also been linked to multiple sclerosis (Koprowski *et al.*, 1985; Reddy *et al.*, 1989; Greenberg *et al.*, 1989). The human immunodeficiency virus (HIV) may cause varied central and peripheral neuropsychiatric symptoms and opportunistic brain infections (Navia *et al.*, 1986a,b). Recently, several reports have described acute schizophrenia-like symptoms occurring in HIV-seropositive patients (Jones *et al.*, 1987; Maccario and Scharre, 1987).

When serum from chronic schizophrenic patients was tested for antibodies to the retrovirus-specific enzyme, reverse transcriptase, and to HTLV-I and HIV antigens, no antibodies were found (DeLisi and Sarin, 1985). This finding, as pointed out by Crow (1985), does not exclude a retroviral etiology of schizophrenia, as reverse transcriptase is only weakly antigenic. In another study, sera from patients with schizophrenia and schizoaffective disorder were tested for antibodies to the retroviruses HTLV-I, -II, and -III with negative results (Robert-Guroff *et al.*, 1985).

In light of the increasing evidence of interactions between human retroviruses and the CNS (Shaw *et al.*, 1985; Gartner *et al.*, 1986; Koenig *et al.*, 1986), we pursued the retroviral hypothesis in schizophrenia. Using techniques developed for the discovery and isolation of the human lymphotropic retroviruses, HTLV-I, -II, and HIV (Poiesz *et al.*, 1980a, 1981; Gallo *et al.*, 1984; Salahuddin *et al.*, 1985), we investigated the possibility that schizophrenia is associated with an until now unknown retrovirus.

REVERSE TRANSCRIPTASE ACTIVITY IN LYMPHOCYTES OF PATIENTS WITH SCHIZOPHRENIA

In the first study, we established peripheral blood lymphocyte (PBL) cultures from 17 schizophrenic patients and 10 normal controls under conditions favoring the growth of T cells (Feenstra *et al.*, 1989). Lymphocytes were isolated by Ficoll density gradient centrifugation, stimulated with phytohemagglutinin (PHA), and then cultured in the presence of T-cell growth factor (TCGF). Culture supernatant samples were collected at 3- to 4-day intervals, and the particulate fraction tested for reverse transcriptase (RT) and DNA polymerase activity. RT is a viral RNA-directed DNA polymerase essential in the retroviral life cycle (Kacian, 1977; Varmus and Swanstrom, 1984). *In vitro* the enzyme is able to use RNA:DNA, and DNA:DNA hybrids as templates. The relative preference of RT for the RNA:DNA template oligo(dT):poly(rA) is used to distinguish RT from cellular DNA polymerases that favor the DNA:DNA hybrid oligo(dT):poly(dA) as a template. RT and DNA polymerase activity were determined simultaneously, and a sample was considered to be RT positive if the RT activity was higher than the DNA polymerase activity. The cell line HUT102B2, a low-level producer of HTLV-I (Poiesz *et al.*, 1980b; kindly provided by Dr. S. Salahuddin), was used as a positive control.

As shown in Fig. 1, there was no significant difference between the peak activity of RT of the patient group and the normal control group, which was also true at all other sampling points in culture ($F = 0.03, p = 0.85$). At all time points the DNA polymerase activity was higher than the RT activity for patient and control samples ($F = 9.13$, $p = 0.0049$).

There is evidence in the literature of an effect of neuroleptic treatment on lymphocyte function (Fieve *et al.*, 1966; Ferguson *et al.*, 1987). We compared the RT activity in PBL cultures from patients on neuroleptic medication ($n = 11$) with those off medication ($n = 6$) and found no differences at any time ($F = 0.61, p = 0.44$; Table 1). Thus, in this first effort to find direct evidence for a link between retroviruses and schizophrenia, we could not detect T-cell-associated RT activity, our retroviral marker, in PBL cultures from patients with schizophrenia. One explanation of this negative result, however, might be that a virus was present, but not expressing RT in these cultured lymphocytes.

REVERSE TRANSCRIPTASE ACTIVITY IN 5-AZACYTIDINE-TREATED LYMPHOCYTE CULTURES

In a second study, lymphocyte cultures of schizophrenic patients and normal controls were treated with 5-azacytidine, a compound widely used to reactivate viral genes (Groudine *et al.*, 1981; Hoffmann *et al.*, 1982). After isolation and

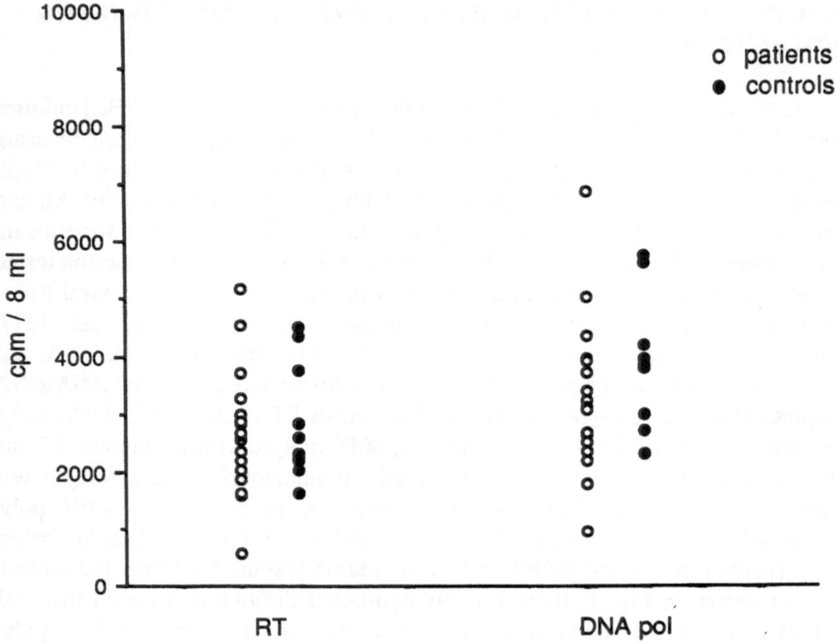

Figure 1. Peak polymerase activity in the particulate fraction of PBL cultures of chronic schizophrenic patients (○) and normal controls (●). Activity is expressed as [^{3}H]-TTP (cpm) incorporated/8 ml culture supernatant, using polyrA·dT_{12-18} for RT and polydA·dT_{12-18} for DNA polymerase as template. The HUT102B2 cell line, a low-level producer of HTLV-I (Poiesz *et al.*, 1981), tested positive for RT at [^{3}H]-TTP incorporation levels of 3000–13,000 cpm/8 ml with a DNA polymerase activity of 600–3000 cpm/8 ml.

All patients (n = 17) met DSM-III criteria for the diagnosis of chronic schizophrenia. The mean age of the patient group was 32.9 years (range 20–47), and the mean duration of illness was 11.4 years (range 3–27). The control group (n = 10) consisted of healthy volunteers, the mean age of this group being 31.6 years (range 29–37), with 6 men and 4 women. All subjects provided informed consent for venipuncture, and all tested HIV antibody negative.

Table 1. Effect of Medication on Reverse Transcriptase Activity in Cultures of Schizophrenic

	Day 10	Day 15	Day 18	Day 21	Day 28
Medicated patients (n = 11)	2840[a]	2169	2200	1307	1200
Nonmedicated patients (n = 6)	2373	2066	1770	1191	1020

[a]Values are the mean of the group; activity is expressed as cpm incorporated/8 ml culture fluid.

stimulation of the lymphocytes with PHA, the cultures were treated with 2.5 and/or 5 μM 5-azacytidine for 24 hr and subsequently screened for the retroviral marker RT, as previously described (Feenstra *et al.*, 1988). The RT activity in the culture supernatant from cultures treated with 5-azacytidine was compared with the RT activity in untreated cultures from the same individual. Consistent with the first study, no increase of RT activity was found in the untreated PBL cultures of our schizophrenic patients compared with normal controls. Supernatants of cultures treated with 2.5 or 5 μM 5-azacytidine were also negative for RT activity in both the patient and control groups (Fig. 2). No significant difference was found between the azacytidine-treated and untreated cultures in both groups.

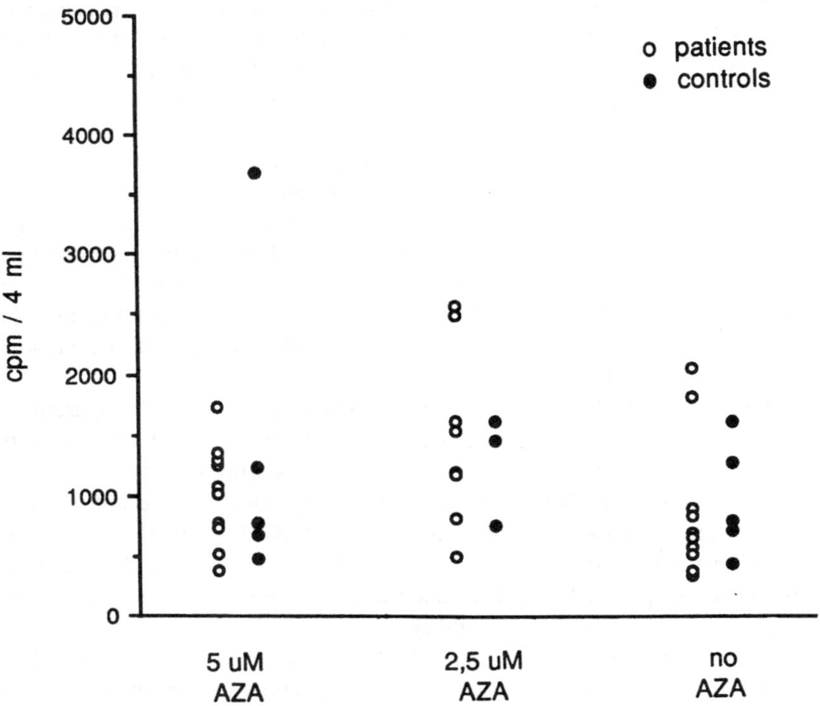

Figure 2. Peak RT activity in azacytidine (AZA)-treated lymphocyte cultures of schizophrenic patients (○) and controls (●). Activity is expressed as [^{3}H]-TTP (cpm) incorporated/4 ml culture supernatant.

All patients (n = 11) met DSM-III criteria for the diagnosis of schizophrenia. The mean age of the patient group was 29.6 years (range 20–47) and their mean duration of illness was 10.8 years (range 3–27). The group consisted of 7 men and 4 women. The control group consisted of 6 healthy volunteers, the mean age of this group being 29.8 years (range 24–36), with 4 men and 2 women. Patients and controls provided informed consent for venipuncture and all tested HIV antibody negative.

DISCUSSION

We screened for the presence of a retrovirus in lymphocyte cultures of schizophrenic patients by using techniques that have been successfully used to uncover evidence for retroviral involvement in illnesses including leukemia, AIDS, and possibly Kawasaki disease (Burns *et al.*, 1986; Melish *et al.*, 1989). In our first screening effort, we showed that no T-cell-associated retroviral RT activity could be detected in PBL from schizophrenic patients. In the second study, we attempted to activate a retrovirus in the PBL cultures of schizophrenic patients by treating the cells with 5-azacytidine. Azacytidine, a nucleoside analogue of cytidine, is widely used to reactivate viral genes (Groudine *et al.*, 1981; Hoffmann *et al.*, 1982) by reducing the methylation state of the genome (Taylor and Jones, 1982; Santi *et al.*, 1983). DNA methylation is thought to play a role as a modulator in the latency of HIV (Bednarik *et al.*, 1987) and has been associated with the inactive state of many retroviral, viral, and cellular genes (Doerfler, 1983). This approach, however, failed to provide evidence for a retroviral presence in the lymphocytes of patients with schizophrenia.

Some caution is indicated prior to excluding a retroviral etiology of schizophrenia on the basis of these results. As Crow (1984) suggested, schizophrenia might be the result of a retroviral integration in which the virus is either endogenous to the human genome or acquired *in utero*. The culture conditions used might not have been adequate to elicit expression of an integrated retroviral genome. Agents such as 5-iodo-2′-deoxyuridine (Poiesz *et al.*, 1981) and cocultivation with PHA-activated lymphocytes from cord blood (Salahuddin *et al.*, 1985) are among other techniques used to activate retroviral genes.

Our studies were limited to peripheral lymphocytes. As schizophrenia is considered a brain disorder, an obvious explanation of our negative results might be that the virus is located in the brain and not in PBL. Attempts to transmit a virus from CSF or brain tissue from schizophrenic patients *in vivo* have not provided definitive results (Baker *et al.*, 1983; Mered *et al.*, 1983; Kaufmann *et al.*, 1988). Cocultivation of postmortem brain material with PHA-activated lymphocytes from cord blood or peripheral blood (Salahuddin *et al.*, 1985) may provide a more sensitive method to study this possibility.

We studied schizophrenic patients who had been chronically ill, all of whom had previous neuroleptic treatment. Although neuroleptics are known to affect the expression of certain viruses (Wunderlich *et al.*, 1980; Patou *et al.*, 1986), we showed that the medication status of the patient at the time of blood sampling did not appear to influence RT activity. It is conceivable, however, that a virus can only be isolated from patients early in their illness and perhaps prior to any neuroleptic treatment.

In conclusion, the lymphocyte cultures of patients with schizophrenia were negative for RT activity, despite activation with 5-azacytidine. Therefore, our findings do not provide evidence for the presence of a retrovirus in PBL of these patients, and do not support a retroviral etiology of schizophrenia. They do not exclude, however, such an etiology. It may emerge that viral exposure is a causal factor in only a small subset of cases of schizophrenia. In addition, if viruses are implicated in schizophrenia, it is possible that the pathogenesis involves an early (i.e., pre- or perinatal) exposure leaving little residual genomic evidence. Other approaches, such as gene amplification techniques (Saiki *et al.*, 1988) to identify small quantities of viral DNA, have been successfully used to detect evidence of retroviral involvement in some cases of multiple sclerosis (Reddy *et al.*, 1989; Greenberg *et al.*, 1989) and may provide new avenues to probe a viral etiology of schizophrenia.

REFERENCES

Baker, H. F., Ridley, R. M., Crow, T. J., Bloxham, C. A., Parry, R. P., and Tyrrell, D. A. J., 1983, An investigation of the effects of intracerebral injection in the marmoset of cytopathic cerebrospinal fluid from patients with schizophrenia or neurological disease, *Psychol. Med.* **13**:499–511.

Bednarik D. P., Mosca, J. D., and Raj, N. B. K., 1987, Methylation as a modulator of expression of human immunodeficiency virus, *J. Virol.* **61**:1253–1257.

Burns, J. C., Geha, R. S., Schneeberger, E. E., Newburger, J. W., Rosen, F. S., Glezen, L. S., Natale, J., and Huang, A. S., 1986, Polymerase activity in lymphocyte culture supernatants from patients with Kawasaki disease, *Nature* **323**:814–816.

Coffey, C. E., Sullivan, J. L., and Rice, J. R., 1983, T lymphocytes in schizophrenia, *Biol. Psychiatry* **18**:113–119.

Cook, S. D., and Dowling, P. C., 1980, Multiple sclerosis and viruses: An overview, *Neurology* **30**:113–119.

Crow, T. J., 1983, Is schizophrenia an infectious disease? *Lancet* **1**:173–175.

Crow, T. J., 1984, A re-evaluation of the viral hypothesis: Is psychosis the result of retroviral integration at a site close to the cerebral dominance gene? *Br. J. Psychiatry* **145**:243–253.

Crow, T. J., 1985, *Br. J. Psychiatry* **146**:674–675.

DeLisi, L. E., 1986, Neuroimmunology: Clinical studies of schizophrenia and other psychiatric disorders, in: *Handbook of Schizophrenia: The Neurology of Schizophrenia* (H. A. Nasrallah and D. R. Weinberger, eds.), Elsevier, Amsterdam, p. 674.

DeLisi, L. E., and Sarin, P. S., 1985, Lack of evidence for retrovirus infection in schizophrenic patients, *Br. J. Psychiatry* **146**:674.

DeLisi, L. E., Goodman, S., Neckers, L. M., and Wyatt, R. J., 1982, An analysis of lymphocyte subpopulations in schizophrenic patients, *Biol. Psychiatry* **17**:1003–1009.

Doerfler, W., 1983, DNA methylation and gene activity, *Annu. Rev. Biochem.* **52**:93–124.

Feenstra, A., Kirch, D. G., Coggiano, M. A., and Wyatt, R. J., 1988, Reverse transcriptase activity in 5-azacytidine-treated lymphocyte cultures of patients with schizophrenia, *Schiz. Res.* **1**:385–389.

Feenstra, A., Kirch, D. G., Bracha, H. S., and Wyatt, R. J., 1989, Lack of evidence for a role of T-cell-associated retroviruses as an etiology of schizophrenia, *Biol. Psychiatry* **25**:421–430.

Ferguson, R. M., Schmidtke, J. R., and Simmons, R. L., 1987, Effects of psychoactive drugs on in vitro lymphocyte activation, in: *Neurochemical and Immunological Components of Schizophrenia* (D. Bergsma and A. L. Goldstein, eds.), Liss, New York, pp. 379–402.

Fieve, R. R., Blumenthal, B., and Little, B., 1966, The relationship of atypical lymphocytes, phenothiazines and schizophrenia, *Arch. Gen. Psychiatry* **15**:529–534.

Gallo, R. C., Salahuddin, S. Z., Popovic, M., Shearer, G. M., Kaplan, M., Haynes, B. F., Palker, T. J., Redfield, R., Oleske, J., Safai, B., White, G., Foester, P., and Markham, P. D., 1984, Frequent detection and isolation of cytopathic retroviruses (HTLV-III) from patients with AIDS and at risk for AIDS, *Science* **224**:500–503.

Ganguli, R., Rabin, B., Raghu, U., and Ulrich, R. S., 1987, T-lymphocytes in schizophrenics and normals and the effects of varying antipsychotic dosage, in: *Viruses, Immunity and Mental Disorders* (E. Kurstak, Z. J. Lipowski, and P. V. Morozov, eds.), Plenum Press, New York, pp. 321–326.

Gartner, S., Markovits, P., Markovitz, D. M., Betts, R. F., and Popovic, M., 1986, Virus isolation from and identification of HTLV-III/LAV-producing cells in brain tissue from a patient with AIDS, *J. Am. Med. Assoc.* **256**:2365–2371.

Gessain, A., Vernant, J. C., Maurs, L., Barin, F., Gout, O., Calender, A., and De The, G., 1985, Antibodies to human T-lymphotropic virus type-I in patients with tropical spastic paraparesis, *Lancet* **2**:407–409.

Greenberg, S. J., Ehrlich, G. D., Abbott, M. A., Hurwitz, B. J., Waldmann, T. A., and Poiesz, B. J., 1989, Detection of sequences homologous to human retroviral DNA in multiple sclerosis by gene amplification, *Proc. Natl. Acad. Sci. USA* **86**:2878–2882.

Groudine, M., Eisenman, R., and Weintraub, H., 1981, Chromatin structure of endogenous retroviral genes and activation by an inhibitor of DNA methylation, *Nature* **292**:311–317.

Hoffmann, J. W., Steffen, D., Gusella, J., Tabin, C., Bird, S., Cowing, D., and Weinberg, R. A., 1982, DNA methylation affecting the expression of murine leukemia proviruses, *J. Virol.* **44**:144–157.

Jones, G. H., Kelly, C. L., and Davies, J. A., 1987, HIV and onset of schizophrenia, *Lancet* **1**:982.

Kacian, D. L., 1977, Methods for assaying reverse transcriptase, in: *Methods in Virology*, (K. Maramorosch and H. Koprowski, eds.), Academic Press, New York, p. 143.

Kaufmann, C. A., Weinberger, D. R., Yolken, R. H., Torrey, E. F., and Potkin, S. G., 1983, Viruses and schizophrenia, *Lancet* **2**:1136–1137.

Kaufmann, C. A., Weinberger, D. R., Stevens, J. R., Asher, D. M., Kleinman, J. E., Sulima, M. P., Gibbs, C. J., and Gadjusek, D. C., 1988, Intracerebral inoculation of experimental animals with brain tissue from patients with schizophrenia: Failure to observe consistent or specific behavioral and neuropathological effects, *Arch. Gen. Psychiatry* **45**:648–652.

King, D. J., Cooper, S. J., Earle, J. A. P., Martin, S. J., McFerran, N. V., and Wisdom, G. B., 1985, Serum and CSF antibody titres to seven common viruses in schizophrenic patients, *Br. J. Psychiatry* **147**:145–149.

Kirch, D. G., Kaufmann, C. A., Papadopoulus, N. M., Martin, B., and Weinberger, D. R., 1985, Abnormal cerebrospinal fluid protein indices in schizophrenia, *Biol. Psychiatry* **20**:1039–1046.

Koenig, S., Gendelman, H. E., Orenstein, J. M., Dal Conto, M. C., Pezeshkpour, G. H., Yungbluth, M., Janotta, F., and Aksamit, A., 1986, Detection of AIDS virus in macrophages in brain tissue from AIDS patients with encephalopathy, *Science* **233**:1089–1093.

Koprowski, H., DeFreitas, E. C., Harper, M. E., Sandberg-Wollheim, M., Sheremata, W. A., Robert-Guroff, M., Saxinger, C. W., and Feinberg, M. B., 1985, Multiple sclerosis and human T-cell lymphotropic retroviruses, *Nature* **318**:154–160.

Maccario, M., and Scharre, D. W., 1987, HIV and acute onset of psychosis, *Lancet* **2**:342.

Melish, M. E., Marchette, N. J., Kaplan, J. C., Kihira, S., Ching, D., and Ho, D. D., 1989, Absence of significant RNA-dependent DNA polymerase activity in lymphocytes from patients with Kawasaki syndrome, *Nature* **337**:288–290.

Mered, B., Albrecht, P., Torrey, E. F., Weinberger, D. R., Potkin, S. G., and Winfrey, C. J., 1983, Failure to isolate virus from CSF of schizophrenics, *Lancet* **11**:919.

Navia, B. A., Jordan, B. D., and Price, R. W., 1986a, The AIDS dementia complex: I. Clinical features, *Ann. Neurol.* **19**:517–524.

Navia, B. A., Cho, E. S., Petito, C. K., and Price, R. W., 1986b, The AIDS dementia complex: II. Neuropathology, *Ann. Neurol.* **19:**525–535.

Osame, M., Matsumoto, M., Usuku, K., Izumo, S., Ijichi, N., Amitani, H., Tara, M., and Igata, A., 1987, Chronic progressive myelopathy associated with elevated antibodies to human T-lymphotropic virus type I and adult T-cell leukemia-like cells, *Ann. Neurol.* **21:**117–122.

Patou, G., Crow, T. J., and Taylor, G. R., 1986, The effects of psychotropic drugs on synthesis of DNA and the infectivity of herpes symplex virus, *Biol. Psychiatry* **21:**1221–1225.

Poiesz, B. J., Ruscetti, F. W., Gazdar, A. F., Bunn, P. A., Minna, J. D., and Gallo, R. C., 1980a, Detection and isolation of C retrovirus particles from fresh and cultured lymphocytes of a patient with cutaneous T-cell lymphoma, *Proc. Natl. Acad. Sci. USA* **77:**7415–7419.

Poiesz, B. J., Ruscetti, F. W., Mier, J. W., Woods, A. M., and Gallo, R. C., 1980b, T-cell lines established from human T-lymphocytic neoplasias by direct response to T-cell growth factor, *Proc. Natl. Acad. Sci. USA* **77:**6815–6819.

Poiesz, B. J., Ruscetti, F. W., Reitz, M. S., Kalyanaraman, V. S., and Gallo, R. C., 1981, Isolation of a new type C retrovirus (HTLV) in primary uncultured cells of a patient with Sezary T-cell leukemia, *Nature* **294:**268–271.

Ravenholt, R. T., and Foege, W. H., 1982, 1918 influenza, encephalitis lethargica, parkinsonism, *Lancet* **2:**860–864.

Reddy, E. P., Sandberg-Wollheim, M., Mettus, R. V., Ray, P. E., DeFreitas, E., and Koprowski, H., 1989, Amplification and molecular cloning of HTLV-I sequences from DNA of multiple sclerosis patients, *Science* **243:**529–533.

Robert-Guroff, M., Torrey, E. F., and Brown, M., 1985, Retroviruses and schizophrenia, *Br. J. Psychiatry* **146:**326.

Roos, R. P., Davis, K., and Meltzer, H. Y., 1985, Immunoglobulin studies with psychiatric diseases, *Arch. Gen. Psychiatry* **42:**124–128.

Saiki, R. K., Gelfand, D. H., Stoffel, S., Scharf, S. J., Higuchi, R., Horn, G. T., Mullis, K. B., and Ehrlich, H. E., 1988, Primer-directed enzymatic amplification of DNA with a thermostable DNA polymerase, *Science* **239:**487–491.

Salahuddin, S. Z., Markham, P. D., Popovic, M., Sarngadharan, M. G., Orndorff, S., Fladagar, A., Patel, A., Gold, J., and Gallo, R. C., 1985, Isolation of infectious human T-cell leukemia/lymphotropic virus type-III (HTLV-III) from patients with acquired immunodeficiency syndrome (AIDS) or AIDS-related complex (ARC) and from healthy carriers: A study of risk groups and tissue sources, *Proc. Natl. Acad. Sci. USA* **82:**5530–5534.

Santi, D. V., Garret, C. E., and Barr, P. J., 1983, On the mechanism of inhibition of DNA-cytosine methyltransferases by cytosine analogs, *Cell* **33:**9–10.

Shaw, G. M., Harper, M. E., Hahn, B. E., Epstein, L. G., Gajdusek, D. C., Price, R. W., Navia, B. A., Pitito, C. K., O'Hara, C. J., Groopman, J. E., Cho, E. S., Oleske, J. M., Wong-Staal, F., and Gallo, R. C., 1985, HTLV-III infection in brains of children and adults with AIDS encephalopathy, *Science* **277:**177.

Stevens, J. R., Albrecht, P., Godfrey, L., and Krauthammer, E., 1983, Viral antigen in the brain of schizophrenic patients? A preliminary report, *Adv. Biol. Psychiatry* **12:**76–96.

Taylor, S. M., and Jones, P. A., 1982, Mechanism of action of eukariotic DNA methyltransferase. Use of 5-azacytosine-containing DNA, *J. Mol. Biol.* **162:**679–692.

Terry, R. D., and Davies, P., 1980, Dementia of the Alzheimer type, *Annu. Rev. Neurosci.* **3:**77–95.

Torrey, E. F., 1987, Prevalence studies in schizophrenia, *Br. J. Psychiatry* **150:**598–608.

Torrey, E. F., and Kaufmann, C. A., 1986, Schizophrenia and neuroviruses, in: *Handbook of Schizophrenia*, Volume I (H. A. Nasrallah and D. R. Weinberger, eds.), Elsevier, Amsterdam, p. 361.

Torrey, E. F., and Peterson, M. R., 1976, The viral hypothesis of schizophrenia, *Schiz. Bull.* **2:**136–137.

Torrey, E. F., Torrey, B. B., and Peterson, M. R., 1977, Seasonality of schizophrenic births in the United States, *Arch. Gen. Psychiatry* **34:**1065.

Torrey, E. F., Yolken, R. H., and Winfrey, C. J., 1982, Cytomegalovirus antibody in cerebrospinal fluid of schizophrenic patients detected by enzyme immunoassay, *Science* **216**:892–894.

Tyrrell, D. A. J., Crow, T. J., Parry, R. P., Johnstone, E., and Ferrier, I. N., 1979, Possible virus in schizophrenia and some neurological disorders, *Lancet* **1**:839–841.

Varmus, R., and Swanstrom, R., 1984, Replication of retroviruses, in: *RNA Tumor Viruses* (R. Weiss, N. Teich, H. Varmus, and J. Coffin, eds.), Cold Spring Harbor Laboratory, Cold Spring Harbor, N.Y., p. 369.

Vartanian, M. E., Kolyaskina, G. I., Lozovsky, D. V., Burbaeva, G. S. A., and Ignatov, S. A., 1987, Aspects of humoral and cellular immunity in schizophrenia, *Birth Defects* **18**:339–364.

Vernant, J. C., Maurs, L., Gessain, A., Barin, F., Gout, O., Delaporte, J. M., Sanhadji, J., and Buisson, G., 1987, Endemic tropical spastic paraparesis associated with human T-lymphotropic virus type I: A clinical study and seroepidemiological study of 25 cases, *Ann. Neurol.* **21**:123–130.

Wunderlich, V., Vey, F., and Sydow, G., 1980, Antiviral effect of haloperidol on Rauscher murine leukemia virus, *Arch. Geschwulstforsch.* **50**:758–762.

Wyatt, R. J., and DeLisi, L. E., 1984, Future research directions in the treatment of schizophrenia, in: *Guidelines for the Use of Psychotropic Drugs* (H. D. Stancer, P. E. Garfunkle, and V. M. Rakoff, eds.), Medical and Scientific Books, New York, pp. 277–293.

Chapter **12**

Lymphocyte Subsets in Schizophrenic Patients

Cinzia Masserini, Pasquale Ferrante, Antonio Vita, and Carlo Lorenzo Cazzullo

INTRODUCTION

Several immune system abnormalities have been described in schizophrenic patients. Evidence for the presence of antibrain antibodies in serum (Lehmann-Facius, 1937), morphological changes of lymphocytes (Hirata-Hibi *et al.*, 1982), abnormal distribution of serum and CSF immunoglobulins (Zarrabi *et al.*, 1979; DeLisi *et al.*, 1984), decreased *in vitro* function of lymphocytes (Vartanian *et al.*, 1978) and of natural killer cells (DeLisi *et al.*, 1983), and deficient Interleukin-2 production (Villemain *et al.*, 1989) have been reported. With regard to the distribution of lymphocyte subsets in peripheral blood, there is evidence either of T suppressor cell decrease (Muller *et al.*, 1987; Kolyaskina *et al.*, 1987), or of T helper increase (Ganguli *et al.*, 1987), or of T total, T suppressor, and B lymphocyte increase (DeLisi and Wyatt, 1982), or of no changes at all (Kaufmann *et al.*, 1987; Villemain *et al.*, 1987, 1989).

These contradictory results have been mainly achieved in chronic schizophrenic patients, with a long history of disease and of neuroleptic treatment. An exception to this issue is the recent work by Villemain (Villemain *et al.*, 1989) who studied the immune status of a group of untreated schizophrenic patients.

Cinzia Masserini, Antonio Vita, and Carlo Lorenzo Cazzullo • *Institute of Clinical Psychiatry, University of Milan, 20122 Milan, Italy.* Pasquale Ferrante • *Multiple Sclerosis University Center "Don C. Gnocchi," 20148 Milan, Italy.*

Since abnormal immune functioning may suggest the presence of an infectious agent, several authors have searched for specific viral antibodies in sera and CSF from schizophrenic patients. The data from these studies are controversial and contradictory.

There is a suggestion that antibodies to some types of herpes-class viruses may be increased in schizophrenic patients (Rimon and Halonen, 1969; Cappell and Sprecher, 1983; Libikova, 1983).

Torrey (Torrey *et al.*, 1982) showed the presence of specific IgM antibodies to cytomegalovirus in serum and CSF of some schizophrenic patients. So far the greater number of advanced hypotheses and researches made have concerned viruses such as Herpesviridae, being able to produce latent and persistent infections with or without frequent reactivations.

On the basis of these findings, we considered in our study four Herpesviridae and the measles virus, an agent having marked neurotropism and able to stimulate a very large antibody response.

In the present study, we collected a population of patients affected by schizophrenia or schizophrenic spectrum disorders, a third of whom had never been treated with neuroleptic drugs, and we studied the lymphocyte subsets, the immunoglobulin distribution, and the antibody levels to viruses in peripheral blood, dividing the patient group according to the presence or absence of neuroleptic medication.

PATIENTS AND METHODS

Peripheral blood subsets of T and B lymphocytes were determined, using the immunoperoxidase staining method described by Hofman (Hofman *et al.*, 1982), in 42 schizophrenic patients. No patient had clinical evidence of a medical or neurological illness, nor history of alcohol or drug abuse, head trauma with loss of consciousness, seizure disorder, or electroconvulsive therapy. No recent infections or diseases associated with immunological abnormalities had been reported.

Twenty-four patients (20 males and 4 females; mean age ± S.D., 22 ± 4 years) were drug-free: 15 patients had never been treated with neuroleptic medication before, and 9 patients had been free from neuroleptic medication for at least 3 months. Eighteen patients (12 males and 6 females; mean age ± S.D., 24 ± 4 years) had been on neuroleptic medication for a period lasting from 1 month to 3 years, with daily doses ranging from 2 to 13 mg of haloperidol. The mean age of illness onset was 20 ± 4 years in either drug-free or drug-treated patients. The illness duration was 2.7 ± 2.2 years in the drug-free group and 3.6 ± 2.9 years in the drug-treated group. Twenty-seven patients fulfilled the DSM-III criteria for the diagnosis of schizophrenia (12 disorganized, 8 undifferentiated, and 7 paranoid types) and 15 patients had a schizophrenic spectrum disorder (4 schizophreniform, 7 schizotypic, and 4 schizoid disorders).

Thirty-seven healthy subjects, age and sex matched to patients, served as the control group. The sera from 22 patients were tested, at 1:40 dilution, for the presence of specific IgG against measles virus (MV), varicella–zoster virus (VZV), herpesvirus type 1 (HSV1) and type 2 (HSV2), and cytomegalovirus (CMV) by mean of an enzyme-linked immunosorbent assay (ELISA), prepared in our laboratory (Ferrante *et al.*, 1987), and the results expressed as mean optical density (O.D.).

Twenty-six patients underwent computed tomographic (CT) scan examination of the brain. CT scans were performed to assess the presence of neuromorphological alterations. Ventricular size was measured on the tomographic slice which showed the greatest extension of the lateral ventricles by manual planimetric method (Sacchetti *et al.*, 1987) and expressed as ventricular brain ratio (VBR) (Synek and Reuben, 1976).

Cortical atrophy was measured using a four-point visual scale, assessing increasing degrees of atrophy (Vita *et al.*, 1988).

The values of IgA, IgG, and IgM serum immunoglobulins were assessed by commercially available radial immunodiffusion plates.

IMMUNOLOGICAL RESULTS

The drug-free patient group showed an increase of percentage of T total ($p < 0.05$), T suppressor ($p < 0.001$), and B lymphocytes ($p < 0.05$) as compared with control values (Table 1). This difference is also evident by comparing the absolute number of T total ($p < 0.001$), T suppressor ($p < 0.001$), and B ($p < 0.05$) lymphocytes per cubic milliliter of blood. The absolute number ($p < 0.001$), but not the percentage of T-helper lymphocytes significantly differed between drug-free patients and healthy controls.

The drug-treated patients differed from normal controls for a T-helper cell increase either as a percentage ($p < 0.01$) or as an absolute number ($p < 0.001$). They differed also from healthy subjects in having a higher number per cubic milliliter of T total lymphocytes ($p < 0.005$).

The drug-free versus drug-treated patients showed higher values of T suppressor cells either as a percentage ($p < 0.02$) or as an absolute number per cubic millimeter ($p < 0.005$).

No significant difference could be found in immunoglobulin values between patients and healthy subjects but we observed a significant decrease of IgM values in drug-treated patients versus drug-free ones ($p < 0.05$).

By separating the patients with schizophrenia from those with schizophrenic

Table 1. Lymphocyte Subsets in Patients and Healthy Subjects

	Healthy subjects (n = 37)	Drug-free patients (n = 24)	Patients on drugs (n = 18)
Lymphocytes/mm³	1958 ± 62*a*	2424 ± 721**	2273 ± 728*
T total			
%	64 ± 9	70 ± 7*	65 ± 12
Cells/mm³	1214 ± 406	1888 ± 660**	1603 ± 561*
T helper			
%	43 ± 6	43 ± 7	48 ± 7*
Cells/mm³	833 ± 274	1153 ± 383**	1208 ± 439*
T suppressor			
%	31 ± 6	37 ± 9**	29 ± 6§
Cells/mm³	619 ± 208	993 ± 404**	713 ± 213§
B			
%	14 ± 3	17 ± 4*	17 ± 8
Cells/mm³	268 ± 112	441 ± 155*	417 ± 275

*a*Values are means ± S.D. Statistical analysis by student's t test. *$p < 0.05$ and **$p > 0.001$ patients versus healthy subjects. §$p < 0.02$ drug-treated versus drug-free patients.

spectrum disorders and the schizophrenic patients into the different clinical subtypes, we found that the significance of some differences mainly depends on the disorganized subtype of schizophrenia: (1) Considering T total and T suppressor values, the difference persists for the drug-free disorganized-type patients versus healthy controls ($p < 0.005$ and $p < 0.02$, respectively), but it disappears for the other patients. (2) Considering B lymphocyte values, the difference persists for healthy controls versus drug-free spectrum disorders ($p < 0.01$), undifferentiated ($p < 0.05$) and paranoid ($p < 0.05$) subtypes, but it disappears for disorganized subtype. (3) Considering T helper values, the difference persists comparing healthy controls with drug-treated disorganized subtype ($p < 0.01$), but it disappears in the other groups. (4) The significant differences of T suppressor cells and IgM values between drug-free and drug-treated patients are present again even after the division into subgroups.

We then controlled for any differences, as for sex, age, age of onset, duration of illness, family history, neuropathological findings on CT scans, among our diagnostic subtypes: the only difference we could find was an earlier age of illness onset in the disorganized type versus the other forms of schizophrenia with a p value less than 0.05. Nevertheless, the immunological alterations did not correlate with age of illness onset.

We checked finally for a correlation between immunological parameters and clinical or neuromorphological characteristics by comparing patients with and without immunological values above the mean of control values plus two standard deviations.

We found an increase of obstetric complications of birth in drug-free patients ($p < 0.05$) and an increase of percent deterioration in drug-treated patients ($p < 0.05$) without immunological alterations compared with patients showing immunological alterations.

VIROLOGICAL RESULTS

Results regarding the titration of viral antibodies are reported in Table 2, for each group of subjects as mean OD and standard deviation.

No significant difference could be found between patients and controls with regard to anti-MV and anti-CMV antibodies.

The schizophrenic group showed a significantly ($p < 0.05$) higher value of VZV antibodies compared with the control group. Among schizophrenic patients, the drug-free ones had a mean OD of anti-VZV antibodies higher than that of on-drug ones. In fact, the difference between drug-free patients and healthy controls was statistically significant ($p < 0.02$), while that between patients on drug and controls was not.

Another interesting result was that regarding anti-HSV1 and anti-HSV2 antibodies: drug-free patients showed the lowest levels of antibodies to these two agents. At the statistical analysis, drug-free patients showed antibodies to HSV1 significantly lower ($p < 0.02$) than on-drug patients, which otherwise had the highest mean OD among all groups considered.

With regard to HSV2, the drug-free group had significantly lower titers of antibodies either versus patients on drug ($p < 0.001$) or versus controls ($p < 0.025$).

It is important to underline that schizophrenic patients, when considered as a

Table 2. Viral Antibodies in Schizophrenic Patients and Controls

	Mean OD ± S.D.				
	Measles	HSV 1	HSV 2	VZV	CMV
Controls ($n = 10$)	1.02 ± 0.3	0.7 ± 0.56	0.44 ± 0.27	0.23 ± 0.22	0.65 ± 0.41
All patients ($n = 22$)	1.12 ± 0.3	0.6 ± 0.49	0.34 ± 0.27	0.49 ± 0.33	0.45 ± 0.24
Drug-free ($n = 15$)	1.2 ± 0.4	0.4 ± 0.46	0.21 ± 0.19	0.55 ± 0.32	0.47 ± 0.27
In drugs ($n = 7$)	0.95 ± 0.2	1.0 ± 0.26	0.61 ± 0.20	0.36 ± 0.34	0.42 ± 0.20

VZH $p < 0.05$ all patients versus controls.
HSV1 $p < 0.025$ drug-free versus controls; $p < 0.02$ drug-free versus drug treated.
HSV2 $p < 0.001$ drug-free versus drug-treated.

group, did not show significant differences in anti-HSV1 and anti-HSV2 antibodies versus healthy subjects.

The drug-free patients had significantly lower values of HSV 2 ($p < 0.025$) antibodies and significantly higher values of VZV ($p < 0.02$) antibodies compared with the controls. The drug-free patients differed also from drug-treated patients for lower values of HSV 1 ($p < 0.02$) and HVS 2 ($p < 0.001$) antibodies.

DISCUSSION

Several immunological alterations have been found in schizophrenic patients. To our knowledge, our study presents the largest number of drug-free schizophrenic patients, tested for lymphocyte subsets, with the exception of the recent work by Villemain (Villemain *et al.*, 1989). Mean age of patients is lower and the duration of illness shorter than those of patients referred to in previous studies (DeLisi and Wyatt, 1982; Muller *et al.*, 1987; Ganguli *et al.*, 1987; Kaufmann *et al.*, 1987). No patient had a history of long-term hospitalization and patients with schizophrenic spectrum disorders were included as well.

The four groups of schizophrenic patients—drug-free and drug-treated and schizophrenia and schizophrenic spectrum disorders—are highly matched for sex, age, age of illness onset, family history, and duration of illness; in the drug-free group are 15 patients never treated with neuroleptic drugs and the remaining had a withdrawal period longer than those referred to in the literature.

We found an increase of T total, T suppressor, and B lymphocytes, either as a percentage or as an absolute number of cells per cubic millimeter of blood, in the drug-free schizophrenic group as compared with healthy subjects. Similar results were obtained by DeLisi (DeLisi and Wyatt, 1982) in a group of 38 chronic schizophrenic inpatients, 7 of whom had been free from neuroleptics for at least 1 month.

The T total and T suppressor increase in our study seems to be dependent on disorganized type of schizophrenia.

Patients on drugs differed from healthy controls for higher T-helper lymphocytes, the difference being dependent also in this case on values of disorganized type of schizophrenic patients.

Differences between drug-free and drug-treated schizophrenic patients are present in (1) the distribution of lymphocytes bearing the receptor for OKT8 monoclonal antibody, which detects the T subpopulation with suppressor/cytotoxic function, and in (2) the IgM values. These results are equally distributed in all subtypes of diagnosis and might depend on drug effect. With regard to the latter, our findings are similar to those of Kolyaskina (Kolyaskina *et al.*, 1987), who reported a significant decrease of the T suppressor subpopulation in 53 chronic schizophrenic patients, diagnosed as suffering from malignant form according to the ICD9 and free from drug medication for 3 weeks only.

In agreement with Kolyaskina's hypothesis that psychotropic drugs are responsible for immunological changes, we also found a lower IgM value in drug-treated patients versus drug-free ones.

The report of immunological abnormalities in schizophrenic patients is not new: several earlier published studies found such changes. A difference in the immunological assessment between drug-free and drug-treated schizophrenic patients has never been reported so clearly before.

The neuroleptic drugs either directly or by modulation of neurotransmitter function might be responsible for the immunological alterations present in some drug-treated schizophrenic patients (Ferguson *et al.*, 1978; Ganguli *et al.*, 1987; Kerepcic *et al.*, 1987), but they might also mask an abnormal immunological picture preceding the pharmacological treatment.

The T suppressor/cytotoxic elevation found in the drug-free patients may be linked with a previous or recent infection by some viruses, such as CMV which, as is known, may produce T suppressor elevation lasting for 10 or more months after the clinical outcome of infection (Carney *et al.*, 1981).

Otherwise a T suppressor increase, not checked through *in vitro* functionality tests, could hide a decreased activity of T suppressor/cytotoxic cells, as observed by Muller (Muller *et al.*, 1987) in a population of previously drug-treated schizophrenic patients.

A T suppressor increase could also express the dopamine immunosuppressive activity in those schizophrenic patients with a dopaminergic hyperfunction.

With regard to virological results, it is interesting to note that schizophrenic patients, as a group, did not differ from healthy subjects for herpesvirus effects, contrary to previous reports based on patients mainly treated with neuroleptic drugs (Pogady *et al.*, 1979; Libikova, 1983).

If we compare the results, separating drug-free patients from patients on drug, we can show that the latter have the higher antibody titer.

This observation may suggest that HSV1 and HSV2 are not involved in the early stage of the disease, but that they tend to give infection, reinfection, or reactivation in subsequent times of the disease.

The VZV results are different and very interesting. Drug-free patients had the greatest levels of antibodies against this virus. This finding, new to us, is particularly important because it is emerging in drug-free patients.

VZV is a virus that certainly can produce neuropathological alterations, either acute or subacute, and it may persist latent in the nervous system at the level of the trigeminal ganglion.

REFERENCES

Cappell, R., and Sprecher, S., 1983, Are herpes viruses responsible for neuropsychiatric diseases? in: *Research on the Viral Hypothesis of Mental Disorders* (P. V. Morozov, ed.), Karger, Basel, pp. 168–173.

Carney, W. P., Rubin, R. H., Hoffman, R. A., Hansen, W. P., Healey, K., and Hirsch, M. S., 1981, Analysis of T lymphocyte subsets in cytomegalovirus mononucleosis, *J. Immunol.* **126:**2114–2116.

DeLisi, L. E., and Wyatt, R. J., 1982, Abnormal immune regulation in schizophrenic patients, *Psychopharmacol. Bull.* **18:**158–163.

DeLisi, L. E., Ortaldo, J. R., Maluish, A. E., and Wyatt, R. J., 1983, Deficient natural killer cell (NK) activity and macrophage functioning in schizophrenic patients, *J. Neural Transm.* **58:**96–106.

DeLisi, L. E., King, A. K., and Targum, S., 1984, Serum immunoglobulin concentrations in patients admitted to an acute psychiatric inpatient service, *Br. J. Psychiatry* **145:**661–664.

Ferguson, R. M., Schmidtke, J. R., and Simmons, R. L., 1978, Effects of antipsychotic drugs on in-vitro lymphocyte activation, *Birth Defects* **14:**379–405.

Ferrante, P., Achilli, G., Gerna, G., and Bergamini, F., 1987, Subacute sclerosing panencephalitis: Detection of measles antibody in serum and cerebrospinal fluid by enzyme-linked immunosorbent assay, complement fixation and hemagglutination inhibition, *Microbiologica* **10:**111–118.

Ganguli, R., Rabin, B., Raghu, U., and Ulrich, R. S., 1987, T lymphocytes in schizophrenics and normal and the effects of varying antipsychotic dosage, in: *Viruses, Immunity and Mental Disorders* (E. Kurstak, Z. Lipowski, and P. Morozov, eds.), Plenum Medical, New York, pp. 321–326.

Hirata-Hibi, M., Higashi, S., Tachibana, T., and Watanabe, N., 1982, Stimulated lymphocytes in schizophrenia, *Arch. Gen. Psychiatry* **39:**82–87.

Hofman, F. M., Billing, R. J., Parker, J. W., and Taylor, C. R., 1982, Cytoplasmatic as opposed to surface Ia antigens expressed on human peripheral blood lymphocytes and monocytes, *Clin. Exp. Immunol.* **49:**355–363.

Kaufmann, C. A., DeLisi, L. E., Torrey, E. F., Folstein, S. E., and Smith, W. J., 1987, T lymphocytes subsets and schizophrenia, in: *Viruses, Immunity and Mental Disorders* (E. Kurstak, Z. Lipowski, and P. Morozov, eds.), Plenum Medical, New York, pp. 307–320.

Kerepcic, I., Bamburac, J., and Jurin, M., 1987, Is dopamine related to immunologic changes in schizophrenic patients? *Ann. N.Y. Acad. Sci.* **496:**737–739.

Kolyaskina, G. I., Sekirina, T. P., Zozulya, A. A., Kushner, S. G., Zuzulkovskaya, M. Y., and Abramova, L. I., 1987, Some aspects of immunologic studies in schizophrenia, in: *Viruses, Immunity and Mental Disorders* (E. Kurstak, Z. Lipowski, and P. Morozov, eds.), Plenum Medical, New York, pp. 285–294.

Lehmann-Facius, H., 1937, Uber die liquordiagnose der schizophrenien, *Klin. Wochenschr.* **16:**1646–1648.

Libikova, H., 1983, Schizophrenia and viruses: Principles of etiologic studies, in: *Research on the Viral Hypothesis of Mental Disorders* (P. V. Morozov, ed.), Karger, Basel, pp. 20–51.

Muller, N., Ackenmeil, M., Eckstein, R., Hofschuster, E., and Mempel, W., 1987, Reduced suppressor cell function in psychiatric patients, *Ann. N.Y. Acad. Sci.* **486:**686–689.

Pogady, J., Libikova, H., and Breier, S., 1979, Immunitats-Reaktionen gegen Herpesvirus hominis Typ 1(HSV1) by Psychosen im hoheren Lebensalter, in: *19 Neuropsychiatrisches Symposium, Referate* (G. Grinschgl, ed.), Kuratorium der Neuropsychiatrischen Symposien, Pula, p. 205.

Rimon, R., and Halonen, P., 1969, Herpes simplex virus infection and depressive illness, *Dis. Nerv. Syst.* **30:**338–340.

Sacchetti, E., Vita, A., Calzeroni, A., Invernizzi, G., and Cazzullo, C. L., 1987, Neuromorphological correlates of schizophrenic disorders: Focus on cerebral ventricular enlargement, in: Cazzullo, C. L., Invernizzi, G., Sacchetti, E., and Vita, A. (eds.), *Etiopathogenetic Hypotheses of Schizophrenia*, MTP Press, Lancaster, pp. 67–93.

Synek, V., and Reuben, J. R., 1976, The ventricular brain ratio, using planimetric measurement of EMI scans, *Br. J. Radiol.* **49:**233–237.

Torrey, E. F., Yolken, R. H., and Winfrey, C. J., 1982, Cytomegalovirus antibodies in cerebrospinal fluid of schizophrenic patients detected by enzyme immunoassay, *Science* **216**:892–894.

Vartanian, M. E., Kolyaskina, G. L., Lozovsky, D. V., Burbaeva, G. S., and Ignatov, S. A., 1978, Aspects of humoral and cellular immunity in schizophrenia, *Birth Defects* **18**:339–365.

Villemain, F., Chatenoud, L., Guillbert, E., Pelicier, Y., and Bach, J. F., 1987, Decreased production of interleukin-2 in schizophrenia, *Ann. N.Y. Acad. Sci.* **496**:669–675.

Villemain, F., Chatenoud, L., Galinowski, A., Homo-Delarche, F., Ginestet, D., Loo, H., Zarifian, E., and Bach, J. F., 1989, Aberrant T cell-mediated immunity in untreated schizophrenic patients: Deficient interleukin-2 production, *Am. J. Psychiatry* **146**:609–615.

Vita, A., Sacchetti, E., Calzeroni, A., and Cazzullo, C. L., 1988, Cortical atrophy in schizophrenia: Prevalence and associated features, *Schiz. Res.* **1**:329–337.

Zarrabi, M. N., Zucker, S., Miller, F., Derman, R. M., Romano, G. S., Martinett, Y. A., and Varma, A. O., 1979, Immunologic and coagulation disorders in clorpromazine treated patients, *Ann. Intern. Med.* **91**:194–199.

Chapter 13

Immunological Studies in Schizophrenia

Critical Analysis of Data Obtained

G. Kolyaskina, T. Sekirina, T. Voronkova, T. Micheeva, M. Shchurin, A. Ivanushkin, P. Morozov, and M. Tsutsulkovskaya

INTRODUCTION

This chapter presents the current state of knowledge, the problems and prospects of immunological research into schizophrenia.

The development of immunological research in psychiatry has run parallel to that of immunology, reflecting the methodological and theoretical advances made in the latter field. The 1970s and 1980s have seen a resurgence of activity in this area and the appearance of new centers in which impairment of immunity in schizophrenia is being examined. These matters are being studied at present by experts from Yugoslavia, the United States, France, the Soviet Union, Finland, Canada, and many other countries. It should be emphasized that the active development of immunological research in psychiatry was largely promoted by the

G. Kolyaskina, T. Sekirina, T. Voronkova, T. Micheeva, M. Shchurin, A. Ivanushkin, P. Morozov, and M. Tsutsulkovskaya • *All Union Mental Health Research Center of the USSR Academy of Medical Sciences, 113152 Moscow, USSR.*

Division of Mental Health of WHO which, since 1978, has organized one or two symposia as part of the World Congress of Biological Psychiatry, at which the results of research in that field are discussed. In recent years, three conferences devoted entirely to "Viruses, Immunity and Mental Disorders" were organized with the help of WHO (Louvain, Belgium, 1983; Montreal, Canada, 1984; Mont-Gabriel, Canada, 1988), and the results have been published in two monographs (Morozov, 1983; Kurstak *et al.*, 1987).

Of late, specialists in the immunology of mental illness have been focusing their attention on peripheral blood lymphocytes. Blood tests on schizophrenic patients have revealed unusual quantities of the morphologically altered cells known as atypical lymphocytes (Hirata-Hibi *et al.*, 1982, 1987). Detailed studies have identified them as T lymphocytes and shown that they have unusually high adhesive properties and are spontaneously transformed into lymphoblasts in culture (Kolyaskina, 1967; Liedeman and Prilipko, 1978). Atypical lymphocytes are thymus-dependent, and given their high proportion in schizophrenia, it has been suggested that the process of involution of the thymus which normally occurs in the adult is retarded in those patients; this points to a similarity between the immune system of the schizophrenic patient and that of the child, whose thymus gland is still active and whose peripheral blood also contains a high proportion of atypical lymphocytes (Hirata-Hibi *et al.*, 1987). However, careful study of the population of T lymphocytes in schizophrenic patients has produced completely contradictory results. Some authors (Vartanian *et al.*, 1978; Zarrabi *et al.*, 1979) have found significantly less T lymphocytes in the blood of patients compared to normals.

The reason for the appearance of immunological disturbances in schizophrenia is not known. Some scientists assign a certain role in their development to the lymphotropic activity of viruses, others consider the breakage of the blood–brain barrier to be one of the mechanisms provoking their appearance, and still others find the reason for the development immunopathological reaction in the hereditary deficiency in the functioning of the immunologically competent cells.

However, it is not possible now to explain precisely the appearance of these immunological disturbances and to determine their role and place in the pathogenesis of schizophrenia. The attempts to do so have encountered contradictory results obtained by different authors in the study of the same immunological parameters in schizophrenia. In fact, some authors studying the population of T lymphocytes, for example, have found significantly less T lymphocytes (Vartanian *et al.*, 1978; Zarrabi *et al.*, 1979) in the blood, while others (DeLisi *et al.*, 1982; Ganguli *et al.*, 1987) have found them in higher proportion and the third group (Bessler *et al.*, 1987; Kovaleva *et al.*, 1977) could find no difference whatsoever in this indicator between schizophrenic patients and healthy donors. It is clear that such discrepancies can be attributed to many factors.

This report presents the analysis of some factors which can have an influence on obtained data in the study of immunological peculiarities in schizophrenic patients. We have not attempted to provide an inventory of all of the work in this field, but have concentrated on those factors which we consider vital to the understanding of immunological shifts in schizophrenia.

MATERIAL AND METHODS

A total of 168 patients with different forms of schizophrenia were included in the present study. The number of persons examined in each experiment is showed in the tables. Their age varied between 18 and 55 years. According to clinical characteristics, the patients were distributed into five groups:

1. Malignant form (according to ICD-9 295.10 and 295.20).
2. Paranoid form (according to ICD-9 295.31 and 295.32).
3. Slow-progressive form (according to ICD-9 295.51 and 295.52).
4. Shift-like form (according to ICD-9 295.41 and 295.42).
5. Recurrent form (according to ICD-9 295.70).

In addition, 89 healthy individuals aged between 18 and 48 were included as normal controls for blood cell studies.

Several generally accepted methods were used to describe the quantitative correlations and functional activity of T and B lymphocytes: rosette-forming test, immunofluorescence method using polyclonal and monoclonal antibodies, cultivation of blood lymphocytes under conditions of stimulation by nonspecific mitogens (PHA, Con A, PWM).

RESULTS AND COMMENTS

It is clear that such discrepancies in the data obtained in immunological studies of schizophrenia can be attributed to insufficient differentiation in the clinical description of patients under examination. In our laboratory, for example, the need for a differentiated approach to clinical assessment of patients has been demonstrated in the study of immunity of schizophrenic patients.

It was shown that change in the studied immunological parameters did not occur in all patients and depended on the form of schizophrenia.

The study of T lymphocytes and T-lymphocyte subpopulations (helpers and suppressors) in the total group of schizophrenic patients did not allow detection of any differences between patients and normals. But the analysis of different T-lymphocyte number carried out in two groups of schizophrenic patients—paranoid and slow-progressive schizophrenia—allowed us to demonstrate that there is an increase of T helpers and a decrease of T suppressors in the patients with paranoid schizophrenia and a decrease of T lymphocytes in the patients with slow-progre-

Table 1. T Lymphocytes in Schizophrenia

		Number of			
Group examined	*n*	T3 (OKT3)	T4 (OKT4)	T8 (OKT8)	T4/T8
Schizophrenia (ICD-295)	45	61.86 ± 1.1	38.2 ± 1.2	23.5 ± 0.88	1.8
Paranoid form (ICD-295.31; 295.32)	15	64.99 ± 2.02	45.2 ± 2.24*	18.9 ± 0.99*	2.5*
Slow-progressive form (ICD-295.51; 295.52)	30	60.2 ± 1.83	35.3 ± 1.77	23.98 ± 1.26	1.6
Normals	28	63.34 ± 1.8	39.9 ± 1.47	22.64 ± 1.1	1.83

*p to normals < 0.05.

dient form. Thus, this analysis showed the need for a differentiated approach to clinical assessment of schizophrenic patients (Table 1).

The same situation was found in the study of interleukin 2 (IL-2) production in the blood lymphocyte cultures of patients with different forms of schizophrenia and healthy donors (Table 2). It can be seen that there is no difference in IL-2 production between the total group of schizophrenic patients and normals. But detailed clinical and immunological analysis after distribution of the schizophrenic patients into four groups according to their form of disease showed the following.

IL-2 production was decreased in the patients with recurrent, shiftlike, and slow-progressive forms of schizophrenia compared to normals. The patients with paranoid form had a tendency to increase IL-2 production compared to normals.

It is not possible presently to explain the above-mentioned data on IL-2

Table 2. Interleukin 2 (IL-2) Production in Schizophrenia

Group examined	*n*	Il-2 (U/ml)
Schizophrenia (ICD-295)	52	1.20 ± 0.13
Paranoid form (ICD-295.31; 295.32)	12	2.06 ± 0.38
Slow-progressive form (ICD-295.51; 295.52)	22	1.14 ± 0.16*
Shift-like form (ICD-295.42; 295.41)	10	0.86 ± 0.25**
Recurrent form (ICD-295.7)	8	0.53 ± 0.19**
Normals	57	1.63 ± 0.23

*p to normals < 0.05
**p to normals < 0.001

production in the patients with different forms of schizophrenia. But it is possible to suppose that the changed IL-2 production in some forms of schizophrenia is the result of several factors—the number of cell-producers, the difference in their activity, the level of mediator utilization, and others—which can be different in different forms of disease.

An application of the immunofluorescence technique demonstrated that the proportion of B lymphocytes in schizophrenic patients significantly increased in peripheral blood compared to that of normal subjects (Table 3). The same situation was found in the patients with different forms of schizophrenia. Perhaps such homogeneous results obtained for all schizophrenic patients are the explanation for agreement of different authors studying this immunological parameter in schizophrenia.

Studies on the ability of B lymphocytes to produce immunoglobulins demonstrated (Table 4) that the functional activity of these cells in schizophrenia was increased. In this case the number of B cells in peripheral blood of schizophrenic patients markedly increased in parallel with accumulation of cytoplasmic immunoglobulins. This phenomenon persisted when lymphocytes in culture were incubated for 7 days with a polyclonal B-cell mitogen (PWM) known to cause differentiation of B cells and to induce immunoglobulin synthesis in them. The number of immunoglobulin-synthesizing cells in PWM-stimulated blood lymphocytes in culture rose markedly, being statistically significantly higher in schizophrenics than normal subjects.

These results indicate that the observed reduction of suppressor T lymphocytes in schizophrenia is concomitant with hyperactivation of the B system of immunity. Similar changes in the immune system are often due to the development

Table 3. B Lymphocytes in Schizophrenia

Group examined	n	Number of B lymphocytes by OKT7	sIg$^+$
Schizophrenia (ICD-295)	68	17.39 ± 0.58*	19.51 ± 0.54
Paranoid form (ICD-295.31; 295.32)	15	18.08 ± 1.17*	21.04 ± 1.08*
Slow-progressive form (ICD-295.51; 295.52)	29	15.62 ± 0.75*	17.8 ± 0.77*
Shiftlike form (ICD-295.42; 295.41)	12	18.59 ± 1.6*	22.25 ± 1.75*
Recurrent form (ICD-295.7)	12	18.57 ± 1.29*	20.0 ± 1.34*
Normals	57	13.36 ± 1.06	14.4 ± 0.86

*p to normals < 0.001

Table 4. Number of Immunoglobulin-Synthesizing Cells

		PWM stimulation				
		Before	After			
	n	cΣIg	cΣIg	cIgA	cIgG	cIgM
Schizophrenic patients	16	0.4 ± 0.06*	4.4 ± 0.06*	1.56 ± 0.3	2.67 ± 0.5*	0.9 ± 0.15
Normals	19	0.2 ± 0.05	2.6 ± 0.4	1.3 ± 0.1	1.47 ± 0.2	1.0 ± 0.2

*p to normals < 0.05

of autoimmune disorders or diseases whose pathogenesis is aggravated by an autoimmune component; therefore the above results can be regarded as additional evidence of the interrelationship between schizophrenia and autoimmune diseases.

It is not possible to check any of the theories of the disease course without having reliable and adequate scales for evaluating the clinical data. The patients' biological indicators can be compared only when the same approach to the assessment of their clinical state is used.

The interest of psychiatrists in the classification and diagnosis of mental disorders has considerably increased in recent years. This progress is associated with the progress in the field of psychiatric epidemiology and biological psychiatry, where further advance is possible only if improved and uniform diagnostic approaches are used. While it is evident that the traditional diagnostic classifications are very useful in many other respects (mainly for statistical purposes), they do not give the complete story about the state of a particular patient.

The WHO has done a tremendous amount of work in developing uniform approaches toward the clinical evaluation of patients within the framework of the multinational and multilateral projects. A complicated mechanism of the multicenter studies in biological psychiatry, and particularly in mental disease immunology, has been worked out and tested in practice over the last 15 years. The correct choice of clinical assessment scales, the comprehensive training of clinicians, the organization of international courses for teaching the scales using videotechnology and computerized statistical analysis of the results, enabled professionals from many countries to obtain highly reliable data. A certain consensus reached by the representatives of 26 WHO collaborative centers on using uniform methods contributed considerably to this success. The significance of this consensus cannot be overestimated, for despite a great number of already existing scales and questionnaires, many researchers created new devices instead of using and testing the already known methods. At a certain point the method requiring the use of scales and based on the principle of international communication, became a menace to carrying out the international comparative research. Bech *et al.* (1984)

and Morozov (1985) came out with the following set of scales, used both as criteria for including a patient in the study and as indices for evaluating the treatment results.

The above-mentioned scales were used primarily for studying inpatients. Neither personal scales nor social adjustment scales were used in the WHO programs on biological psychiatry. The majority of scales were translated into several languages, including English, French, Russian, German, Spanish, and Japanese. It is important to use the internationally known scales in biological psychiatry. However, these scales need to be checked locally by training the specialists before engaging them in the research.

One more factor which can have an influence on the immunological data in the study of schizophrenic patients is psychotropic drugs.

Problems connected with the immunomodulation by psychotropic preparations must always be approached with special care since long-term consumption of such preparations in high doses can cause a whole range of alterations in the humoral and cellular immunity of schizophrenic patients. It is known that neuroleptics can reduce the blood serum concentration of IgM and the quantity of T lymphocytes, give rise to atypical lymphocytes, modify the proliferation of T lymphocytes under the influence of mitogens, and reduce or increase capping when blood lymphocytes are stimulated with Con A. It is also possible that these indicators will not return to normal when use of neuroleptics on the patient is discontinued, which testifies to the involvement of other mechanisms in immunological impairment in schizophrenia. In such cases the delayed effects of neuroleptics must also be taken into account, since they can appear long after the patient has stopped taking the preparation.

We studied the psychotropic drug effect on the number of T suppressors and antithymic immunoglobulins IgG and IgM in the patients with a malignant form of schizophrenia (Fig. 1). These results were obtained in the study of schizophrenic patients who were examined three times—when they were treated with psychotropic drugs more than a year; free of any medication for at least 3 weeks; and treated again with psychotropic drugs for 3 weeks. It was demonstrated that prolonged psychotropic drug therapy decreased significantly the number of T suppressors in the patients. Their number was partly restored in the same patients free of any medication for 3 weeks. The number of these cells decreased again when the psychotropic drug treatment was renewed for 3 weeks. It was demonstrated also that the antithymic IgG level ranged considerably and depended highly on the moment at which a patient was investigated. This level was very high in patients who were under psychotropic treatment for a long time; it became distinctly lower in untreated patients and appeared to be high again when the treatment resumed. The range of antithymic IgM was less significant, though the tendency shown by antithymic IgG remained: the level of antithymic IgM was higher in patients under treatment and lower when they became free of medication.

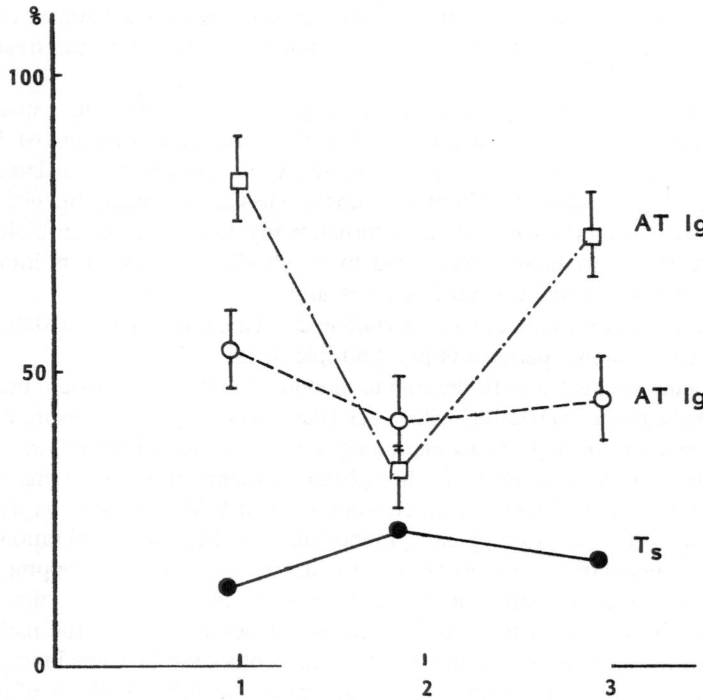

Figure 1. Suppressor T lymphocytes (T_s), antithymic IgG (AT IgG), and antithymic IgM (AT IgM) in schizophrenic patients during therapy with psychotropic drugs. 1, psychotropic drug therapy for more than a year; 2, no therapy; 3, psychotropic drug therapy for 3 weeks.

The interpretation of obtained data depends not only on the form of schizophrenia or psychotropic drug treatment but also on the method used for the study of immunological parameters in patients.

The functional activity of T lymphocytes in schizophrenia as evinced by proliferative activity level in response to stimulation by mitogen, is variously assessed by different authors, as is the case with most other immunological parameters. Some researchers find no change in this indicator among schizophrenic patients (Surman *et al.*, 1986) while others find a higher (Kronfol *et al.*, 1983) or lower (Kronfol *et al.*, 1984; Vartanian *et al.*, 1978) functional activity in such patients.

There are at least two causes for the contradictions in these data. The first concerns the enormous individual fluctuations of the lymphocyte response to mitogens (see Fig. 2). The second relates to the dose-dependent mitogen effect (Fig. 3) (Pivovarova and Kolyaskina, 1980). The dependence of the lymphocyte

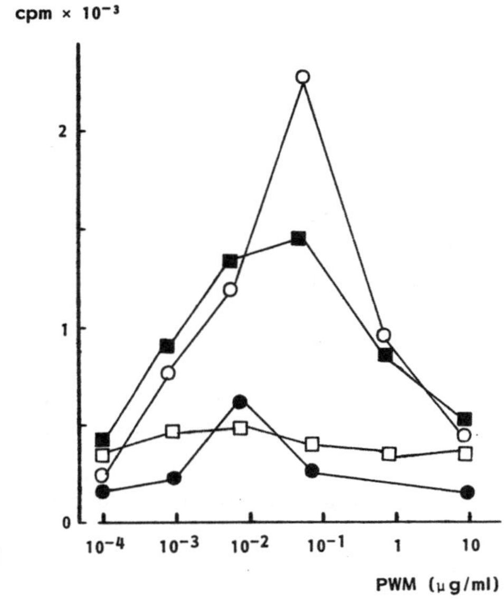

Figure 2. Individual variation of blood lymphocyte mitogen response in normals.

response on mitogen dose used in experiments was found in the study of the functional activity of lymphocytes in cultures with each mitogen used: PHA, Con A, PWM. It is important to stress that the difference between schizophrenic patients and healthy donors may be found only when using certain doses while at other doses the lymphocyte response will be similar in patients and normals. To understand the actual situation in the response of lymphocytes to mitogens in schizophrenia, it is very important to use four or five doses of mitogen in each experiment.

Finally, the results may depend on the method used to produce them. It is well known that the indicator which shows the relative proportions of different T lymphocytes changes considerably in accordance with the method employed. We demonstrated that the difference between the schizophrenic patients as a group and normals which was found by rosette-forming test disappears when these cells are studied by immunofluorescence using monoclonal antibodies to surface markers of these cells (Table 5). In view of the above, it would be preferable for clinical studies of proportions of T-lymphocyte subpopulations to consider fluctuations of the indicator in an individual patient during different periods (or ranges) of disease, rather than conducting an analysis based on comparisons of average proportions in groups of sick and healthy people.

Moreover, there are many unanswered theoretical questions in clinical immunology. It is known that the number of T lymphocytes with different functional

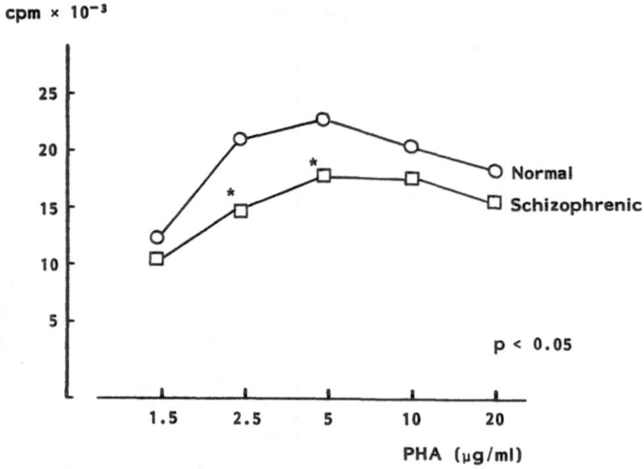

Figure 3. PHA response of blood lymphocytes in schizophrenia.

ability can be tested by rosette-forming test, by theophylline-sensitivity test, and by immunofluorescence using monoclonal antibodies to surface structures on lymphocytes. All of these tests are based on the determination of unique surface structures on lymphocytes with different functional activity. However, there are many theoretical aspects in fundamental immunology which have been worked out insufficiently at present and this sometimes does not allow precise determination of

Table 5. T Lymphocytes in Shizophrenia Tested by Different Methods

		Number of			
		T lymphocytes		T suppressors	
	n	E rosettes	OKT3	E rosettes	OKT8
Schizophrenia (ICD-295)	86	56.1 ± 0.8	61.86 ± 1.1	17.6 ± 0.4*	23.5 ± 0.83
Maligant and paranoid forms (ICD-295.00; 295.10; 295.20; 295.31; 295.32)	35	57.64 ± 0.97	64.99 ± 2.02	18.04 ± 0.46*	18.9 ± 0.99*
Slow progressive form (ICD-295.51; 295.52)	51	51.3 ± 0.97*	60.2 ± 1.83	16.24 ± 0.61*	23.99 ± 1.26
Normals	73	56.5 ± 0.05	63.34 ± 1.89	21.03 ± 0.02	22.64 ± 1.1

*p to normals < 0.05

the affiliation of cells tested to subpopulations. Moreover, the careful studies allowed the demonstration that the surface marker expression on the lymphocytes is not stable and can change in the process of immune response. As a result, the disturbance between phenotype and function of the cell appears. Therefore, use of any of the above methods gives only a general impression about the number of lymphocytes with different function.

There are many other factors which can affect the results in a study of immunological parameters in patients; e.g., their age, sex, biological rhythms, stress factors, and others.

Summing up the above, it is important to stress that to understand the real situation in the study of immunity in schizophrenia it is necessary to consider all of the mentioned factors; in connection with this expedient, to unite the efforts of scientists of different countries who worked out this problem and created the collaborative program. It will help to collect enough material over a shorter period, use various tests for the study of immunity in schizophrenia and produce new data. Moreover, such collaboration will help to standardize both the method for testing of immunological parameters and the clinical assessment scales for patients under examination.

REFERENCES

Bech, P., Gastpar, M., and Morozov, P., 1984, Clinical assessment scale for biological psychiatry to be used in WHO studies, *Prog. Neuropsychopharmacol. Biol. Psychiatry* **1:**190–197.

Bessler, H., Eviator, J., Meshulam, M., Tyano, S., Djaldetti, M., and Sirota, P., 1987, Theophylline-sensitive T-lymphocyte subpopulation in schizophrenic patients, *Biol. Psychiatry* **22:**1025–1028.

DeLisi, L., Goodman, S., Neckers, L., and Wyatt, R., 1982, An analysis of lymphocyte subpopulations in schizophrenic patients, *Biol. Psychiatry* **17:**1003–1007.

Ganguli, R., Rabin, B., Raghu, U., and Ulrich, R., 1987, T-lymphocytes in schizophrenics and normals and the effects of varying antipsychotic dosage, in: *Viruses, Immunity and Mental Disorders* (E. Kurstak, Z. Lipowski, and P. Morozov, eds.), Plenum Medical, New York, pp. 321–326.

Hirata-Hibi, M., Higashi, S., Tachibana, T., and Watanabe, W., 1982, Stimulated lymphocytes in schizophrenia, *Arch. Gen. Psychiatry* **39:**82–87.

Hirata-Hibi, M., Miyauchi, K., and Tachibana, T., 1987, Evidence of lymphocyte abnormality in schizophrenia, in: *Viruses, Immunity and Mental Disorders* (E. Kurstak, Z. Lipowski, and P. Morozov, eds.), Plenum Medical, New York, pp. 327–341.

Kolyaskina, G., 1967, The study of sensitivity of schizophrenic patients by the method of lymphocyte cultivation, *Korsakoff J. Neuropathol. Psychiatry USSR* **2:**284–288.

Kovaleva, E., Bonarcev, P., and Prilipko, L., 1977, Lymphocyte reaction in schizophrenic patients to the phytomitogens: phytohemagglutinin and concanavalin A, *Bull. Exp. Biol. Med. (USSR)* **84:** 182–185.

Kronfol, Z., Silva, J., Greden, J., Dembinski, I., Gardner, R., and Carroll, B. I., 1983, Impaired lymphocyte function in depressive illness, *Life Sci.* **33:**241–247.

Kronfol, Z., Turner, R., Nasrallah, H., and Winokur, G., 1984, Leucocyte regulation in depression and schizophrenia, *Psychiatr. Res.* **13:**13–18.

Kurstak, E., Lipowski, Z., and Morozov, P. (eds.), 1987, *Viruses, Immunity and Mental Disorders*, Plenum Medical, New York.
Liedeman, R., and Prilipko, L., 1978, The behavior of T lymphocytes in schizophrenia, in: *Neurochemical and Immunological Components in Schizophrenia* (D. Bergsma and A. Goldstein, eds.), Liss, New York, pp. 365–377.
Morozov, P. (ed.), 1983, *Research on the Viral Hypothesis of Mental Disorders*, Karger, Basel.
Morozov, P., 1985, Training models in biological psychiatry and psychopharmacology: WHO experience, *Prog. Neuropsychopharmacol. Biol. Psychiatry* **3**:334–340.
Pivovarova, A., and Kolyaskina, G., 1980, The different phytohemagglutinin doses action on the blood lymphocyte proliferation in schizophrenia, *Bull. Exp. Biol. Med. (USSR)* **11**:552–554.
Surman, O., Williams, J., Sheehan, D., Strom, T., Jones, K., and Coleman, J., 1986, Immunological response to stress in agoraphobia and panic attacks, *Biol. Psychiatry* **21**:768–774.
Vartanian, M., Kolyaskina, G., Lozovsky, D., Burbaeva, G., and Ignatov, S., 1978, Aspects of humoral and cellular immunity in schizophrenia, in: *Neurochemical and Immunological Components in Schizophrenia* (D. Bergsma and A. Goldstein, eds.), Liss, New York, pp. 339–364.
Zarrabi, M., Zuker, S., Miller, F., Derman, R., Romano, G., Hartnett, I., Varma, A., 1979, Immunologic and coagulation disorders in chlorpromazine treated patients, *Ann. Intern. Med.* **91**: 194–199.

Chapter **14**

Diagnostic Criteria for Selection of Schizophrenic Patients in the Study of Biological Markers

J. Pogády, J. Rajčáni, D. Martišová, and J. Krajčík

During the last few years, there has been progress into the biological markers of mental diseases, especially in the field of neurochemistry, in spite of the fact that the multifactorial origin and mechanisms of the development of mental disease are not sufficiently understood. That is why, despite unknown etiology and pathogenesis, research into biological markers has great importance not only for diagnostics but also for a better assessment of developmental dynamics and perhaps for enlightenment of up-to-now unknown etiologic and pathogenetic mechanisms of schizophrenia. In this selection, with exactly determined criteria, we try to exclude the possibility of a faulty diagnosis and to eliminate or to reduce subjectivity of evaluation, applied in psychiatric diagnostics in spite of the above-mentioned facts.

According to our point of view, there is a necessity to take advantage of multilevel, widely drawn, and more exact diagnostics. At present this is done at four levels, i.e., symptoms, syndrome, nosologic or nosographic unit diagnosis, confronted with an existing structure of personality. For personality structure diagnosis we use a general theoretic contribution of personality conception of Royce and Powell (1981, 1983) along with our conception of exact personality

---

J. Pogády, J. Rajčáni, D. Martišová, and J. Krajčík • *Regional Psychiatry Hospital, Pezinok, Czechoslovakia.*

structure diagnostics through Thorne's (1965, 1966) integration level test series (ILTS). This is the only way to improve the classic, phenomenologic, psychopathologic diagnostics of schizophrenia.

In addition, we apply the above-mentioned diagnostic method for comparison with schizophrenia diagnostics by means of DSM III and ICD X. This method enables us to eliminate any mistakes related to a four-level, classic, phenomenologic, psychopathologic diagnostics of schizophrenia.

The further diagnostic exactness mainly in the diagnostics of symptoms and syndromes allows us to prepare their functional psychopathologic analysis. The functional analysis is indicated if some principal doubts appear about symptom classification or if we want to penetrate deeper into their substance under the given conditions. The main task is always to determine functions, affected by a given psychopathologic symptom or state. We cannot be limited by a description of determinable symptoms; we have to concentrate on an absence of such symptoms under normal conditions, too. The principles of functional analyses are successfully illustrated by defects of perception, consciousness, depersonalization, transformation, and mainly various forms of delusions. In connection with the functional psychopathologic analysis, it is acceptable to analyze the so-called primary or secondary symptoms of schizophrenia, arising from various psychopathologic diagnostic schools, e.g., Bleuler (1983), Schneider (1976), and others. In differentiated diagnostics of depressions, our own expert system of endogenous and organic psychosis is used in our hospital. It agrees well with our project of a computerized information system in the psychiatric department.

The term of pathochemical markers, both neurochemical and neuroendocrine, has been analyzed in special monographs (Beckmann and Riederer, 1985). The diagnostics of the importance of biologic markers in schizophrenia, mainly neurochemical, immunologic, genetic, molecular-biologic, physicochemical, molecular-pharmacologic, neurophysiologic ones, are at present considerably limited, especially for the low specificity even at a given reproducibility of separate markers in various psychopathologic states. Pathomorphologic markers, aberration of protein metabolism, proteases, amino acids, lipids, membranous endogenous toxins, pathologic immune response to viral and bacterial antigens, and also neurohormonal markers are similarly less specific and less helpful in the diagnostics of schizophrenia. When simultaneously evaluating the results by means of a multidimensional scale for separate biologic markers, their diagnostic value increases with the assumption that the contemporary presence of biological markers can be proved in a larger number of subjects.

Two-dimensional representation of 44 subjects for 17 CSF biochemical parameters was obtained by multidimensional scaling (MDS). The normative region, defined by the 15/16 convex hull of a control group, is quite compact and does not contain a single schizophrenic subject. There is one subject of the control group lying amidst schizophrenic subjects.

With only one exception, all untreated schizophrenic patients are close together, separated from the normative region with respect to dimension 2. The group of schizophrenics and neuroleptics, on the other hand, is on average more distant from the normative region and shows a very wide scattering, indicating a substantial heterogeneity with regard to CSF parameters. The results indicate that a biological heterogeneity between schizophrenic and nonschizophrenic subjects can be detected by a simultaneous analysis of the CSF concentrations of substances related directly or indirectly to the neuronal activity of the brain (W. F. Gattaz *et al.*, 1985).

The multidimensional approach can ensure a significant strategy in a further study of schizophrenia and search for biological markers, resp. biological substance of schizophrenia and its possible viral etiology and by pathogenesis conditioned dependence.

Computers are successfully used for multifactorial research into the disease state and its evaluation. A system of data collection in three stages has been implemented in our hospital as a framework of a complete information system in the psychiatric clinic.

Stage 1 is a formalized determination of the patient's state. First, the physician examines the patient according to the CPRS questionnaire (*Cs. Psychiatrie* No. 6/80). The examined severity score of separate symptoms is then put into the computer. There are complete data in databases concerning the questionnaire and so a further processing of data obtained is possible, e.g., retrieving the state of the patient in a verbal form.

The examination of personality structure is done by a set of tests, the patient responding on a sheet of paper or directly via videoterminal with keyboard. The results of the tests are compared with the symptoms found and with anamnestic data by a psychiatrist, thus contributing to a more exactly established diagnosis and therapy.

Examination of a patient's anamnesis is also substantially computerized. The necessity of automation derives from the need to reduce individually the basic set of anamnestic questions (up to 800) for a single patient due to his or her basic data and due to already obtained information for which many of the questions become irrelevant. Presently, it is secured that no important information escapes the physician's attention. Besides formalized, diagnostic selection of the patients, there are some unexpected or rare clinical facts and observations for assessing, sometimes necessary to express in a form of nonformalized free text. The data formalization makes possible a problemless, mass statistic processing of results.

The computer (SM 4-20) is used for a computerized examination, computer diagnostics, and statistic processing with an operation system (DIAMS-2) being suitable for interactive work with text data. This multiusable system provides the possibility to serve simultaneously up to several tens of various tasks represented mainly by a user working with a videoterminal.

A comprehensive multilevel simultaneous evaluation of various signs and symptoms creates the opportunity to formulate a substantially more exact diagnosis of major psychosis such as schizophrenia, manic-depressive, endogenous or exogenous psychosis.

REFERENCES

Beckmann, H., and Riederer, P., 1985, *Pathochemical Markers in Major Psychoses*, Springer-Verlag, Berlin.

Bleuler, E., 1983, *Lehrbuch der Psychiatrie*, Springer-Verlag, Berlin.

Pogády, J., and Guensberger, E., 1987, *Základy psycholatológie*, Martin, Osveta [in Slovak] English review, pp. 13–78.

Pogády, J., and Nociar, A., 1986, *Osobnosť a choroba*, Veda, Bratislava [in Slovak] English review, pp. 150–180.

Royce, J. R., and Powell, A., 1981, An overview of a multifactor-system theory of personality and individual differences. II. System dynamics and person–situation interactions, *J. Pers. Soc. Psychol.* **41**:1019–1030.

Royce, J. R., and Powell, A., 1983, Individuality and pluralistic images of the nature of man. Impact of science on society, *J. Pers. Soc. Psychol.* **2**:211–223.

Schneider, K., 1976, *Klinische Psychopathologie*, Thieme, Stuttgart.

Thorne, F. C., 1965, *The Integration Level Test Series: Research Edition*, Clinical Psychology Publishing Company, Brandon, VT.

Thorne, F. C., 1966, Theory of the psychological state, *J. Clin. Psychol.* **22**:127–137.

Gattaz, W. F., Gasses, T., and Beckmann, H., 1985, *CSF Studies in Schizophrenia: A Multidimensional Approach*, Springer-Verlag, Berlin, pp. 144–153.

Part **III**

Immunomodulators and Psychiatric Disorders

Chapter 15

Interferon in Schizophrenia

Daniel Becker, Eli Kritschmann, Susy Floru, Yaffa Shlomo-David, and Tamar Gotlieb-Stematsky

INTRODUCTION

The association of schizophrenia and viral infection and/or immune dysfunction was considered and critically summarized by DeLisi and Crow (1986).

Viral infections involving sometimes the central nervous system (CNS) (Raymond and Williams, 1948; Shearer and Finch, 1964; Gotlieb-Stematsky and Arlozoroff, 1976) and recently AIDS (Faulstich, 1987) may present symptoms resembling psychosis or schizophrenia-like disorders.

Epidemiologic observations indicated a seasonal and geographic distribution in the birthrates of schizophrenics, which were explained in terms of a viral etiology (DeLisi and Crow, 1986). Controlled studies have examined the presence of viral antibodies in the serum and spinal fluid (CSF) of schizophrenic patients (Lycke *et al.*, 1974; Albrecht *et al.*, 1980; Gotlieb-Stematsky *et al.*, 1981).

Contradictory findings on a wide spectrum of antibodies to neurotropic viruses led to the search for a nonspecific indicator of viral infection such as interferon (IFN). Raised levels of IFN were demonstrated in schizophrenic patients (Libikova *et al.*, 1979; Preble and Torrey, 1985), although others failed to confirm these results (Rimón *et al.*, 1985; Ahokas *et al.*, 1987).

Daniel Becker, Eli Kritschmann, Susy Floru, Yaffa Shlomo-David, and Tamar Gotlieb-Stematsky • *Department of Psychiatry and The Central Virology Laboratory, Chaim Sheba Medical Center, Tel-Aviv University, Sackler School of Medicine, Tel-Hashomer 52621, Israel.*

RESULTS

In order to eliminate factors such as aging, neuroleptic treatment, or hospitalization, which may modify the immune response, we conducted a study on IFN levels in sera of young adults at their first episode of acute psychotic attack before hospitalization, and before treatment.

The study group included 34 young adults admitted on their first psychotic attack before medication. Clinical diagnosis on the spectrum of schizophrenia was based on RDC and DSM-III. Blood samples were drawn on the same day from patients and 24 age- and sex-matched healthy controls. IFN assay was based on a dye-binding semi-microassay (Negreanu *et al.*, 1983). IFN titers $\geqslant 25$ international units per milliliter (IU/ml) were considered positive.

The results were analyzed by χ^2 test and t test, employing mean and median values.

Table 1 shows the characteristics of the research groups, which represented five diagnostic categories.

The groups were first compared according to the sampling, in which IFN levels were 25 IU/ml or over. No significant difference ($p > 0.20$) was observed between the group of brief psychotic episode (group A) versus prolonged psychosis (groups B and C).

The groups were analyzed for IFN level per group mean titers (Table 2) and no differences were found between the psychotic and nonpsychotic groups (A, B, C versus D, E) or between the brief psychotic episode group (A) versus the second (B) and third (C) schizophrenic groups combined.

DISCUSSION

Our results are similar to those obtained by Ahokas *et al.* (1987) and Rimón *et al.* (1985) who found no significant differences in the level of IFN in the serum of

Table 1. Research Groups

	No. of patients	Sex	
		M	F
Psychotic groups	34	20	14
A. Brief psychotic episode	9	5	4
B. Schizophreniform disorder	15	9	6
C. Schizophenia	10	6	4
Controls	24	13	11
D. Personality disorder	4	2	2
E. Nonpsychotic patients	20	11	9

Table 2. Comparison of Mean Values of Serum IFN in Psychotic (A, B, C) versus Control Groups (D, E) and in Brief Psychotic Episode (A) versus Prolonged Psychosis (B, C)

	A + B + C	D + E	*p*
Mean titers of IFN (IU/ml)	14.97 ± 27.7	21.06 ± 32.3	⩾ 0.457
	A	B + C	*p*
	22.56 ± 35.1	12.24 ± 24.4	⩾ 0.445

The large S.D. are attributed to the method that considers IFN levels below 3.125 as 0.

acute psychiatric patients as compared to nonpsychiatric patients. Their studies were conducted on "functional" psychiatric disorders, and not only on schizophrenic patients as tested in our study.

Preble and Torrey (1985) reported raised IFN levels in the serum of 24% of a group of 82 schizophrenics, as against 3% in a control group, and it was suggested that there were abnormalities of the immune system or viral infections in some of these patients who were treated with neuroleptic drugs, which may have affected their immune response.

Our study is characterized by selection of young adult patients at their initial attack before drug treatment and before hospitalization.

The comparison between groups was done on the assumption that group A (brief psychotic episode) differs from the others by the acuteness of symptoms and the course of disease that may have indicated viral infection rather than a course of slow insidious schizophrenia. However, no differences were found when this group was segregated from the other two prolonged psychotic groups.

Although our study yielded negative results as for the presence of IFN in sera of psychotic patients, it seemed worthwhile to present these results which may contribute to the controversy regarding possible viral etiology in schizophrenia. We also stress the importance of selection of acute psychotic patients and conducting simultaneous testing with matched controls. The causes of research discrepancies regarding the presence of IFN in sera of psychotic patients could have been age, drug treatment, length of hospitalization, research methodologies, and diagnostic modalities.

Our results suggest further research on carefully grouped psychotic patients with defined specific characteristics and evaluation of a variety of immunologic and virologic parameters.

Acknowledgments We thank Mrs. M. Modan and Mrs. A. Lusky of the Department of Clinical Epidemiology, Ch. Sheba Medical Center, for statistical evaluation.

REFERENCES

Ahokas, A., Rimón, R., Koskiniemi, M., Vaheri, A., Julkunen, I., and Sarna, S., 1987, Viral antibodies and interferon in acute psychiatric disorders, *J. Clin. Psychiatry* **48:**194–196.

Albrecht, P., Torrey, E. F., Boone, E., Hicks, J. T., and Daniel, N., 1980, Raised cytomegalovirus antibody level in cerebrospinal fluid of schizophrenic patients, *Lancet* **2:**769–772.

DeLisi, L. E., and Crow, I. J., 1986, Is schizophrenia a viral or immunologic disorder? *Psychiatr. Clin. North Am.* **9:**115–132.

Faulstich, M. E., 1987, Psychiatric aspects of AIDS, *Am. J. Psychiatry* **144:**551–556.

Gotlieb-Stematsky, T., and Arlozoroff, A., 1976, EBV in neurological disease, *J. Neurol. Sci.* **28:** 115–120.

Gotlieb-Stematsky, T., Zonis, J., Arlozoroff, A., Mozes, T., Sigal, M., and Szekeley, A. G., 1981, Antibodies to Epstein–Barr virus, herpes simplex type 1, cytomegalovirus and measles virus in psychiatric patients, *Arch. Virol.* **67:**333–339.

Libikova, H., Breier, S., and Kocisove, M., 1979, Assay of interferon and viral antibodies in the cerebrospinal fluid in clinical neurology and psychiatry, *Acta Biol. Med. Germ.* **38:**879–893.

Lycke, E., Norrby, R., and Rosse, B. E., 1974, A serological study on mentally ill patients with particular reference to the prevalence of herpes virus infections, *Br. J. Psychiatry* **124:**273–279.

Negreanu, J., Shif, I., and Gotlieb-Stematsky, T., 1983, Interferon assay in patients suspected of viral infections as a tool for rapid diagnosis, *Arch. Virol.* **78:**103–107.

Preble, O. T., and Torrey, E. F., 1985, Serum interferon in patient with psychosis, *Am. J. Psychiatry* **142:**1184–1186.

Raymond, R., and Williams, R., 1948, Infectious mononucleosis with psychosis, *N. Engl. J. Med.* **239:**542–544.

Rimón, R., Ahokas, A., Hintikka, J., and Meikkila, L., 1985, Serum interferon in schizophrenia, *Ann. Clin. Res.* **17:**139–140.

Shearer, M. L., and Finch, S. M., 1964, Periodic organic psychosis associated with recurrent herpes simplex, *N. Engl. J. Med.* **271:**494–497.

Chapter **16**

Interferon Production in Acute Psychiatric Disorders

Heikki Katila, Ranan Rimón, Kari Cantell, Björn Appelberg, and Heikki Nikkilä

INTRODUCTION

Interferons (IFNs) have marked antiviral, cytostatic, and immunomodulatory activities and represent potent modulators of several cell membrane functions including regulation of the excitability of neurons (De Maeyer and De Maeyer-Guignard, 1988). Changes in the production of these mediators may result in disturbed function of immune responses as well as neuronal transmission mechanisms.

Various stresses have been found to affect IFN production. Solomon *et al.* (1967) found enhancement of IFN production in electric shock-stressed mice. On the other hand, Chang and Rasmussen (1965) and Jensen (1968) reported stress-induced transitory suppression of IFN production in mice. In humans, Palmblad *et al.* (1974, 1976) showed that stress exposure and sleep deprivation increased lymphocyte IFN production. Contrarily, Pavlidis and Chirigos (1980) maintained that acute short-term stress may reduce IFN-related immune functions. Glaser *et al.* (1986) demonstrated a significant decrease of IFN production by Con A-stimulated leukocytes from students stressed by their examinations when compared to baseline values obtained 6 weeks earlier.

Heikki Katila, Ranan Rimón, Björn Appelberg, and Heikki Nikkilä • *Department of Psychiatry, University of Helsinki, SF-00180 Helsinki, Finland.* Kari Cantell • *National Public Health Institute, Helsinki, Finland.*

In psychiatric disorders, IFN production has so far been studied only in schizophrenia. Based on three recent studies it seems evident that schizophrenic patients are poorer producers of both IFN-α and -γ than healthy controls (Moises *et al.*, 1985; Inglot *et al.*, personal communication 1988; Katila *et al.*, 1989).

The aim of the present study was to elucidate the IFN production by leukocytes from psychiatric patients other than schizophrenics.

PATIENTS AND METHODS

Patients

The series consisted of 34 (16 f, 18 m; age 16–63, mean 32.4) consecutive non-schizophrenic patients admitted acutely to the Department of Psychiatry, University of Helsinki, Helsinki, Finland. For each patient an age- and sex-matched healthy control from the hospital staff was selected (age 19–51, mean 32.6).

The diagnoses were made applying the DSM-III diagnostic criteria. Thirteen (8 f, 5 m; age 18–63, mean 35.9) patients met the criteria for paranoid or other brief reactive psychosis. For 9 of these psychotic patients this was the first admission to a psychiatric hospital and none of them had received antipsychotic drug treatment prior to hospital admission. The remaining 4 reentry patients in this group all had 1–12 (mean 4.7) weeks of washout prior to the first blood sampling. The mean duration of illness for these patients was 11.9 (range 2–48) weeks. For 12 of these patients a second blood sample was drawn following 5 to 6 weeks of treatment. Of the remaining 21 patients (8 f, 13 m; age 16–59, mean 30.2), 15 were diagnosed as suffering from affective disorder and 6 from borderline disturbances. For 12 of these nonpsychotic patients, this was their first admission to a psychiatric hospital and 4 of them had never been on psychotropic medication. For patients on psychoactive substances, a washout period (mean 3.6 weeks) was applied prior to the first blood sampling. Due to the relatively short hospital stay of the patients, a second blood sample was drawn only from 3 patients (results not reported in this study). Informed consent for the research procedure was given by all patients.

Procedure

Paired blood samples (15 ml) from both patients and controls were handled simultaneously. Our techniques aimed at optimum production of IFN-α and -γ. The isolated and washed leukocytes were suspended in 4 ml of Iscove's modified Dulbecco's medium supplemented with 0.6% $NaHCO_3$ and 10% human serum. The final cell suspension was divided to two plastic dishes. For induction we used the most potent inducers of IFN-α and -γ: Sendai virus and *Lens culinaris* lectin (LCL), respectively (Cantell *et al.*, 1981, 1986). The dish with Sendai virus for

IFN-α and the dish with LCL for IFN-γ production were then incubated in 8.5% CO_2 atmosphere at 36.5°C for 24 and 72 hr, respectively. After incubation, the cell suspension was diluted 1/3 with the medium used, the cells were removed by centrifugation, and the supernatants were stored at −70°C.

Both IFNs were later blindly assayed by the plaque reduction of vesicular stomatitis virus in HEp2 cells. Reference preparations were included in each assay. All activities are expressed as international units (IU) of IFN-α and -γ per milliliter. The techniques used are described in more detail elsewhere (Katila *et al.*, 1989).

Statistics

The results of the production of IFNs by leukocytes from the patients and the controls were analyzed by the Mann–Whitney U-test and for the psychotic group the effect of medication was analyzed by the Wilcoxon matched pairs signed-ranks test. All significance levels are expressed by two-tailed p values.

RESULTS

The mean values of IFN-α and γ production by leukocytes from the patients and the controls are given in Tables 1 and 2.

The mean values of IFN-α are consistently lower for the patients than for the controls in all diagnostic groups, though statistical significance is reached only when all patients are compared with the controls ($p = 0.02$). For IFN-γ production the same trend is seen in nonpsychotic patients. The posttreatment value of IFN-γ in the group of psychotic patients is greater than the corresponding value of the

Table 1. Production of IFN-α (IU, Log Mean) by Leukocytes from 34 Psychiatric Patients and 34 Controls

	n	Patients	Controls	
Paranoid and reactive psychoses				
Before treatment	13	2038	3456	N.S. ($p = 0.14$)
After treatment	12	2611	5581	N.S. ($p = 0.08$)
Mood and borderline disturbances				
On admission	21	3378	5190	N.S. ($p = 0.08$)
Depression				
On admission	15	3620	5058	N.S. ($p = 0.27$)
All patients				
On admission	34	2784	4442	$p = 0.02$[a]

[a]Mann–Whitney U-test $N = 34$; $R1 = 1360$; $R2 = 986$; $z = 2.29$; two-tailed $p = 0.02$.

Table 2. Production of IFN-γ (IU, Log Mean) by Leukocytes from 34 Psychiatric Patients and 34 Controls

	n	Patients	Controls	
Paranoid and reactive psychoses				
Before treatment	13	3829	3,857	N.S. ($p = 0.76$)
After treatment	12	9699	4,696	$p = 0.054^a$
Mood and borderline disturbances				
On admission	21	5196	8,502	N.S. ($p = 0.41$)
Depression				
On admission	15	5346	10,250	N.S. ($p = 0.70$)
All patients				
On admission	34	4624	6,284	N.S. ($p = 0.37$)

[a]Mann–Whitney U-test $N = 12$; $R1 = 116.5$; $R2 = 183.5$; $z = 1.93$; two-tailed $p = 0.054$.

controls. Nevertheless, the neuroleptic treatment in the present series did not reveal a significant effect on IFN production (Table 3).

DISCUSSION

Taking all patients together, the production of IFN-α was significantly lower in psychiatric patients than in healthy medical personnel. The differences for IFN-α in the diagnostic subgroups, however, did not reach statistical significance. Likewise, the production of IFN-γ was not significantly reduced. This may be due to the relatively small number of subjects studied and to great interindividual variations. According to our experience, interindividual variations are especially large for the production of IFN-γ, yet the trend of decreased IFN production is seen for IFN-γ as well.

The results of the present study and those of previous reports may be taken to suggest that decreased IFN production is not specific to any psychiatric disorder, but reflects a general impairment of immune responses in psychiatric crisis

Table 3. Production of INF-α and -γ (IU, Log Mean) by Leukocytes from 12 Patients with Paranoid and Reactive Psychoses before (a) and after 5 to 6 Weeks of treatment with Neuroleptics (b)

	a	b	
IFN-α	2262	2611	N.S. ($p = 0.51$)
IFN-γ	3997	9699	N.S. ($p = 0.10$)

Statistics by the Wilcoxon matched pairs signed-ranks test.

situations. The patients in this study were, indeed, in an acute psychiatric crisis as the duration of the psychotic state or psychiatric decompensation which led to hospital treatment was relatively short (mean 11.9 weeks for reactive psychoses and 24.7 weeks for mood and borderline disturbances). Different forms of stress (Chang and Rasmussen, 1965; Jensen, 1968; Pavlidis and Chirigos, 1980; Glaser *et al.*, 1986) and corticosteroid administration (Mendelson and Glascow, 1966) have been shown to cause a transitory decrease in the production of IFN. Furthermore, depression, psychosocial stress situation, and difficult life events seem to have a decreasing impact on a number of different facets of the immune responses (Bartrop *et al.*, 1977; Schleifer *et al.*, 1985; Glaser *et al.*, 1985; Irwin *et al.*, 1987; Kiecolt-Glaser *et al.*, 1987). The results of the present study are in keeping with the findings of partial immunosuppression in states of psychic distress.

CONCLUSION

Production of IFN-α and -γ by leukocytes from 34 patients with acute nonschizophrenic reactive psychoses and mood and borderline disturbances and 34 controls was measured by using Sendai virus as IFN-α inducer and lentil lectin as inducer for IFN-γ production.

The mean values of IFN-α were consistently lower for the patients than for the controls in all diagnostic groups, though statistical significance was reached only when all patients were compared with the controls ($p = 0.02$). For IFN-γ the same trend was seen in nonpsychotic patients. Neuroleptic treatment did not reveal a significant effect on IFN production.

The results of the present study and those of previous reports indicate a partial immunosuppression in states of acute psychiatric decompensation.

ACKNOWLEDGMENT This study was financially supported by the Medicinska Understödsföreningen Liv och Hälsa r.f. and by the Jalmari ja Rauha Ahokkaan Säätiö.

REFERENCES

Bartrop, R. W., Luckhurst, E., Lazarus, L., Kiloh, L. G., and Penny, R., 1977, Depressed lymphocyte function after bereavement, *Lancet* **2**:834–836.

Cantell, K., Hirvonen, S., Kauppinen, H. L., and Myllylä, G., 1981, Production of interferon in human leukocytes from normal donors with the use of Sendai virus, *Methods Enzymol.* **78**:29–38.

Cantell, K., Hirvonen, S., and Kauppinen, H. L., 1986, Production and partial purification of human immune interferon, *Methods Enzymol.* **119**:54–63.

Chang, S., and Rasmussen, A. F., 1965, Stress induced suppression of interferon production in virus-infected mice, *Nature* **205**:623–624.

De Maeyer, E., and De Maeyer-Guignard, J., 1988, *Interferons and Other Regulatory Cytokines*, Wiley, New York.

Glaser, R., Kiecolt-Glaser, J. K., Stout, J. C., Tarr, K., Speicher, C. E., and Holliday, J. E., 1985, Stress-related impairments in cellular immunity, *Psychiatr. Res.* **16**:233–239.

Glaser, R., Rice, J., Speicher, C. E., Stout, J. C., and Kiecolt-Glaser, J. K., 1986, Stress depresses interferon production by leukocytes concomitant with a decrease in natural killer cell activity. *Behav. Neurosci.* **100**:675–678.

Irwin, M., Daniels, M., Bloom, E. T., Smith, T. L., and Weiner, H., 1987, Life events, depressive symptoms and immune function, *Am. J. Psychiatry* **144**:437–441.

Jensen, M. M., 1968, Transitory impairment of interferon production in stressed mice, *J. Infect. Dis.* **118**:230–234.

Katila, H., Cantell, K., Hirvonen, S., and Rimón, R., 1989, Production of interferon alpha and gamma by leukocytes from patients with schizophrenia, *Schiz. Res.* **2**:361–365.

Kiecolt-Glaser, J. K., Fisher, D., Georges, J., Messick, G., Speicher, C. E., and Glaser, R., 1987, Marital quality, marital disruption, and immune function, *Psychosom. Med.* **49**:13–34.

Mendelson, J., and Glascow, L. A., 1966, The *in vitro* and *in vivo* effects of corticol on interferon production and action, *J. Immunol.* **96**:345–349.

Moises, H. W., Schindler, L., Leroux, M., and Kirchner, H., 1985, Decreased production of interferon alpha and interferon gamma in leukocyte cultures of schizophrenic patients, *Acta Psychiatr. Scand.* **72**:45–50.

Palmblad, J., Cantell, K., Strander, H., Fröberg, J., Karlsson, C. G., and Levi, L., 1974, Stressor exposure and human interferon production, Reports from Laboratory for Clinical Stress Research, Department of Medicine and Psychiatry, Karolinska sjukhuset, Stockholm, No. 35.

Palmblad, J., Cantell, K., Strander, H., Fröberg, J., Karlsson, C. G., Levi, L., Granström, M., and Unger, M., 1976, Stressor exposure and immunological response in man: Interferon-producing capacity and phagocytosis, *J. Psychosom. Res.* **20**:193–199.

Pavlidis, N., and Chirigos, M., 1980, Stress-induced impairment of macrophage tumoricidal function, *Psychosom. Med.* **42**:47–54.

Schleifer, S. J., Keller, S. E., Siris, S. G., Davis, K. L., and Stein, M., 1985, Depression and immunity, *Arch. Gen. Psychiatry* **42**:129–133.

Solomon, G. F, Merigan, T. C., and Levine, S., 1967, Variation in adrenal cortical hormones within physiologic ranges, stress, and interferon production in mice, *Proc. Soc. Exp. Biol. Med.* **126**: 74–79.

Chapter **17**

Interferon and Immunoglobulin G as Immunological Markers in Chronic Schizophrenia

Darrell G. Kirch and Richard Jed Wyatt

INTRODUCTION

The hypothesis that the etiology of schizophrenia may involve a viral infection is certainly not new (Menninger, 1926). One refinement of the hypothesis has led to the concept that the disorder may involve an abnormal immune response, such as production of a central nervous system (CNS) autoantibody, perhaps following exposure to viral antigens (Knight, 1982). While the viral/immunologic hypothesis has generated decades of research, these investigations have failed to yield definitive evidence to support or refute the concept (DeLisi and Crow, 1986; Torrey and Kaufmann, 1986). Nevertheless, the rapid advances being made in understanding the molecular processes involved in viral pathogenesis and immune regulation are presenting dramatic new opportunities to test this hypothesis.

Historically, it was clear to astute clinical observers that psychosis could be induced by infection of the brain, as seen when *Treponema pallidum* infection of the CNS was found to be the cause of general paralysis of the insane and also noted in certain postencephalitic states (Menninger, 1919). Relatively crude measures of

Darrell G. Kirch and Richard Jed Wyatt • *Neuropsychiatry Branch, Intramural Research Program, National Institute of Mental Health, Washington, D.C. 20032.*

immune response, e.g., fever or an increased white blood cell count (Bruce and Peebles, 1903), were among the first biological markers studied and thought by some to be abnormal in schizophrenic patients. Early in this century, qualitative and quantitative examinations of cerebrospinal fluid (CSF) proteins not only were the tools that allowed appropriate diagnosis of the psychosis associated with tertiary neurosyphilis (Wasley and Wong, 1988), but also subsequently revealed abnormalities in extensive studies of patients diagnosed as having schizophrenia (Bruetsch *et al.*, 1942).

As more sophisticated approaches to epidemiology have been developed, the body of indirect evidence supporting a viral/immunologic hypothesis for the etiology of at least some cases of schizophrenia has increased. Among the more interesting findings are observations of an increased number of late winter and early spring births among patients (reviewed by Torrey and Kaufmann, 1986), an excess of cases among those exposed *in utero* to an influenza type A2 epidemic during the second trimester (Mednick *et al.*, 1988), and possible geographic pockets of high and low prevalence (Eaton, 1985; Torrey, 1987). In addition, more direct laboratory approaches have also yielded data in support of viral or immunologic pathogenesis in schizophrenia. Some studies of humoral immunity in serum and CSF have indicated increased antibody titers to neurotropic viruses such as herpes simplex (Libikova, 1983) and cytomegalovirus (Kaufmann *et al.*, 1983). Examinations of cellular immune function have shown alterations in lymphocyte subpopulations (DeLisi *et al.*, 1982; Nyland *et al.*, 1980) and function (Hirata-Hibi *et al.*, 1982), as well as the function of immune regulators such as interferon (Preble and Torrey, 1985) and interleukin (Ganguli and Rabin, 1989; Rapaport *et al.*, 1989). Further, albeit circumstantial, evidence of a possible viral or autoimmune insult is provided by studies identifying gliosis, a possible marker of prior infection, in postmortem brain tissue from schizophrenic patients (Stevens, 1982), and by reports of other signs of subtle CNS structural pathology as revealed by histology (Kirch and Weinberger, 1986) and brain imaging techniques (Suddath *et al.*, 1989). It must be emphasized, however, that many studies of humoral and cellular immunity in schizophrenia have been negative, and the ultimate proof of identification (Feenstra *et al.*, 1988) and/or definitive transmission (Baker *et al.*, 1983; Kaufmann *et al.*, 1988) of a virus, has not been forthcoming (see DeLisi and Crow, 1986; Torrey and Kaufmann, 1986, for reviews).

Given these mixed results, it becomes increasingly important for studies of schizophrenia to utilize newly developed techniques that may serve as general biological markers of viral infection and/or immune dysfunction. While not directly identifying a specific virus, these techniques could provide additional evidence in support of a viral/immunologic hypothesis and, assuming that schizophrenia may have multiple causes, would also provide mechanisms for identifying a specific subset of patients meriting more focused study. Two such markers, interferon and immunoglobulin G (IgG), are discussed in this chapter.

INTERFERON AS AN IMMUNOLOGIC MARKER IN SCHIZOPHRENIA

The immune response is not only composed of varied cellular elements, but also involves multiple mediators that serve to induce or suppress cellular functions. One such regulatory factor is interferon, a glycoprotein that may induce antiviral activity (Grossberg, 1987; Preble *et al.*, 1982). Interferon is produced in three classes, α, β and γ, and the primary cellular sources of these proteins are peripheral leukocytes, fibroblasts, and stimulated lymphocytes, respectively. An apparent primary function of interferon is the induction of an antiviral state via inhibition of DNA/RNA synthesis. Elevated levels of interferon may indicate enhanced immune activity and be correlated with either a state of infection and/or an active immune response, including autoimmunity. Accordingly, increased interferon has been associated with varied disorders, not only viral infections including the acquired immunodeficiency syndrome (AIDS), but also autoimmune disorders such as systemic lupus erythematosus (SLE) (Preble *et al.*, 1982). It would seem that detection of elevated interferon production would represent an excellent general marker for the presence of an infectious/immune pathogenic process.

Prior studies of interferon in schizophrenia have yielded mixed results. Libikova (1983) reported increased interferon in a study of CSF, and Preble and Torrey (1985) noted increased interferon in serum (but not in CSF) in some patients with psychosis, reporting also that increased interferon seemed to be associated with more acute symptoms in unmedicated patients. Other investigators, however, failed to detect significant increases in interferon production in schizophrenic patients using both serum and CSF samples (Ahokas *et al.*, 1987; Rimón and Ahokas, 1987; Rimón *et al.*, 1983, 1985; Roy *et al.*, 1985; Schindler *et al.*, 1986), and others reported decreased interferon production in peripheral lymphocyte cultures from schizophrenic patients (Moises *et al.*, 1985, 1986). Nevertheless, it is important to note that a failure to detect interferon does not rule out the possibility that a latent infection or autoimmune process is present, but simply not active at the time of sampling.

INTERFERON DATA

In an attempt to replicate an earlier finding of increased serum interferon in schizophrenia (Preble and Torrey, 1985) and to also assess the relationship, if any, between elevated interferon and severity of symptoms, we have collected data (unpublished) on 19 schizophrenic patients (13 males and 6 females) before and after at least 2 weeks of withdrawal from chronic neuroleptic treatment. A total of 48 blood samples were collected from the 19 patients for determinations of interferon titers. There were two samples each (one drawn while on chronic neuroleptic treatment and the second at least 2 weeks after withdrawal from neuroleptics) from 14 subjects. In 5 subjects who underwent two different periods of withdrawal, there were four samples each. Psychopathology in the patients was rated daily using the Psychiatric Symptom Assessment Scale (PSAS) (Bigelow and Berthot, 1989), a modified version of the Brief Psychiatric Rating Scale (Overall and Gorham, 1962), and the mean of the ratings for the week prior to each blood sample was calculated.

Interferon was measured in plasma using a semi-micromethod on continuous cell lines of bovine kidney cells and human fibroblasts, with determinations of interferon-α antiviral activity on bovine cells and of neutralization by specific anti-interferon antibodies. In general, interferon titers ≤ 4 IU/ml are not considered to be significant. Among normal individuals, less than 5% have circulating interferon titers ≥ 8 IU/ml (Preble *et al.*, 1982).

Of the 48 patient samples, 16 (33%) showed interferon-α titers ≥ 8 IU/ml. The patients were clearly more symptomatic after withdrawal from neuroleptic treatment, showing a 37% increase in PSAS scores. However, 11 of 24 samples before withdrawal and 5 of 24 samples after withdrawal showed elevated interferon ($p = 0.13$; Fisher-exact). Thus, although a subset of patients showed elevations in this immunologic marker, no evidence for a direct association with severity of psychopathology was seen. In fact, these data showed a nonsignificant trend toward elevated interferon being more likely during chronic neuroleptic treatment. Another important point is that all the elevations observed in these patients were quite modest, and in no case did titers exceed 20 IU/ml. This is in contrast to interferon-α titers of 100–1000 IU/ml observed in acute influenza infection and up to 100 IU/ml associated with SLE (Preble *et al.*, 1982).

CSF PROTEINS AS AN IMMUNOLOGIC MARKER IN SCHIZOPHRENIA

Immunoglobulins, the key effectors of humoral immunity, are proteins that represent another potential general marker of immune response. The various classes of immunoglobulins, IgA, IgE, IgG, and IgM, vary structurally in their heavy chain constituents and functionally in the timing of their production and their specific role in the immune response. IgG is the immunoglobulin present in the highest concentration in serum and is the major antibody involved in the secondary immune response. As proteins, the immunoglobulins are measured together with albumin and other constituents in assays of the total protein content of biological fluids. In the first half of this century, investigators examining the CSF of schizophrenic patients noted increases in total protein in some schizophrenic patients (Bruetsch *et al.*, 1942). Subsequent technological advances have allowed the quantification not only of specific immunoglobulin classes but also of virus-specific antibodies. The assessment of immunoglobulins is an area of schizophrenia research that has also been marked by a diversity of findings, and increases, decreases, and no change in CSF immunoglobulins have been observed by different investigators (see Bock and Rafaelsen, 1974; DeLisi and Crow, 1986; Pearson, 1973; Torrey and Kaufmann, 1986; van Kammen and Sternberg, 1980, for reviews).

Recent refinements have taken place in the assessment of CSF proteins. It has become clear that, given the fact that the concentration of any given protein in blood may be several hundred times greater than in CSF, some assessment of and correction for variability in blood–brain barrier permeability is required in order to determine whether CSF immunoglobulins are of CNS origin or have entered the CSF from the periphery. A key advance in this area was the development of quantitative indices to assess blood–brain barrier permeability and CNS immunoglobulin production (Killingsworth, 1982). Insofar as there is a gradient of albumin across the blood–brain barrier, permeability is reflected by the quotient: [(CSF albumin/serum albumin) × 1000]. In turn, IgG production in the CNS, corrected for variance in blood–brain barrier permeability that would allow peripheral IgG to enter the CSF, is reflected by the index [(CSF IgG/serum IgG)/(CSF albumin/serum albumin)]. Several studies using these indices in populations of control subjects have revealed consistent reference values (Killingsworth, 1982; Papadopoulos *et al.*, 1984; Tibbling *et al.*, 1977). A mathematical formula for actually quantifying the rate of endogenous CNS synthesis of IgG has also been developed (Tourtellotte *et al.*, 1980) using these same serum and CSF protein variables.

With regard to the application of these techniques to schizophrenia and other psychoses, we and others have reported apparent increases in blood–brain barrier permeability in some patients as defined by the CSF/serum albumin quotient (Axelsson *et al.*, 1982; Bauer and Kornhuber, 1987; Kirch *et al.*, 1985; Torrey *et al.*, 1985). Using the Tourtellotte formula, one group reported no increase in CSF IgG synthesis in a group of schizophrenic patients (Roos *et al.*, 1985). Using the IgG index as described above, we noted that a third of patients showed elevations in CNS IgG production above previously established reference values (Kirch *et al.*, 1985), while others observed no increase (Bauer and Kornhuber, 1987). In addition, some have noted an increased frequency of oligoclonal IgG bands in CSF from schizophrenic patients (Ahokas *et al.*, 1985).

CSF IGG DATA

Believing that the CSF IgG index represents a useful tool for screening patients for endogenous CNS IgG production, we have expanded upon our earlier analysis of CSF proteins (Kirch *et al.*, 1985), and now have data (unpublished) on a total cohort of 46 patients (31 male, 15 female) and 20 healthy control subjects (16 male, 4 female). The mean (± S.D.) age of the patients was 29.9 ± 5.9 years and that of the control subjects was 54.1 ± 20.5 years, the latter group having been recruited for a study (Papadopoulos *et al.*, 1984) analyzing CSF proteins across the age span for comparison with reference values established by other investigators.

All patients were diagnosed as having chronic schizophrenia by DSM-III criteria. Eight of the patients underwent two separate lumbar punctures in order to allow assessment of proteins on and off neuroleptic treatment, yielding a total of 54 samples from the 46 schizophrenic patients. Protein quantification was performed by rate nephelometry (Papadopoulos *et al.*, 1984).

The group values for the individual CSF and serum variables and the calculated albumin quotient and IgG index are listed in Table 1. The group mean CSF albumin and albumin quotient for the 20 control samples are significantly higher than those for the 54 patient samples, reflecting the fact that the control subjects included a number of elderly individuals. The previously observed (Tibbling *et al.*, 1977) increase in blood–brain barrier permeability with age is replicated in these older control subjects. When the data obtained regarding blood–brain barrier permeability are assessed taking into account patient age, 12 of the patient samples and only 1 of the control samples exceeded previously established age-specific reference values (Tibbling *et al.*, 1977) ($p = 0.08$; chi-square). In this sense, some of the schizophrenic patients who were in their third and fourth decade had an albumin quotient that was at or above the normal range for the sixth, seventh, and eighth decade in control subjects, a finding consistent with reports by other observers (Axelsson *et al.*, 1982; Bauer and Kornhuber, 1987; Torrey *et al.*, 1985). This not only confirms that some younger schizophrenic patients have apparent increases in blood–brain barrier permeability, but also highlights the importance of correcting for this in any studies of CSF proteins or other CSF variables for which a blood–brain gradient may exist. For studies of IgG, this is accomplished by using the IgG index as defined in the preceding section with its internal correction for the CSF/serum albumin quotient. With this correction, the reference

Table 1. Group Values (Mean ± S.D.) in 54 Samples from Schizophrenic Patients and 20 Control Samples for Concentrations of Albumin and IgG in CSF and Serum, and for the Calculated Albumin Quotient and IgG Index, Indicators of Blood–Brain Barrier Permeability and Endogenous CNS IgG Production, Respectively

	Patients	Controls
CSF albumin (mg/dl)	19.7 ± 7.9*	24.2 ± 4.5*
Serum albumin (g/dl)	4.03 ± 0.42	4.05 ± 0.50
CSF IgG (mg/dl)	2.44 ± 1.33	2.56 ± 0.83
Serum IgG (mg/dl)	989 ± 222	970 ± 174
Albumin quotient	4.85 ± 1.77*	6.09 ± 1.47*
IgG index	0.53 ± 0.23**	0.44 ± 0.10**

*$p < 0.01$ (t test).
**$p < 0.05$ (t test).

range for the IgG index appears to be constant across the adult age span (Papadopoulos *et al.*, 1984; Tibbling *et al.*, 1977).

The data regarding the CSF IgG index in the 54 samples from 46 schizophrenic patients also revealed abnormalities. Although most were clearly in the normal range, the group mean IgG index for the patient samples did show a statistically significant increase compared with the control samples. In addition, the variance was greater in the schizophrenic subjects, and of the 54 patient samples, 12 showed the IgG index higher than that observed in any of the control subjects.

When the paired samples collected from eight schizophrenic subjects on and off neuroleptics were compared by a matched-pairs *t* test, no significant differences in either albumin quotient or IgG index were observed on versus off neuroleptic. Thus, the apparent increase in CNS IgG production observed in at least a subset of these schizophrenic patients does not appear to be attributable simply to a neuroleptic effect.

CONCLUSIONS

Taken as a whole, the studies and data reviewed here seem to converge on three important points. First, examinations of immunologic function using advanced methods continue to reveal *abnormalities in some, but not all, cases of schizophrenia*, which may or may not result in modest group differences compared with controls. Second, *even when abnormalities are observed, they are usually relatively modest* when compared with active cases of known viral infections or "classical" autoimmune disorders such as SLE. The data outlined above on interferon-α are instructive, with the highest titers observed in schizophrenic patients at a level of 20 IU/ml, while in acute viral infection titers may be 50 times higher and in SLE patients 5 times higher (Preble *et al.*, 1982). Likewise, the CSF IgG index data from schizophrenic patients summarized in the preceding section show that few patients have indices as high as commonly observed in active cases of multiple sclerosis, another disorder thought to involve a viral infection and/or a subsequent autoimmune response (Link and Tibbling, 1977; Papadopoulos *et al.*, 1984). Third, the *potential role of neuroleptic treatment in altering immune response* must always be considered. For example, in the interferon data summarized above, the trend is toward elevated interferon being more frequently associated with neuroleptic treatment than with the neuroleptic withdrawal state, even though the patients were significantly more symptomatic in the latter state. Few studies of immunologic markers in schizophrenia have avoided this potential methodological source of variance by examining cohorts of never-treated patients.

These cautionary observations are in no way meant to "rule out" the viral/immunologic hypothesis of schizophrenia. Rather, they simply call for revisions in the hypothesis that take these facts into account. The most obvious conclusion is that, insofar as viral/immunologic data typically show marked variance between patients, the probability of etiologic heterogeneity in schizophrenia remains high. Only some cases, perhaps those with an underlying genetic susceptibility, may involve viral/immune pathogenesis. In addition, it is possible that even the subset of cases showing viral/immunologic abnormalities may be heterogeneous, with different viral agents or even different autoantibodies acting on a common CNS pathway to create similar psychopathology. This might explain the fact that associations have been proposed between schizophrenia and a variety of specific DNA and RNA viruses of disparate classes, such as influenza, herpes simplex, cytomegalovirus, and retroviruses.

That observed immunologic abnormalities are subtle rather than marked, that attempts at viral isolation and transmission have met with no definitive success, and that no clear evidence of active inflammation or progressive cell death is seen in neuropathological studies of schizophrenia are facts that must be reconciled with the viral/immunologic hypothesis. These observations certainly militate against the idea that the illness involves an active infection or cytopathic immune response. Rather, it becomes much more compelling to consider the possibility of an early, i.e., pre- or perinatal, insult leaving minimal residual evidence. In this regard, the ideas now being advanced regarding expanded notions of virally induced pathology are important (Oldstone, 1984). Viruses (and the immune response that accompanies them) are capable of effects that are much more subtle than overt inflammation and cell death. In particular, the ability of viruses to utilize endogenous cellular receptors, including neurotransmitter receptors, as attachment points (Co *et al.*, 1985) makes it possible that they may significantly alter selective aspects of CNS development and function, especially in the fetal or neonatal brain, without the more blatant neuropathological signs typical of an active encephalitis. The capacity of many viruses to remain latent or, in the case of retroviruses, to be actually incorporated into the host genome and transmitted vertically, makes it entirely possible that viral agents could affect neuronal function and gene expression while eliciting minimal or no immune response.

The need, therefore, is not for abandonment of the viral hypothesis, but rather for the development of new techniques by which it may be tested. Clinically, these might include improved methods for the definition of lymphocyte subpopulations, for the identification and measurement of molecular immune regulators, and for the determination of viral antigen, virus-specific antibodies, and CNS autoantibodies in patients. For example, newly developed gene amplification techniques (Saiki *et al.*, 1988) have great potential for allowing identification of extremely small quantities of viral genomic material in tissue samples, including the brain. Most importantly, as these new techniques are developed, studies should be focused on the subset of schizophrenic patients who demonstrate immunologic abnormalities on multiple tests, a technique that is likely to assist in overcoming the apparent etiologic heterogeneity of the disorder.

However, even with the application of advanced techniques to patient studies, clinical heterogeneity still might make it extremely difficult to prove directly the involvement of a specific virus (or the immune response to a specific virus) in investigations of schizophrenia. Thus, it might also be productive to more actively pursue further development of animal models of CNS viral/immunologic pathogenesis. For example, it seems reasonable to design animal studies of nonlethal pre- and perinatal exposure to low titers of the specific viruses that have been implicated in schizophrenia, following the animals to adult life while examining them not only for behavioral changes, but also for CNS neuropathological and neurochemical abnormalities parallel to those reported in clinical studies of the disorder. Such studies would at least clarify the potential for subtle early viral infection and/or an autoimmune response to pathogenically establish a CNS substrate that, in humans, may be involved in schizophrenia.

ACKNOWLEDGMENTS The following have contributed significantly to the projects described in this chapter: Drs. R. C. Alexander, U. Choudhry, C. A. Kaufmann, B. Martin, N. M. Papadopoulos, O. T. Preble, R. L. Suddath, and E. F. Torrey.

REFERENCES

Ahokas, A., Koskiniemi, M., Vaheri, A., and Rimón, R., 1985, Altered white cell count, protein concentration and oligoclonal IgG bands in the cerebrospinal fluid of many patients with acute psychiatric disorders, *Neuropsychobiology* **14**:1–4.

Ahokas, A., Rimón, R. Koskiniemi, M., Vaheri, A., Julkunen, I., and Sarna, S., 1987, Viral antibodies and interferon in acute psychiatric disorders, *J. Clin. Psychiatry* **48**:194–196.

Axelsson, R., Martensson, E., and Alling, C., 1982, Impairment of the blood–brain barrier as an aetiological factor in paranoid psychosis, *Br. J. Psychiatry* **141**:273–281.

Baker, H. F., Ridley, R.M., Crow, T. J., Bloxham, C. A., Parry, R. P. and Tyrrell, D. A. J., 1983, An investigation of the effects of intracerebral injection in the marmoset of cytopathic cerebrospinal fluid from patients with schizophrenia or neurological disease, *Psychol. Med.* **13**:499–511.

Bauer, K., and Kornhuber, J., 1987, Blood–cerebrospinal fluid barrier in schizophrenic patients, *Eur. Arch. Psychiatry Neurol. Sci.* **236**:257–259.

Bigelow, L. B., and Berthot, B., 1989, The Psychiatric Symptom Assessment Scale (PSAS), *Psychopharmacol. Bull.* **25**:168–179.

Bock, E., and Rafaelsen, O. J., 1974, Schizophrenia: Proteins in blood and cerebrospinal fluid, *Dan. Med. Bull.* **21**:93–105.

Bruce, L. C., and Peebles, A. M. S., 1903, Clinical and experimental observations on catatonia, *J. Ment. Sci.* **49**:614–628.

Bruetsch, W. L., Bahr, M. A., Skobba, J. S., and Dieter, W. J., 1942, The group of dementia praecox patients with an increase of the protein content of the cerebrospinal fluid, *J. Nerv. Ment. Dis.* **95**:669–679.

Co, M. S., Gaulton, G. N., Tominaga, A., Homcy, C. J., Fields, B. N., and Greene, M. I., 1985, Structural similarities between the mammalian beta-adrenergic and reovirus type 3 receptors, *Proc. Natl. Acad. Sci. USA* **82**:5315–5318.

DeLisi, L. E., and Crow, T. J., 1986, Is schizophrenia a viral or immunologic disorder? *Psychiatr. Clin. North Am.* **9**:115–132.

DeLisi, L. E., Goodman, S., Neckers, L. M., and Wyatt, R. J., 1982, Lymphocyte subpopulations in schizophrenic patients, *Biol. Psychiatry* **17**, 1003–1007.

Eaton, W. W., 1985, Epidemiology of schizophrenia, *Epidemiol. Rev.* **7**:105–126.

Feenstra, A., Kirch, D. G., Coggiano, M. A., and Wyatt, R. J., 1988, Reverse transcriptase activity in 5-azacytidine-treated lymphocyte cultures of patients with schizophrenia, *Schiz. Res.* **1**:385–389.

Ganguli, R., and Rabin, B. S., 1989, Increased serum interleukin 2 receptor concentration in schizophrenic and brain-damaged subjects, *Arch. Gen. Psychiatry* **46**:292.

Grossberg, S. E., 1987, Interferons: An overview of their biological and biochemical properties, in: *Mechanisms of Interferon Actions*, Volume I (L. M. Pfeffer, ed.), CRC Press, Boca Raton, pp. 1–32.

Hirata-Hibi, M., Higashi, S., Tachibana, T., and Watanabi, N., 1982, Stimulated lymphocytes in schizophrenia, *Arch. Gen. Psychiatry* **39**:82–87.

Kaufmann, C. A., Weinberger, D. R., Yolken, R. H., Torrey, E. F., and Potkin, S. G., 1983, Viruses and schizophrenia, *Lancet* **2**:1136.

Kaufmann, C. A., Weinberger, D. R., Stevens, J. R., Asher, D. M., Kleinman, J. E., Sulima, M. P., Gibbs, C. J., and Gadjusek, D. C., 1988, Intracerebral inoculation of experimental animals with brain tissue from patients with schizophrenia: Failure to observe consistent or specific behavioral and neuropathological effects, *Arch. Gen. Psychiatry* **45**:648–652.

Killingsworth, L. M., 1982, Clinical applications of protein determinations in biological fluids other than blood, *Clin. Chem.* (Winston-Salem, N.C.) **28**:1093–1102.

Kirch, D. G., and Weinberger, D. R., 1986, Anatomical neuropathology in schizophrenia: Post-mortem findings, in: *The Neurology of Schizophrenia* (H. A. Nasrallah and D. R. Weinberger, eds.), Elsevier, Amsterdam, pp. 325–348.

Kirch, D. G., Kaufmann, C. A. Papadopoulos, N. M., Martin, B., and Weinberger, D. R., 1985, Abnormal cerebrospinal fluid protein indices in schizophrenia, *Biol. Psychiatry* **20**, 1039–1046.

Knight, J. G., 1982, Dopamine-receptor-stimulating autoantibodies: A possible cause of schizophrenia, *Lancet* **2**:1073–1076.

Libikova, H., 1983, Schizophrenia and viruses: Principles of etiologic studies, in: *Research on the Viral Hypothesis of Mental Disorders* (P. Morozov, ed.), Karger, Basel, pp. 20–51.

Link, H., and Tibbling, G., 1977, Principles of albumin and IgG analyses in neurological disorders. III. Evaluation of IgG synthesis within the central nervous system in multiple sclerosis, *Scand. J. Clin. Lab. Invest.* **37**:397–401.

Mednick, S. A., Machon, R. A., Huttunen, M. O., and Bonett, D., 1988, Adult schizophrenia following prenatal exposure to an influenza epidemic, *Arch. Gen. Psychiatry* **45**:189–192.

Menninger, K. A., 1919, Psychoses associated with influenza, *J. Am. Med. Assoc.* **72**:235–241.

Menninger, K. A., 1926, Influenza and schizophrenia: An analysis of post-influenzal "dementia praecox" as of 1918 and five years later, *Am. J. Psychiatry* **5**:469–529.

Moises, H. W., Schindler, L., Leroux, M., and Kirchner, H., 1985, Decreased production of interferon alpha and interferon gamma in leucocyte cultures of schizophrenic patients, *Acta Psychiatr. Scand.* **72**:42–50.

Moises, H. W., Beck, J., Schindler, L., and Kirchner, H., 1986, Decreased interferon in schizophrenic patients, *Pharmacopsychiatry* **19**:226–227.

Nyland, H., Naess, A., and Lunde, H., 1980, Lymphocyte subpopulations in peripheral blood from schizophrenic patients, *Acta Psychiatr. Scand.* **61**:313–318.

Oldstone, M. B. A., 1984, Viruses can alter cell function without causing cell pathology: Disordered function leads to imbalance of homeostasis and disease, in *Concepts in Viral Pathogenesis* (A. L. Notkins and M. B. A. Oldstone, eds.), Springer-Verlag, Berlin, pp. 269–276.

Overall, J. E., and Gorham, D. R., 1962, The Brief Psychiatric Rating Scale, *Psychol. Rep.* **10**:799–812.

Papadopoulos, N. M., Costello, R., Kay, A. D., Cutler, N. R., and Rapaport, S. I., 1984, Combined immunochemical and electrophoretic determinations of proteins in paired serum and cerebrospinal fluid samples, *Clin. Chem.* (Winston-Salem, N.C.) **30**:1814–1816.

Pearson, E. K., 1973, Study of cerebrospinal fluid in schizophrenics: A review of the literature, *Psychopharmacol. Bull.* **9**:59–62.

Preble, O. T., and Torrey, E. F., 1985, Serum interferon in patients with psychosis, *Am. J. Psychiatry* **142**:1184–1186.

Preble, O. T., Black, R. J., Friedman, R. M., Klippel, J. H., and Vilcek, J., 1982, Systemic lupus erythematosus: Presence in human serum of an unusual acid-labile leukocyte interferon, *Science* **216**:429–431.

Rapaport, M. H., McAllister, C. G., Pickar, D., Nelson, D. L., and Paul, S. M., 1989, Elevated levels of soluble interleukin 2 receptors in schizophrenia, *Arch. Gen. Psychiatry* **46**:291–292.

Rimón, R., and Ahokas, A., 1987, Interferon in schizophrenia, in: *Viruses, Immunity, and Mental Disorders* (E. Kurstak, Z. J. Lipowski, and P. V. Morozov, eds.), Plenum Medical, New York, pp. 379–382.

Rimón, R., Halonen, P., Lebon, P., Heikkila, L., Frey, H., Karhula, P., Hintikka, J., and Salmela, L., 1983, Antibrain antibodies and interferon in the serum and cerebrospinal fluid of patients with schizophrenia, in: *Research on the Viral Hypothesis of Mental Disorders* (P. Morozov, ed.), Karger, Basel, pp. 161–167.

Rimón, R., Ahokas, A., Hintikka, J., and Heikkila, L., 1985, Serum interferon in schizophrenia, *Ann. Clin. Res.* **17**:139–140.

Roos, R. P., Davis, K., and Meltzer, H. Y., 1985, Immunoglobulin studies in patients with psychiatric diseases, *Arch. Gen. Psychiatry* **42**:124–128.

Roy, A., Pickar, D., Ninan, P., Hooks, J., and Paul, S. M., 1985, A search for interferon in the CSF of chronic schizophrenic patients, *Am. J. Psychiatry* **142**:269.

Saiki, R. K., Gelfand, D. H., Stoffel, S., Scharf, S. J., Higuchi, R., Horn, G. T., Mullis, K. B., and Ehrlich, H. E., 1988, Primer-directed enzymatic amplification of DNA with a thermostable DNA polymerase, *Science* **239**:487–491.

Schindler, L., Leroux, M., Beck, J., Moises, H. W., and Kirchner, H., 1986, Studies of cellular immunity, serum interferon titers, and natural killer cell activity in schizophrenic patients, *Acta Psychiatr. Scand.* **73**:651–657.

Stevens, J. R., 1982, Neuropathology of schizophrenia, *Arch. Gen. Psychiatry* **39**:1131–1139.

Suddath, R. L., Casanova, M. F., Goldberg, T. E., Daniel, D. G., Kelsoe, J. R., and Weinberger, D. R., 1989, Temporal lobe pathology in schizophrenia: A quantitative magnetic resonance imaging study, *Am. J. Psychiatry* **146**:464–472.

Tibbling, G., Link, H., and Ohman, S., 1977, Principles of albumin and IgG analyses in neurological disorders. I. Establishment of reference values, *Scand. J. Clin. Lab. Invest.* **37**:385–390.

Torrey, E. F., 1987, Prevalence studies in schizophrenia, *Br. J. Psychiatry* **150**:598–608.

Torrey, E. F., and Kaufmann, C. A., 1986, Schizophrenia and neuroviruses, in: *The Neurology of Schizophrenia* (H. A. Nasrallah and D. R. Weinberger, eds.), Elsevier, Amsterdam, pp. 361–376.

Torrey, E. F., Albrecht, P., and Behr, D. E., 1985, Permeability of the blood–brain barrier in psychiatric patients, *Am. J. Psychiatry* **142**:657–658.

Tourtellotte, W. W., Potvin, A. R., Fleming, J. O., Murthy, K. N., Levy, J., Syndulko, K., and Potvin, J. H., 1980, Multiple sclerosis: Measurement and validation of central nervous system IgG synthesis rate, *Neurology* **30**:240–244.

van Kammen, D. P., and Sternberg, D. E., 1980, Cerebrospinal fluid studies in schizophrenia, in: *Neurobiology of Cerebrospinal Fluid* (J. H. Wood, ed.), Plenum Press, New York, pp. 719–742.

Wasley, G. D., and Wong, H. H. Y., 1988, *Syphilis Serology: Principles and Practice*, Oxford University Press, Oxford, pp. 1–4.

Chapter **18**

Immune Modulation in Major Depressive Patients in Remission

Eli Kritschmann, Daniel Becker, Susy Floru, and Tamar Gotlieb-Stematsky

INTRODUCTION

Compromised immunologic function has been demonstrated in psychological stress, bereavement, and depression (Calabrese *et al.*, 1987). Lymphocyte function has been assessed *in vitro* by proliferative response to nonspecific mitogenic agents such as phytohemagglutinin (PHA), concanavalin A (Con A), and pokeweed mitogen (PWM), yielding blunted stimulation with the three mitogens in the bereaved subjects (Bartrop *et al.*, 1977; Schleifer *et al.*, 1983). In addition, Schleifer *et al.* (1983) studied prospectively bereaved individuals for white blood cell counts and T and B lymphocyte subpopulations and found no changes in the parameters tested.

Glaser and Kiecolt-Glaser (1986) and Kiecolt-Glaser *et al.* (1987) showed that loneliness and stress, as well as marital disruption were associated with poor qualitative and quantitative immune function. Three measures of immune function

Eli Kritschmann, Daniel Becker, Susy Floru, and Tamar Gotlieb-Stematsky • *Department of Psychiatry and The Central Virology Laboratory, Chaim Sheba Medical Center, Tel-Aviv University, Sackler School of Medicine, Tel-Hashomer 52621, Israel.*

presented reduced natural-killer cell (NK) and helper cell activity and poor blastogenic response to mitogens.

Naor *et al.* (1983) studied women in depression after spontaneous or induced abortion and found that the intensity of the depressive reaction was correlated with a decrease in lymphocyte response to mitogenic agents.

The impact of depressive illness on the immune response was studied by Kronfol *et al.* (1983) who found impaired lymphocyte function to mitogen stimulation with Con A, PHA, and PWM. Similar results were found by Schleifer *et al.* (1984). They also found that absolute T and B cell counts were reduced although the relative percentages were unchanged. In a subsequent study, Schleifer *et al.* (1985) found that ambulatory patients with major depressive disorder presented normal immune response, while the number of T lymphocytes was decreased. Sengar *et al.* (1982) studied several immune parameters in major affective disorder, in which manic-depressive patients were in a state of remission. They found that lymphocyte sub-populations and mitogenic responses were normal and there were no differences between patients who were treated prophylactically by lithium carbonate and a control of nontreated patients.

The aim of our study was to define a group of major depressive patients in a state of remission, and evaluate lymphocytic proliferative response to nonspecific mitogen stimulation, in order to determine whether impaired immune response was trait or state dependent. In addition, subpopulations of T lymphocytes (absolute and relative counts) and the ratio between T4 (helper/inducer cells) and T8 (suppressor/cytotoxic cells) in patients and healthy controls were simultaneously assayed.

STUDY GROUP AND METHODS

The research group included ambulatory patients fulfilling the diagnostic criteria for major depression, as required by RDC (Spitzer *et al.*, 1978) and DSM-III (1980) in a state of remission verified by clinical criteria and a Hamilton Rating Score below 7 points (Endicott *et al.*, 1981). The group of patients (Table 1) included 4 males and 16 females, mean age 54.95 ± 10.73 years. The control group included 3 males and 7 females with mean age 49.90 ± 9.43. Past depressive

Table 1 Characteristics of Study Group of Patients and Controls

Group	No.	Age (years) (mean)	Sex	No. of depressive episodes (mean)	Drug treatment (lithium, TCA)
Major depression	20	54.95 ± 10.73	4 M, 16 F	4.15 ± 1.3	16
Control	10	49.90 ± 9.43	3 M, 7 F	—	—

episodes for the group of patients were defined by a Hamilton Rating Score above 25 points and mean number was 4.15 ± 1.3. Maintenance treatment with lithium or antidepressive drugs was administered to 16 of the patients, while the other 4 were drug-free. None of the patients were on neuroleptic drugs or received other psychotropic treatment. Patients were excluded from the research group if affected by acute or chronic diseases presented by impaired cellular immunity.

Lymphocyte proliferative response was tested with three mitogens: PWM (10 μg/ml, Sigma), PHA (1:100, final concentration 0.25 μg/ml, Wellcome), Con A (5 μg/ml, Bio-Yedah). Determination of subpopulations of T lymphocytes was carried out with monoclonal antibodies (Ortho Diagnostic Systems, Raritan, N.J.). The relative numbers of T4 and T8 lymphocytes were determined as a percentage of the total lymphocyte population.

The lymphocyte proliferative response of every subject was established by two methods:

1. Δcpm—the cpm difference between the culture that was stimulated by mitogen and the unstimulated culture.
2. Stimulation index (SI)—The ratio between the counts in the stimulated and the nonstimulated culture.

The comparison between the two groups was calculated by paired *t*-test with logarithmic transformation of Δcpm and SI, and Wilcoxon signed ranks test.

RESULTS

The results of lymphocyte proliferative response tests yielded no significant difference between patients and controls. On the other hand, a descending linear correlation between age and lymphocytic proliferative response to each of the mitogens was observed in both groups (Fig. 1A-C).

Table 2 presents the absolute and relative counts of lymphocyte subpopulations in patients and controls. The differences between the total number of white blood cells, total lymphocytes and percentages, as well as total T3 lymphocytes and T4 subgroup counts were not significantly different, as determined by analysis of variance (ANOVA).

A statistically significant difference was demonstrated in the percentage of T8 cells. The mean count was $17.20 \pm 2.46\%$ for the group of patients versus $25.55 \pm 1.37\%$ for the control group ($p = 0.0039$). The ratio of T4/T8 was significantly higher ($p = 0.0359$) in the group of patients (3.44 ± 0.80), as compared to controls (2.16 ± 0.21).

Analysis of severity of illness and lymphocyte subpopulations yielded an ascending linear correlation between the number of repeated past depressive episodes and the percentage of T4 helper/inducer lymphocytes (Fig. 2).

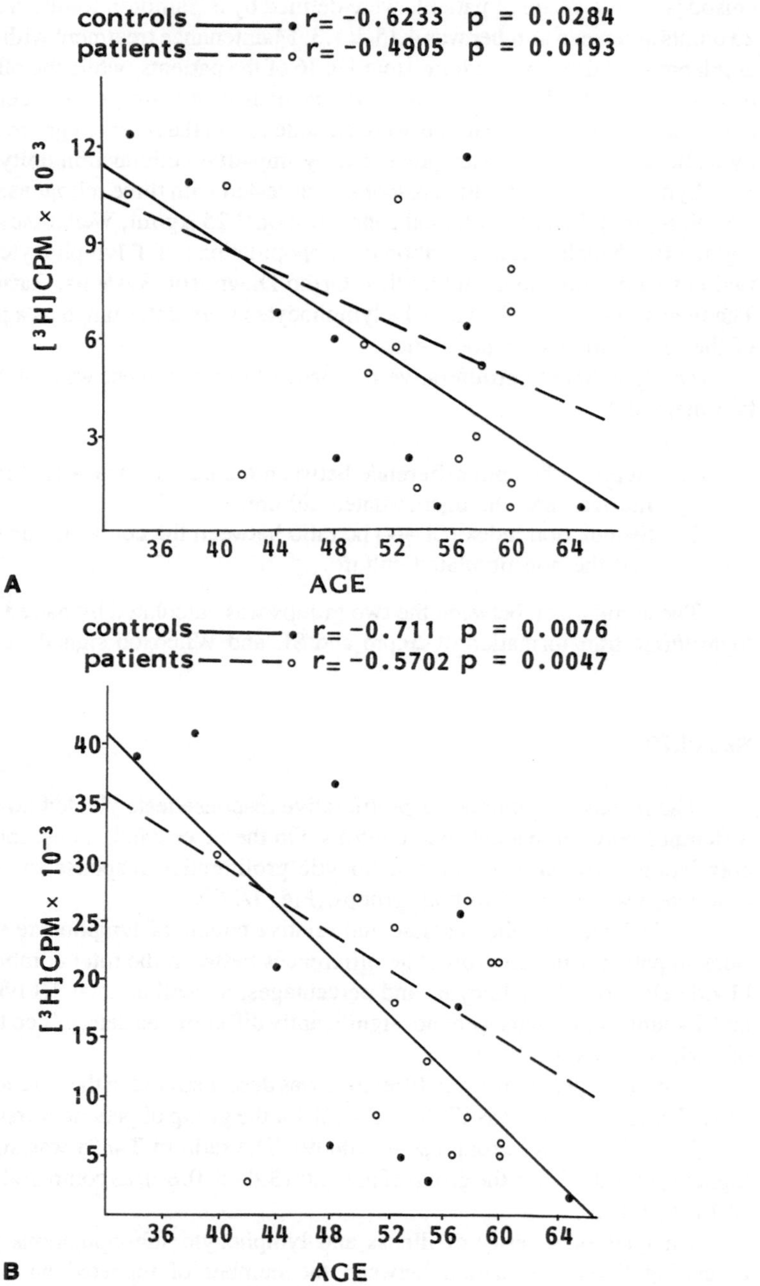
controls ● r= -0.6233 p = 0.0284
patients ○ r= -0.4905 p = 0.0193
[3H]CPM × 10⁻³
12
9
6
3
36 40 44 48 52 56 60 64
AGE
A
controls ● r= -0.711 p = 0.0076
patients ○ r= -0.5702 p = 0.0047
[3H]CPM × 10⁻³
40
35
30
25
20
15
10
5
36 40 44 48 52 56 60 64
AGE
B

Figure 1.

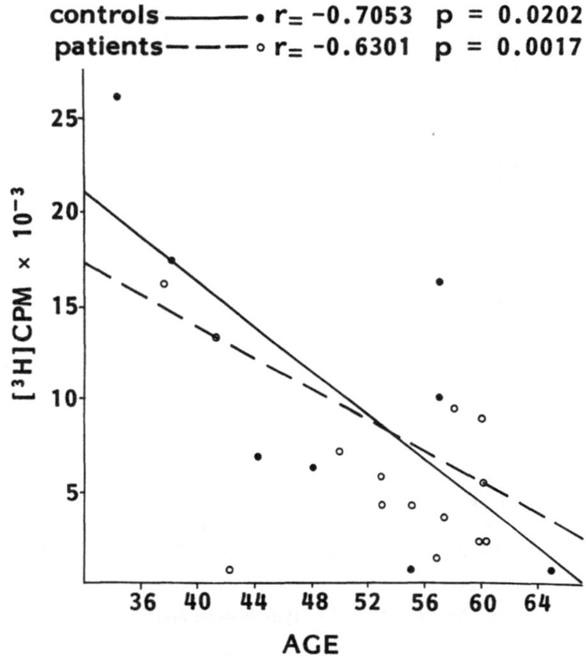

Figure 1. Lymphocyte proliferative response to (A) pokeweed mitogen, (B) phytohemagglutinin, and (C) concanavalin A. Regression line of cpm versus age.

Table 2. Lymphocytes and T Cell Subpopulations in Major Depressive Patients in Remission and Age/Sex-Matched Healthy Controls

	Controls (n = 27)	Patients (n = 10)	p (ANOVA)
WBC × 10^6/l	5968 ± 619[a]	6960 ± 684	N.S.
Lymphocytes × 10^6/l	1992 ± 133	1954 ± 218	N.S.
%	36.58 ± 4.80	29.30 ± 2.60	N.S.
T3 × 10^6/l	1356 ± 123	1276 ± 167	N.S.
%	66.37 ± 2.33	63.80 ± 2.43	N.S.
T4 × 10^6/l	1004 ± 60	859 ± 124	N.S.
%	49.14 ± 1.69	43.90 ± 4.10	N.S.
T8 × 10^6/l	462 ± 43	355 ± 76	N.S.
%	25.55 ± 1.37	17.20 ± 2.46	0.0039
T4/T8	2.16 ± 0.21	3.44 ± 0.80	0.0359

[a]Values are mean ± S.E.M.

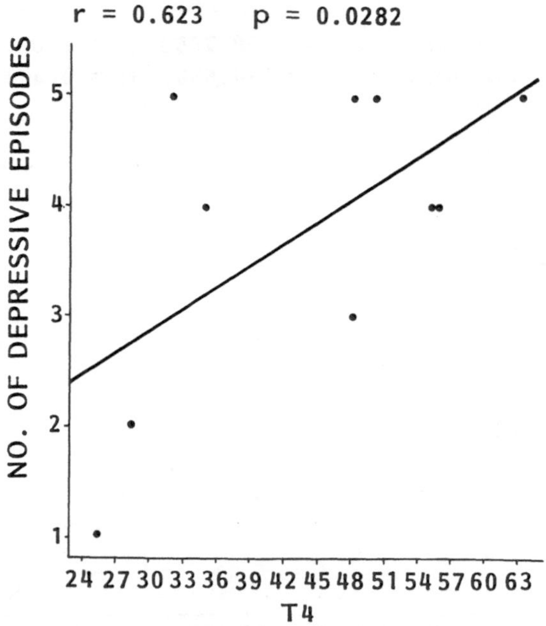

Figure 2. Regression line of the percentage of T4 lymphocytes and the number of depressive episodes in ten patients.

DISCUSSION

In order to clarify whether impaired immune response in major depressive patients was state or trait dependent, we chose a group of patients in full remission as determined by clinical evaluation. Our results did not point to altered cellular immune response, as tested by lymphocyte stimulation, in patients in remission. Most of these patients received psychopharmacologic prophylactic treatment, which included lithium and/or antidepressant drugs.

Although it would have been preferable to examine drug-free patients, our choice of patients with severe illnesses excluded intermission or termination of drug use. The most consistent hematological effect of lithium is a benign, reversible leukocytosis consisting primarily of an increase in mature neutrophils, while basophils, eosinophils, and lymphocytes are unaffected (Murphy *et al.*, 1971; Rossof and Fehir, 1978). Also, Sengar *et al.* (1982) claimed that lithium treatment did not affect cellular immune response, when parameters similar to those tested in our study were considered. As far as we know, tricyclic antidepressive agents do not affect cellular immune response.

The percentage of T8 subgroups of T lymphocytes was significantly reduced and the ratio of T4/T8 was significantly high among the depressive patients (Table 2). T lymphocytes were found to be affected by neurotransmitters of the CNS, by hormones of the pituitary gland, and by endorphins (Besedovsky *et al.*, 1979; Mathews *et al.*, 1983; Jackson *et al.*, 1985; Berczi *et al.*, 1986). These substances were also found to be involved in depressive illnesses.

Our study revealed a correlation between lymphocyte stimulation and age in the group of patients, similar to the correlation found in normal populations (Murasko *et al.*, 1987). This observation points to the importance of consideration of age in studies of the immune response. The ascending linear correlation which was found between the number of repeated past depressive episodes and the percentage of T4 lymphocytes, seems of interest, although the small number of patients tested requires further study.

Our results point to the complexity of the immune response in depressive states and emphasize the requirements for carefully defined groups of patients and controls when testing for the variety of components of the immune system.

ACKNOWLEDGMENTS We thank Mrs. Y. Shlomo-David, of The Central Virology Laboratory, Mrs. M. Biniaminov and Mrs. E. Rosenthal of The Hematologic Institute, for their assistance in performing the tests, and Mrs. R. Golan of the Department of Clinical Epidemiology, for statistical analysis.

REFERENCES

Bartrop, R. W., Luckhurst, E., Lazarus, L., Kiloh, L. G., and Penny, R., 1977, Depressed lymphocyte function after bereavement, *Lancet* **1**:834–836.

Berczi, I., Nagy, E., and Mckenzie, C. E., 1986, Pituitary control of hemolymphopoietic tissue and immune function, Abstracts 6th International Congress Immunology, Toronto, Canada.

Besedovsky, H. O., del Rey, A. E., Sorkin, E., Da Prada, M., and Keller, H. H., 1979, Immunoregulation mediated by the sympathetic nervous system, *Cell. Immunol.* **48**:346–355.

Calabrese, J. R., Kling, M. A., and Gold, P. W., 1987, Alterations in immunocompetence during stress, bereavement, and depression, *Am. J. Psychiatry* **144**:1123–1134.

Endicott, J., Cohen, J., Neel, J., Fleiss, J., and Sarantakos, S., 1981, Hamilton depression rating scale, *Arch. Gen. Psychiatry* **38**:98–103.

Glaser, R., and Kiecolt-Glaser, J. K., 1986, Stress and the immune function, *Clin. Neuropharmacol. Suppl.* **4**:485–487.

Jackson, J. C., Cross, R. G., Walker, R. F., Markesberg, W. R., Brooks, W. H., and Roszman, T. L., 1985, Influence of serotonin on the immune response, *Immunology* **54**:505–506.

Kiecolt-Glaser, J. K., Fisher, L. D., Ogrocki, P., Stout, J. C., Speicher, C. E., and Glaser, R., 1987, Marital quality, marital disruption, and immune function, *Psychosom. Med.* **49**:13–34.

Kronfol, Z., Silva, J., Greden, J., Dembinski, S., Gardner, R., and Carroll, B., 1983, Impaired lymphocyte function in depressive illness, *Life Sci.* **33**:241–247.

Mathews, P. M., Forelick, C. J., Sibbitt, W. L., and Bankhurst, A. D., 1983, Enhancement of natural cytotoxicity by beta endorphin, *J. Immunol.* **130**:1658–1662.

Murasko, D. M., Weiner, P., and Kaye, D., 1987, Decline in mitogen induced proliferation of lymphocytes with increasing age, *Clin. Exp. Immunol.* **70**:440–448.

Murphy, D. L., Groodwin, F. K., and Bunney, W. E., 1971, Leukocytosis during lithium treatment, *Am. J. Psychiatry* **127**:1559–1561.

Naor, S., Assael, M., Pecht, M., Trainin, N., and Samuel, D., 1983, Correlation between emotional reaction to loss of an unborn child and lymphocyte response to mitogenic stimulation in women, *Isr. J. Psychiatry Relat. Sci.* **20**:231–239.

Rossof, A. H., and Fehir, K. M., 1978, Lithium stimulation of granulopoiesis, *N. Engl. J. Med.* **298**:280–281.

Schleifer, S. J., Keller, S. E., Camerino, M., Thornton, J. C., and Stein, M., 1983, Suppression of lymphocyte stimulation following bereavement, *J. Am. Med. Assoc.* **250**:374–377.

Schleifer, S. J., Keller, S. E., Meyerson, A. T., Raskin, M. J., Davis, K. L., and Stein, M., 1984, Lymphocyte function in major depressive disorder, *Arch. Gen. Psychiatry* **41**:484–486.

Schleifer, S. J., Keller, S. E., Siris, S. G., Davis, K. L., and Stein, M., 1985, Depression and immunity, *Arch. Gen. Psychiatry* **42**:129–133.

Sengar, D. P. S., Waters, B. G. H., Dunne, J. V., and Bouer, I. M., 1982, Lymphocyte subpopulations and mitogenic responses of lymphocytes in manic depressive disorders, *Biol. Psychiatry* **17**:1017–1022.

Spitzer, R. L., Endicott, J., and Robins, E., 1978, Research diagnostic criteria, rationale and reliability, *Arch. Gen. Psychiatry* **35**:773–782.

Chapter 19

Lymphokine-Activated Killer (LAK) Cell Activity in Psychiatric Illness

Ziad A. Kronfol, Madhavan P. N. Nair, Kavita Goel, Joann Goodson, and Stanley A. Schwartz

INTRODUCTION

There is now a great deal of evidence that the central nervous system and the immune system are closely interrelated (Ader, 1981). Messengers from the brain are now known to affect immune regulation. Similarly, secretory products of immune cells and tissues can affect brain function. A number of investigators have recently studied the integrity of the immune response in patients with psychiatric disorders. Several immune abnormalities were identified in patients with major depression. These include lymphocytopenia (Kronfol *et al.*, 1984), reduction in circulating T cell numbers (Schleifer *et al.*, 1984), impairment in mitogen-induced lymphocyte proliferation (Kronfol *et al.*, 1983), and a decrease in natural killer (NK) cell activity (Kronfol *et al.*, 1989). Similarly, abnormalities in immune regulation in schizophrenia have also been reported. These include an increase in the number of B lymphocytes, a decrease in NK cell activity, and an increase in the

Ziad A. Kronfol, Kavita Goel, and Joann Goodson • *Department of Psychiatry, University of Michigan Medical Center, Ann Arbor, Michigan 48109.* Madhavan P. N. Nair • *Departments of Psychiatry, Pediatrics, and Epidemiology, University of Michigan Medical Center, Ann Arbor, Michigan 48109.* Stanley A. Schwartz • *Departments of Pediatrics and Epidemiology, University of Michigan Medical Center, Ann Arbor, Michigan 48109.*

level of specific immunoglobulins and/or specific antibrain antibodies (DeLisi, 1984).

Cytotoxic immune systems constitute an important part of the host defense mechanisms and provide protection against a variety of pathogens including virus-infected cells and neoplasm. In addition to NK and cytotoxic T lymphocytes, a new cytotoxic immune system has recently been identified: lymphokine-activated killer (LAK) cytotoxicity. In the present study, we report our preliminary data on LAK cell activity in two psychiatric conditions: major depression and schizophrenia.

MATERIALS AND METHODS

Subjects

Subjects for the study were eight psychiatric patients and eight age- and sex-matched normal controls. Five patients suffered a major affective disorder, while three patients were diagnosed as having schizophrenia. Subjects were excluded from the study if they had a history of medical illness or were taking drugs known to interfere with immune regulation, including psychoactive medications. Diagnoses were made blindly by certified psychiatrists in accordance with Research Diagnostic Criteria (Spitzer *et al.*, 1977).

Methods

Blood was drawn from each patient and his/her matched control at the same time of the day (9:00 a.m.) to control for possible diurnal variation. LAK cell activity assays were run *in vitro* on fresh blood samples as previously described (Nair and Schwartz, 1988). Briefly, blood was centrifuged over Ficoll–Hypaque and run over a G-10 Sephadex column to isolate peripheral blood lymphocytes. A fixed number of lymphocytes was then incubated for 5 days in a complete medium to which 10 units of recombinant interleukin 2 was added to generate LAK cells. LAK cell cytotoxicity was then measured using a standard 4-hr ^{51}Cr release assay against SB, an NK-resistant cell line. Results are expressed in percent cytotoxicity. Comparisons between patients and matched controls were made using a paired *t*-test analysis.

RESULTS

Figure 1 shows the results of LAK cell activity in psychiatric patients and matched controls. Psychiatric patients had lower ($p < 0.05$) LAK cell cytotoxicity

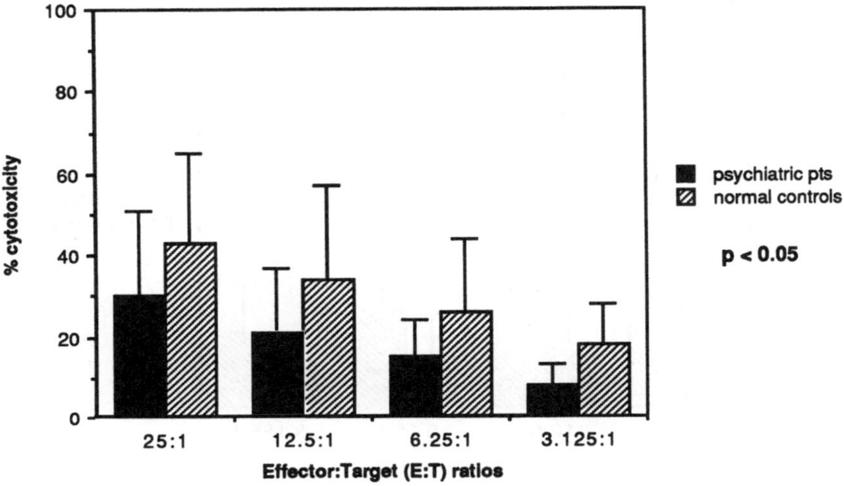

Figure 1. LAK cell activity in psychiatric patients and matched normal controls.

against SB target cells. This pattern was found for all four effector:target (E:T) cell ratios used.

We then examined whether this impairment in LAK cell activity is characteristic of major depression, schizophrenia, or whether it is found in both psychiatric conditions.

Figure 2 shows the results of LAK cell activity in the depressed patients compared to their matched controls. Depressed patients had markedly lower percent cytotoxicites against SB than their matched controls across all E:T ratios used.

Similarly, the LAK cell activity of schizophrenic patients compared to their matched controls is shown in Fig. 3. Again, the LAK cell activity of schizophrenic patients was markedly reduced compared to that of matched normal controls.

CONCLUSION

These results show that LAK cell activity, a cytotoxic immune function, is reduced in patients with severe psychiatric illness compared to age- and sex-matched normal controls. Although the number of patients in each group is small, this reduction in LAK cell activity seems to occur both in major depression and in schizophrenia. Larger samples are needed to confirm these results. An impairment

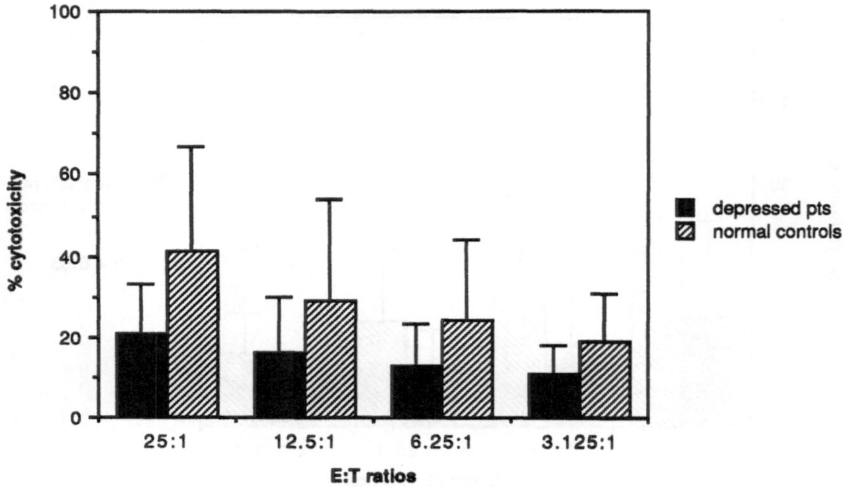

Figure 2. LAK cell activity in depressed patients and their matched controls.

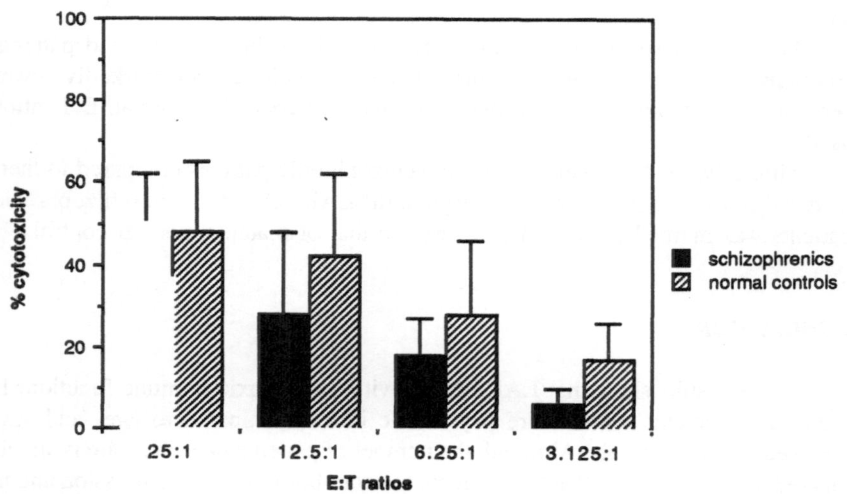

Figure 3. LAK cell activity in schizophrenic patients and their matched controls.

in LAK cell activity in psychiatric patients, if confirmed, provides another example of immune dysregulation in psychiatric illness. The clinical significance of these findings remains to be determined.

ACKNOWLEDGMENTS This work was supported in part by grants from the National Institute of Mental Health (MH42988) and the National Institute of Alcohol Abuse and Alcoholism (AA07378).

REFERENCES

Ader, R., 1981, *Psychoneuroimmunology*, Academic Press, New York.

DeLisi, L., 1984, Is immune dysfunction associated with schizophrenia? A review of the data, *Psychopharmacol. Bull.* **20**:509–513.

Kronfol, Z., Silva, J., Greden, J., Dembinski, S., Gardner, R., and Carroll, B., 1983, Impaired lymphocyte function in depressive illness, *Life Sci.* **33**:241–247.

Kronfol, Z., Turner, R., Nasrallah, H., and Winokur, G., 1984, Leukocyte regulation in depression and schizophrenia, *Psychiatry Res.* **13**:13–18.

Kronfol, Z., Nair, M., Goodson, J., Goel, K., Haskett, R., and Schwartz, S., 1989, Natural killer cell activity in depressive illness: Preliminary report, *Biol. Psychiatry* **26**:753–756.

Nair, M. P. N., and Schwartz, S. A., 1989, Immunoregulation of lymphokine-activated killer (LAK) cells, *Clin. Immunol. Immunopathol.* **49**:28–40.

Schleifer, S. J., Keller, S. E., Meyerson, A. T., Raskin, M. J., Davis, K. L., and Stein, M., 1984, Lymphocyte function in major depressive disorder, *Arch. Gen. Psychiatry* **41**:484–486.

Spitzer, R., Endicott, J., and Robins, E., 1977, *Research Diagnostic Criteria (RDC) for a Selected Group of Functional Disorders*, New York State Psychiatric Institute, New York.

Chapter **20**

Immunity, Cortisol and Psychiatric Disorders

Ziad Kronfol and J. Daniel House

INTRODUCTION

Stress and psychiatric illness are often accompanied by a disturbance in hypothalamic–pituitary–adrenal activity, frequently resulting in the secretion of excessive amounts of cortisol, an immunosuppressive hormone (Carroll *et al.*, 1976). We therefore hypothesized that psychiatric disorders such as depression, mania, and schizophrenia are associated with immune abnormalities, and that many of these abnormalities can be explained on the basis of increased secretion of cortisol. The present study was therefore conducted to characterize several aspects of immune dysfunction in psychiatric illness and to investigate the role of cortisol in such immune dysregulation.

MATERIAL AND METHODS

Subjects

Subjects for the study were patients who were hospitalized for psychiatric illness and normal controls. Psychiatric diagnoses were made by at least two psychiatrists in accordance with DSM-III criteria (APA, 1982). Four groups of subjects were identified: (1) patients with major depressive episode ($n = 40$); (2)

Ziad Kronfol and J. Daniel House • *Department of Psychiatry, University of Michigan Medical Center, Ann Arbor, Michigan 48109 and Northern Illinois University, DeKalb, Illinois 60115.*

manic patients ($n = 11$); (3) schizophrenic patients ($n = 22$); and (4) normal controls ($n = 37$). There were no significant age or sex differences among the groups. Subjects were excluded from the study if they had a coincidental medical illness or were taking drugs known to interfere with immune regulation.

Methods

Blood samples were drawn from patients and controls and the following assays were conducted: (1) total leukocyte (WBC) count; (2) *in vitro* lymphocyte response to the mitogens phytohemagglutinin-P (PHA), concanavalin A (Con A), and pokeweed mitogen (PWM); and (3) plasma cortisol levels. The WBC count was done using standard techniques. Lymphocyte mitogenic responses were assayed as described previously (Kronfol and House, 1989). Cortisol concentrations were obtained using standard radioimmunoassay procedures.

Statistical analyses were done with analyses of variance (ANOVA). Results were considered statistically significant if $p < 0.05$ two-tailed.

RESULTS

Table 1 shows the results of the WBC count, the lymphocyte mitogenic responses, and the plasma cortisol levels in the four groups. The WBC count was significantly higher in all three groups of patients in comparison to the normal controls. There were no significant differences among the groups in the lymphocyte cultures in the absence of mitogen ("blank"), but significant differences emerged when mitogens were added to the cultures. Specifically, patients with affective disorders (either depression or mania) had significantly lower lymphocyte mitogenic responses than either the schizophrenic group or the normal control group. There were no significant differences in mitogenic responses between schizophrenic patients and normal controls. Plasma cortisol values were elevated in all three groups of psychiatric patients and were significantly higher in patients with depression, mania, or schizophrenia compared to normal controls.

Correlations between plasma cortisol values and the immune measures are shown in Table 2. There were no significant associations between cortisol values and total WBC counts or lymphocyte mitogenic responses in the subjects under investigation.

CONCLUSION

This study confirms the existence of immune abnormalities in patients with various psychiatric disorders (DeLisi *et al.*, 1984; Calabrese *et al.*, 1987). Specifi-

Table 1. WBC Counts, Lymphocyte Mitogenic Responses[a], and Cortisol Values in Patients with Different Psychiatric Diagnoses and Normal Controls[b]

	Depression	Mania	Schizophrenia	Normal controls	p
WBC/mm^3	8,556 ± 3,016*	7,867 ± 2,597*	7,797 ± 2,404*	6,786 ± 1,779	0.0313
Blank[a]	1,056 ± 859	718 ± 408	1,031 ± 405	940 ± 702	N.S.
PHA	146,253 ± 60,546	121,957 ± 36,054*†	164,764 ± 64,022	177,772 ± 66,866	0.0665
Con A	88,815 ± 47,037*†	76,501 ± 24,534*	137,843 ± 65,032	151,066 ± 84,373	0.0002
PWM	77,716 ± 28,820*†	70,660 ± 24,398*†	133,370 ± 130,060	109,275 ± 62,558	0.0225
Cortisol (μg/dl)	16.1 ± 4.2*	17.2 ± 4.2*	16.1 ± 2.8*	10.8 ± 5.2	0.0001

[a]Results of the lymphocyte mitogenic responses are expressed in scintillation counts per minute (cpm).
[b]Adapted from Kronfol and House, 1988, and Kronfol and House, 1989.
*Significantly different from controls.
†Significantly different from schizophrenia.

Table 2. Correlation between Plasma Cortisol Values and the Immune Measures

	r	*p*
WBC	0.093	N.S.
Blank	−0.162	N.S.
PHA	−0.091	N.S.
Con A	−0.088	N.S.
PWM	−0.103	N.S.

cally, both depression and mania are associated with leukocytosis and a suppression of mitogen-induced lymphocyte proliferation, while schizophrenia is accompanied by a milder leukocytosis with no evidence of abnormal lymphocyte mitogenic responses. These findings are also in accordance with our previous work (Kronfol *et al.*, 1983) and the work of others (Schleifer *et al.*, 1984). Although plasma cortisol values were significantly elevated in all three groups of psychiatric patients, there were no significant correlations between the cortisol values and the immune variables. This finding also confirms our previously obtained results on a different group of patients where the hormonal variable was urinary free cortisol excretion (Kronfol *et al.*, 1986). We therefore conclude that psychiatric disorders are associated with specific immune abnormalities that cannot be explained solely on the basis of increased cortisol values. Other hormones and/or neurotransmitters are therefore likely to be involved in the immune dysregulation in these patients.

ACKNOLWEDGMENTS This work was supported in part by grants from the National Institute of Mental Health (MH42988) and the National Institute of Alcohol Abuse and Alcoholism (AA07378).

REFERENCES

American Psychiatric Association, 1982, *Diagnostic and Statistical Manual of Mental Disorders*, 3rd ed., Washington, D.C.

Calabrese, J., Kling, M., and Gold, P. W., 1987, Alterations in immunocompetence during stress, bereavement, and depression: Focuses on neuroendocrine regulation, *Am. J. Psychiatry* **144**:1123–1134.

Carroll, B., Curtis, G., Davis, B. M., Mendel, J., Sugerman, A., 1976, Urinary free cortisol excretion in depression. *Psychol. Med.* **6**:43–50.

DeLisi, L. E., King, A. C., and Targum, S., 1984, Serum immunoglobulin concentrations in patients admitted to an acute psychiatric inpatient service, *Br. J. Psychiatry* **145**:661–665.

Kronfol, Z., and House, J. D., 1988, Immune function in mania, *Biol. Psychiatry* **24**:341–343.
Kronfol, Z., and House, J. D., 1989, Lymphocyte mitogenesis, immunoglobulin and complement levels in depressed patients and normal controls, *Acta Psychiatr. Scand.* **80**:142–147.
Kronfol, Z., Silva, J., Greden, J., Dembinski, S., Gardner, R., and Caroll, B., 1983, Impaired lymphocyte function in depressive illness, *Life Sci.* **33**:241–247.
Kronfol, Z., House, J. D., Silva, J., Greden, J., and Caroll, B., 1986, Depression, urinary free cortisol excretion and lymphocyte function, *Br. J. Psychiatry* **148**:70–73.
Schleifer, S. J., Keller, S. E., Meyerson, A. T., Raskin, M. J., Davis, K. L., and Stein, M., 1984, Lymphocyte function in major depressive disorder, *Arch. Gen. Psychiatry* **41**:484–486.

Part **IV**

Viral Fatigue Syndrome and Antivirals

Chapter **21**

Viruses and Fatigue

The Current Status of the Chronic Fatigue Syndrome

Simon Wessely

INTRODUCTION

Perhaps none of the subjects covered in the last edition of this book have changed so quickly as the vexed topic of "postviral" fatigue. When James Jones and Bruce Miller (Jones and Miller, 1987) reviewed the situation, the general theme was one of optimism, and despite an awareness of remaining uncertainties and difficulties, progress in understanding the relationship between viruses and chronic fatigue states was anticipated. Sadly, in the subsequent 3 years little of this optimism has been realized. Even the title of the current contribution is different, reflecting increasing international skepticism concerning the exclusive role of viruses. The new term favored for the condition is "chronic fatigue syndrome" (CFS) (Holmes *et al.*, 1988; Lloyd *et al.*, 1988a), as it is accurate, short, and carries no unproven etiological implications. It will be used in the rest of this chapter to refer to the various illnesses described as "myalgic encephalomyelitis" or "Royal Free Disease" in Britain and Australia, and "chronic Epstein–Barr virus infection" or "chronic mononucleosis" in the United States.

The current hypothesis underlying CFS is simple: that a viral illness is a cause

Simon Wessely • *Department of Psychological Medicine, Institute of Psychiatry, Camberwell, London SE5 8AF, United Kingdom.*

of chronic fatigue. The evidence relevant to the hypothesis is far from simple, and can only be evaluated in the light of the often profound methodological difficulties confronting researchers. These are best illustrated by the confusion concerning the epidemiology of CFS (David *et al.*, 1988). There are few estimates of the occurrence of CFS, and these vary considerably: from 140 cases in 6 months (Calder *et al.*, 1987) in a general practice population of 10,000 (annual rate = 280/10,000) to a hospital estimate of an annual rate of 3–5 per 100,000 (Behan and Behan, 1988). Estimates in the United States vary as widely. What is indisputable is that there is now an epidemic of patients believing they have one or other form of CFS. Self-help organizations are appearing from Alaska (Anonymous, 1986) via Hong Kong (Sinclair, 1988) to New Zealand (Murdoch, 1988). In Britain the main self-help group for patients, the M.E. Association, is the fastest growing charity with 150 new members joining each week (Smith, 1989), and in both Britain and the United States self-help groups are acting as effective political pressure groups.

METHODOLOGICAL DIFFICULTIES

Case–Control Studies and Postviral Fatigue

Nearly all the published work in postviral fatigue uses a case–control design. Cases are selected by disease status, matched with nondisease controls, and then the levels of exposure, which may be any agent the investigator believes of interest, are measured and compared between cases and controls. This is a reputable method of determining relevant associations between pathogens and disease, but is also the most susceptible to bias if performed incorrectly (Rothman, 1986). Unfortunately, the published literature contains many examples in which bias has been inadvertently introduced by poor design.

Case Definition

Problems commence with case definition. Fatigue is part of the human condition, and in certain circumstances all of us have known extreme fatigue. It is a subjective experience, with wide variation according to personality and social desirability (May and Kline, 1988). It is a difficult symptom to record: in one reliability study (Jenkins *et al.*, 1988) the kappa statistic for fatigue was 0.02, indicating agreement only marginally above the chance level. In both normals and depressives, chronic fatigue may be a quantitative rather than a qualitative variable (Monk, 1989; see Wessely and Thomas, 1990). The implication is that future work should adopt a dimensional rather than a categorical approach to the key symptom, fatigue. This is not a new suggestion; Wells (1908) advocated "shifting the viewpoint from the measurement of discrete states of fatigue to continuous determinations of susceptibility."

Furthermore, the symptoms required for diagnosis have changed over time (Archer, 1987; Wessely and Thomas, 1990), especially in the United Kingdom. Originally an acute infective illness with paralytic manifestations, cranial nerve palsies, with fatigue only occurring in half of the cases (Parish, 1978; Compston, 1978), current descriptions are of a noninfective, sporadic condition in which muscular and mental fatigue are now pathognomic (Ramsay, 1986; Behan and Behan, 1988). However, even the current symptoms lack specificity. Wessely and Powell (1989) compared hospital cases of CFS with neuromuscular and affective controls, and found that the symptoms now viewed as characteristic, such as physical fatigue, fatigue after exercise, and muscle pain after exercise, still possess little or no discriminant ability. Only mental fatigue had diagnostic utility, being present in both the CFS and affective disorder groups, but not in neuromuscular disease unless there was coexisting psychiatric disorder. The conclusion, supported by neurophysiological studies (Lloyd *et al.*, 1988b; Stokes *et al.*, 1988), was that the fatigue in CFS is largely of central rather than peripheral origin. Such a conclusion runs contrary to the conclusions of some of those doctors identified with CFS in England, although will be more readily accepted in the United States.

If clinical symptoms are unreliable, what about laboratory tests? Unfortunately, no test exists that is specific for CFS. A variety of biochemical, electromyographic, histopathological, or imaging abnormalities have been proposed, but have either not been replicated or have been found to be due to the effects of disuse (see David *et al.*, 1988; Wessely and Thomas, 1990). Serological criteria will be considered later, but it should be clear that their use introduces a circularity into the definition of the syndrome. The diagnosis of CFS remains a clinical one.

Further problems in case definition are caused by the fact that many groups use the term to describe very different illnesses. For example, there is now little doubt that there exists a small subgroup of patients with clinical evidence of major end organ dysfunction related to persistent viral infection. An example from the British literature is evidence linking enteroviruses in the etiology of cardiac and pericardiac disease (Bowles *et al.*, 1986; Muir *et al.*, 1989). As a consequence, others (Yousef *et al.*, 1988) have included patients with clinical pericarditis within series of CFS patients. In the United States a similar process has resulted in the rare patients with clinical organ dysfunction, extreme elevation of replicative EBV antigens, and a high mortality from cancers of the immune system (Henle *et al.*, 1987; Jones *et al.*, 1988) being included within studies of CFS. This may lead to further confusion, since such patients have a condition that is clinically easily distinguished from chronic fatigue of unknown cause. Including them within research samples will lead to an overestimation of the association between CFS and EBV in the United States, or with Coxsackie in the United Kingdom. Patients with chronic active EBV infection, or viral cardiomyopathy will not be discussed further. Finally, there is now a rapidly growing literature on fibromyalgia, a condition with considerable relevance to CFS, but in Britain at least, largely ignored. This serves further to emphasize the unsatisfactory nature of current case definitions.

Selection Bias

Nearly all published studies suffer from several selection biases, of which the most serious is selection by exposure under investigation. In all case–control studies it is fundamental that the ascertainment of cases of disease is independent of exposure status (Rothman, 1986). In the studies of postviral fatigue, the diagnosis of disease ("postviral fatigue") is frequently influenced by a knowledge of exposure (history of viral infection). In two studies (Yousef *et al.*, 1988; Hotchin *et al.*, 1989) that show an association between serological markers of infection (enterovirus and EBV, respectively) and postviral fatigue, people became cases because of their exposure status. Patients were recruited by the medical adviser to a self-help organization for people with "postviral fatigue." Many of these patients felt they had been exposed to a virus, otherwise they would not have joined that particular organization. The medical adviser recruiting patients (and controls) was also aware of exposure status, so it is possible that further selection took place at this stage, such as the exclusion of those lacking a history suggestive of a viral illness (the opposite occurring for neighborhood controls). Cases are in effect being selected by a risk factor which is then being measured. In view of the overlap between exposure status and ascertainment of cases and controls, the finding of differences between "cases" and "controls" is difficult to interpret.

Selection bias also operates long before the patient reaches the research team. The symptoms of fatigue are common, so general practitioners may be more likely to refer to centers with an interest in postviral fatigue patients with a history of infection, which may or may not be relevant. For example, studies of chronic EBV infection have used "highly selected patients referred to investigators known to have an interest in chronic EBV infection" (Buchwald *et al.*, 1987). Depressed patients with prominent fatigue and sleep difficulties are more likely to be referred to physicians than those presenting with more obvious cognitive features such as guilt and suicidal ideation (Dew *et al.*, 1988).

Bias is also introduced by social class. The symptom of chronic fatigue shows a negative socioeconomic gradient in community studies (Cox *et al.*, 1987). However, nearly all current work on CFS acknowledges a positive socioeconomic gradient, with an overrepresentation of upper social classes, in particular health service professions. Indeed, this has led to the unpleasant term "yuppie flu" (Seligmann *et al.*, 1986). Such a label, even if perjorative, implies that this is a new finding. However, this is not so (Wessely, 1990b). Savage (1875) reported that fatigue was commonest in professions requiring an unflagging devotion to work, or a high degree of emotional stress. Since then, the overrepresentation of higher social classes has been a constant finding (Taylor, 1907; Dowden and Johnson, 1929; Macy and Allen, 1933–1934). Kraepelin (1902) described neurasthenia, the forerunner of CFS, as "one of the products of civilisation, confined largely to the professional and clerical callings, and to women of the middle classes." Such historical evidence disproves the occasional attempt to link this syndrome with various "toxic" agents encountered in modern life (Hall and MacPhee, 1985). It also indicates further bias in published studies based on such samples, which is almost certainly the result of social class differences in health care utilization.

Information Bias

The commonest information bias is the absence of data concerning psychological symptoms. In studies that have looked for them, emotional symptoms, however defined, are intimately associated with fatigue states, for example occurring in 80% of a series of 500 patients (Behan and Behan, 1988). However, many studies make no mention of any psychological variables. Others acknowledge that emotional symptoms are almost invariably present (Fegan *et al.*, 1983; Bell *et al.*, 1988b), but do not collect this information systematically, or use it in a meaningful way. A recent editorial on lassitude (Havard, 1985) stated that "failure to diagnose depression is usually due to failure to seek it rather than to any confusion in diagnostic symptoms."

Further difficulties are the overlap between the symptoms of depression and those of viral infection. If the two occur in sequence (either in consequence or by chance), it is difficult for the doctor, let alone patient, to distinguish between them. In these circumstances it is easy to conclude, often erroneously, that an infective episode is still continuing (Imboden, 1972).

Recall Bias

Recall bias adds further inaccuracy. Patients who believe they have the disease are highly motivated to remember their viral illness, as they attribute this as the cause of their troubles. An inadvertent example of this is provided by Meijer *et al.* (1988). In a study of the relationship between influenza and psychiatric disorder in adolescents, those with greater psychopathology were more likely to report a previous episode of influenza. The authors conclude this is evidence for "post-influenzal psychiatric disorder." However, there were no differences in the levels of influenza antibody between cases and controls. Instead, psychiatric disorder may have caused those affected to be more likely to recall clinical influenza, although this was not confirmed in a new population study (Wessely, unpublished data).

Measurement Bias (Difficulties in Ascertaining Exposure)

If it is difficult to define the disease state, it is almost as difficult to define the presumed exposure, a viral infection. Both within subject variability and observer variability have been noted.

The levels of detectable antibody to many viruses, including EBV, are altered by many confounding factors. Of particular relevance is that stress alone can alter EBV titers (Kiecolt-Glaser *et al.*, 1984). Virtually any chronic stress or intercurrent illness has the capacity to reactivate latent infection or cause an amnestic antibody response, as will any cause of lymphocyte activation (Johnson, 1982). The use of normal controls may be inappropriate in case–control studies of CFS (Straus, 1988; Wessely and Powell, 1989).

Turning to observer variation, many laboratories use different standardizations, and there is evidence of poor reliability within and among laboratories (Holmes *et al.*, 1987). Determination of immunofluoresence depends upon "subjective interpretation of visualised fluorescence" (DeLisi *et al.*, 1986), and is subject to the difficulties in reliability inherent in all bioassays (Merlin, 1986). Finally, it is well known that many clinically apparent viral infections cannot be detected by the available laboratory tests; false-negatives are a problem in addition to false-positives.

Case–Control Studies: Conclusion

Case–control studies are a valid method of estimating the relative risk of an exposure such as a viral illness, provided that both cases and controls are representative of a defined population, and that case selection is independent of exposure. It is clear that neither of these rules has been adhered to in some of the studies reviewed. Most of these biases are not random, and result in overestimation of the relationship between exposure to viruses and fatigue.

Case–control studies, even if correctly executed, may not be the most appropriate for this problem. They are restricted to one particular clinical problem, the disease nominated by the investigator. As it is empirically unlikely that a single infectious agent will be associated with only one outcome, a more powerful design is to define exposure, and then look at a number of possible disease outcomes over time, as in a cohort study. The few studies that conform to this design will be reviewed later.

David *et al.* (1988) have pointed out the problems in case definition, and advocated the use of operational criteria. Since then, although not as a result, at least three case definitions have been published. Unfortunately, problems still remain.

The current operational criteria propose a mixture of clinical and laboratory data, using major and minor criteria analogous to the Duckett–Jones criteria for rheumatic fever (Holmes *et al.*, 1988; Lloyd *et al.*, 1988a). These are useful, as at least they will permit comparisons to be made, but are only as good as the component parts. Already problems have arisen as the rules may be too restrictive: in one study of those who clinically appeared to have chronic fatigue, only 5% of patients fulfilled the criteria (Manu *et al.*, 1988b), the majority being excluded as cases of psychiatric disorder. Recognition that criteria excluding psychiatric disorder may be throwing out the baby with the bath water led to recent alterations in the operational criteria (Komaroff *et al.*, 1989). Operational criteria are an improvement, but to state that the disease is a "common, discrete and easily diagnosable clinical illness" (Bell and Bell, 1988) is both optimistic and inaccurate.

WHAT IS THE RELEVANCE OF EXPOSURE TO DISEASE?

Epidemiology of Viruses and Fatigue

First, the association between viruses and fatigue may be a chance one. Considering just enteroviruses alone, the average individual has between one and four infections per year. Subclinical infections are commoner, and the majority of Coxsackie virus and echovirus infections are not associated with significant clinical problems (Johnson, 1982); indeed, the ratio of infected individuals to known serious clinical cases is 1000:1 (Pallansch, 1988). Commonest of all are self-reported viral infections. Between 25 and 40% of adults felt they had suffered a "cold or 'flu' " in the previous month (Cox *et al.*, 1987), compared with a previous finding of 32% for "cold" and 18% for "influenza" (Dunnell and Cartwright, 1972). The United States National Health Survey listed annual rates of various viral infections: for combined age group 18–44 the total was 90 viral infections per 100 people. In both studies there is a steady fall from peak values in late adolescence (which does not match the age distribution of fatigue).

Turning to fatigue, there is no doubt that the symptom is also widely distributed in the population. Henry Miller (1987) has aptly described "The vague sense of being under the weather is what most people, if asked, will admit to most of the time." Translated into epidemiological terms, this becomes "the fact that a large proportion of the population has the occasional symptom of dysphoria, fatigue or insomnia probably accounts for the high rates reported by earlier surveys" (Goldberg and Huxley, 1980). However, more modern studies have shown that chronic fatigue, arbitrarily defined as more than 1 month in duration, still occurs in between 20 and 30% of the population (Chen, 1986). For example, Kroenke *et al.* (1988) surveyed 1159 consecutive clinic attenders. Cases were those who felt that fatigue was a "major problem" for 1 month, although the mean duration was actually 3.3 years, and the overall prevalence was 24%. As in all other studies, chronic fatigue was commoner in women than men. Buchwald *et al.* (1987) were surprised to find that 21% of all practice attenders satisfied their criteria for "chronic EBV" syndrome. In the first systematic study of psychiatric illness in general practice in the United Kingdom (Shepherd *et al.*, 1981), 16% of males and 24% of females admitted to rising in the morning feeling tired and exhausted, while similar percentages felt that working tired them completely. These figures rose when the sample was restricted to those with psychiatric diagnoses, and rose again in a sample of psychiatric outpatients. Better primary care studies are needed, and although we cannot conclude that all such patients have CFS, but it is already clear that patients with chronic fatigue in both primary care and general hospitals experience personal morbidity and functional impairment similar to that found in chronic medical patients (Kroenke *et al.*, 1988; Wessely and Powell, 1989).

Given the high prevalence of both chronic fatigue and self-reported viral infections, the association of any cause of fatigue and a viral infection will occur by chance in a large number of people. It has also been shown that this figure will be elevated by such factors as selection and recall bias. Samples selected from either self-help groups, or referred to centers with a known interest in CFS, will inevitably contain an overrepresentation of those in whom the association between viruses and fatigue has occurred by chance alone. Such sampling bias will not be corrected by comparison with normal controls.

EBV and CFS

In the United States, but not in the United Kingdom, there has been intense professional and media speculation concerning a possible link between CFS and EBV. However, after initial enthusiasm following the publication of several studies reviewed by Jones and Miller (1987), such optimism is now giving way to pessimism. The marker originally thought to indicate continuing chronic EBV infection was antibody to the early antigen (EBV-EA) (Tobi *et al.*, 1982; Straus *et al.*, 1985). One U.K. study has found antibody to EBV-EA elevation in 20% of selected cases of CFS (Hotchin *et al.*, 1989). However, it is known that many asymptomatic patients continue to show such antibody for 2 to 4 years after full recovery from EBV (Horwitz *et al.*, 1985). Hellinger *et al.* (1988) were unable to find clinical differences between patients with or without EBV-EA antibody, and also found EBV-EA antibody in 18% of asymptomatic blood donors at the Mayo Clinic, with extreme elevation (greater than 1 in 160) in 3%. Similarly, Buchwald *et al.* (1987) found EBV-EA elevation to levels they had previously regarded as abnormal in 43% of controls. The role of EBV nuclear antigen (EBV-NA) is still unclear: lack of antibody to the nuclear antigen remains a possible association of CFS.

Some (Holmes *et al.*, 1987), but not others (Hotchin *et al.*, 1989) report not only elevated titers to EBV, but also to cytomegalovirus, herpes simplex, and measles. There is also no evidence of increased viral burden based on direct assessment of viral load (Schooley, 1988). Finally, there is no evidence of any relationship between clinical symptoms of fatigue and laboratory findings, nor between clinical recovery and the resolution of any serological or immunological abnormalities, even in patients specifically selected for serological abnormalities (Schooley, 1988; Straus *et al.*, 1988; Katon *et al.*, 1988). The current consensus is that EBV serology has no obvious place in the diagnosis of CFS (Straus, 1988; Borysiewicz, 1989).

Coxsackie Viruses and CFS

In the United Kingdom, attention has been focused on the role of the Coxsackie viruses in the etiology of CFS. These are promising candidates, in view of their known myo- and neurotropic actions. Furthermore, interpretation of serological findings is less complex as neither latency nor reactivation has yet been demonstrated. Although previous serological tests have been unsatisfactory, this too has recently changed. The development of an ELISA test for Coxsackie IgM (Bell *et al.*, 1988a) promised a better measure of current or recent infection. It was found in 5–9% of community controls (Bell *et al.*, 1988a). In a hospital series, enterovirus IgM was detected in 31% of cases of CFS, compared to 12% of controls (Banatavala and Muir, personal communication). However, a case–control study of CFS in primary care apparently failed to show any difference in Coxsackie antibody titers between cases and controls (Dawson, 1987).

So far the main evidence is provided by the study of Yousef *et al.* (1988). They reported that 17/76 (22%) of patients referred with postviral fatigue syndrome had enteroviral infection demonstrated by positive stool cultures, which persisted in 5 at 1 year (7%). This is conventional evidence of persistent infection by Coxsackie in 7% of the sample. In a second sample an enteroviral antigen (the VP-1 antigen) was found in 44/87 (51%), persisting in 39 (45%) at 4 months. None was detected in 20 normal controls, although others have found VP-1 antigen in 12% of randomly selected neurological patients (Halpin and Wessely, 1989), while Lynch and Seth (1989) reported equivalent levels of the antigen in CFS patients and depressed controls. The problems of sensitivity and specificity, and the apparent lack of relationship between symptoms and serology, means that the clinical relevance of such findings remains unclear (Wright, 1989).

Perhaps the most exciting possibilities come from new molecular biological techniques. Coxsackie B virus-specific probes have been used to demonstrate viral RNA sequences in the cardiac muscle biopsies of patients with cardiomyopathy (Bowles *et al.*, 1986). Archard *et al.* (1988) reported the results of similar techniques in a sample of muscle biopsies in cases of CFS provided by the Glasgow group. Virus-specific RNA could be detected in 25/96 (26%) of specimens. Four controls were negative, but none of 50 orthopedic specimens previously analyzed were positive. Thus, virus RNA can be demonstrated in a minority of these highly selected patients. Nevertheless, this result shows that the muscles of some patients have been exposed to the virus, although the location of the virus-specific protein is yet to be determined. It does not show whether other tissues are similarly affected, when such exposure occurred (i.e., whether pre- or postmorbid), nor how this is related to the clinical syndrome.

Better clinical studies led to an increased skepticism about the importance of EBV in fatigue states. So far there is less information on the status of enteroviruses, but the realist must expect similar problems. It is already clear that, as in EBV, there is a dissociation between serological findings and clinical status (Calder *et al.*, 1987; Wilson *et al.*, 1989; Halpin and Wessely, 1989).

IMMUNE DYSFUNCTION

There has been a recent interest in possible immune dysfunction in CFS and its relationship to postviral states (Behan *et al.*, 1985; Lloyd *et al.*, 1988a). Straus (1988) has reviewed the immunological studies, and concluded that the findings are inconsistent and difficult to interpret. At present the only finding that has been both replicated and not disproved appears to be an increase in the levels of circulating immune complexes (Straus *et al.*, 1988; Yousef *et al.*, 1988). Most of the reasons for this unsatisfactory state of affairs have been covered in previous sections, in particular observer reliability, subject variability, normative data, and poor experimental design. Again, there is still no convincing evidence of a link between laboratory findings and clinical status, and some evidence to the contrary (Katon *et al*, 1988; Straus *et al.*, 1988).

There has been considerable interest in the role of interferon (IFN) in CFS, commencing with the clinical observation that exogenous IFN-α reproduced the neuropsychiatric features characteristic of CFS (MacDonald *et al.*, 1987), with a dose–response effect on performance measures (Smith *et al.*, 1988) Neither IFN-γ (Straus *et al.*, 1985; Jones *et al.*, 1985; Morte *et al.*, 1988; Lloyd *et al.*, 1988c) nor IFN-α (MacDonald, Burford, and Mann, personal communication) is elevated in CFS. Interest has shifted to the role of leukocyte 2′,5′-oligoadenylate synthetase, modestly increased in two series (Morag *et al.*, 1982; Straus *et al.*, 1985), which may indicate active suppression of IFN production.

Attention has also been given to interleukin 1 (IL-1). In animal studies it has been shown to activate T lymphocytes and induce fever by acting on the hypothalamus, leading to a decrease in REM sleep (Tobler *et al.*, 1984), and in the acute inflammatory response to be associated with changes in muscle metabolism (Baracos *et al.*, 1983; Dinarello, 1984), all of which is potentially relevant to CFS. There is an unpublished report of elevated IL-1β in 13/25 selected chronic fatigue patients (Behan, quoted in Dawson, 1989), although more modest elevations are known to occur in untrained normal men who overexert (Evans *et al.*, 1986). Given that activated T lymphocytes produce IL-2 (Rubin *et al.*, 1985), and that increased serum IL-2 has been associated with both schizophrenia and brain damage (Ganguli and Rabin, 1989), one might predict that reports of elevated IL-2 in CFS will be forthcoming. In the meantime, others have found significant reductions in IL-2 in CFS patients (Kibler *et al.*, 1985; Katon *et al.*, 1988).

A further problem is the role of psychiatric illness as a potential confounder. Readers of this volume will be well aware that psychiatric disorder is associated with immune dysfunction, although both the relevance and specificity of the observed changes are unclear, and perhaps simplistic (King and Cooper, 1989). Since there is no doubt that immune dysfunction causes an increased risk of infection, it is possible that psychiatric illness is associated with an increased risk of both immune disorder and viral infection. Psychiatric illness (like physical inactivity) is a potential confounder of any proposed link between viruses and chronic fatigue, viruses and immune disorder, and immune disorder and chronic fatigue. Just as no researcher into a possible carcinogen would fail to record smoking habits, no researcher in this equally complex field should neglect to measure psychiatric disorder.

CFS AND PSYCHIATRY

Is There a Specific Fatigue Syndrome?

Before CFS, postviral fatigue, or its variants can be accepted as a diagnostic entity, it is necessary to show that it is not identical to known psychiatric disorders. Regrettably, some have chosen to overcome this problem by ignoring it, but recent evidence has shown this to be unacceptable.

There is surprisingly little evidence that a specific fatigue syndrome exists for anything other than a brief period of time after a known viral illness. Perhaps the most convincing evidence comes from the prospective studies of White (1989), who confirmed that a fatigue syndrome does exist after definite EBV infection, as distinct from depression. It was more frequent and lasted longer (mean duration 9 weeks compared to 3 weeks) than post-EBV depression. Barsky *et al.* (1988) studied upper-respiratory-tract infections using both self-report and objective measures, and concluded that the "relationship between objective assessed medical morbidity and patients' subjective experience was surprisingly weak. Medical morbidity did not emerge as an impressive correlate of symptomatology, discomfort and disability." Even in the immediate outcome of minor infection, depression as an independent variable was a weak but significant predictor of the number of days disabled.

Furthermore, these are only short-term studies. By the time most CFS patients are seen in hospital, the mean duration already ranges from 18 months to 13 years (Buchwald *et al.*, 1987; Bell and Bell, 1988; Straus *et al.*, 1988; Wessely and Powell, 1989; Manu *et al.*, 1988a; Katon *et al.*, 1988).

Psychiatric Disorder and CFS

The principal associations of the complaint of chronic fatigue are the symptoms of depression and anxiety. This has been found in studies of the community (Chen, 1986), of students (Montgomery, 1983), and in primary care (Buchwald *et al.*, 1987; Kroenke *et al.*, 1988). The exact relationship between fatigue and psychiatric disorder (as opposed to psychiatric symptoms) has yet to be determined. However, there is strong evidence that most patients complaining of fatigue will have minor psychiatric morbidity, and that the rate of diagnosable psychiatric disorder increases with both the severity and duration of fatigue, as well as the number of accompanying symptoms (Goldberg and Huxley, 1980; Shepherd *et al.*, 1981; Clare and Blacker, 1986).

The only studies that utilize modern research diagnostic interviews in the evaluation of CFS have been conducted in the general hospital setting. There is now convincing evidence that the majority of CFS patients seen in hospital practice (which is where previous research has been based) satisfy criteria for psychiatric disorder. Manu *et al.* (1988a) screened 135 self-referrals to a special fatigue clinic in a university hospital: 67% had psychiatric diagnoses, 3% had medical diagnoses, 5% had operationally defined CFS, and 25% were unexplained. This suggests that further detailed screening of such patients for medical diagnoses has a low yield (Morrison, 1980; Havard, 1985; Hellinger *et al.*, 1988) and most continue to have medically unexplained fatigue.

There are now at least four studies of those referred by their physicians to hospital with chronic fatigue for which no medical explanation can be found. All studies report samples of patients with either physician or self diagnoses of CFS or its local equivalent. A Canadian group interviewed 24 patients with "neuromyasthenia" (Taerk *et al.*, 1987). Two thirds were current cases of major depression, while half had a history of affective disorder prior to the "fatiguing" illness. However, the research diagnostic criteria employed included fatigue as a symptom of psychiatric disorder, thus introducing an unwanted circularity into the results. Wessely and Powell (1989) studied 47 referrals to an English specialist neurology hospital with chronic unexplained fatigue, and found that 72% had a psychiatric diagnosis, using research diagnostic criteria modified to exclude fatigue. Two American studies gave similar figures (Katon *et al.*, 1988; Kruesi *et al.*, 1989). All reported that major depressive disorder was the commonest diagnosis, accounting for more than half of the sample, but it was not the only diagnosis, emphasizing the heterogeneity of CFS. In a separate small sample, Taerk and Abbey (1989) report that over 80% of selected CFS patients had a first-degree relative with psychiatric illness.

Many will be surprised at these high rates of psychiatric disorder, especially since many seem to go unrecognized by the physician. One explanation is provided by Kruesi *et al.*, (1989), who noted the marked dissociation that occurred between the perception of physical and psychological symptoms in these patient groups. This is related to the importance of physical attributions in determining referral patterns and acceptance of treatment (Wessely, 1990a). Wessely and Powell (1989) matched cases of CFS with cases of major depression in a psychiatric hospital. There were no symptomatic differences between the groups, but profound differences emerged in the pattern of responses to questions concerning self-diagnosis and symptom attribution. Physical, as opposed to psychological, explanations of illness, almost invariably to a virus, were the principal reason for the marked differences in referral patterns.

Conclusion

It thus appears that the majority of CFS in hospital practice patients have recognizable psychiatric disorder. In 1904 Charles Dana proposed that neurasthenia was a heterogeneous condition, and many suffered from psychiatric illness, a view echoed in a recent editorial on CFS (Swartz, 1988). However, Dana concluded "I shall be very much disappointed if those who read this paper should flippantly express their interpretation of it by saying 'Well, he justs wants to make out that all neurasthenics are crazy people and ought to be locked up'." Such a warning is appropriate for a variety of reasons.

First, simply because many CFS patients satisfy criteria for affective disorder should not imply that the conditions are identical. In the context of neurasthenia and depression, Shweder (1988) has forcibly argued against this view, and in the social and clinical context it is true that the difference between depression and neurasthenia/CFS may be more important than the similarities (Wessely, 1990b). It is unclear whether such arguments are equally relevant to a discussion of the psychobiological basis of chronic fatigue.

Second, in all the studies reviewed, a minority of patients do not satisfy criteria for psychiatric illness. Such patients may have similar disorders to the majority, or may develop such disorders on follow-up, or alternatively may have a different nosological illness. At present, approximately a quarter of CFS patients encountered in hospital practice have no medical or psychiatric diagnosis.

Third, it is worth emphasizing (although perhaps not to the audience of this book) that psychiatric diagnoses are largely symptomatic descriptions, and convey relatively little information on etiology.

RISK FACTORS FOR CFS

Viral Illness

It has already been demonstrated that it is almost impossible to assess the role of viruses in the etiology of CFS from cross-sectional studies. Instead, valid information can only be gained from longitudinal studies of the outcome of known viral illnesses.

One of the few such studies concerns the outcome of serious enteroviral infections (Lepow *et al.*, 1962), in which 306 cases of aseptic meningitis were followed up. At 3 months, fatigue, poor concentration or motor disturbances (usually tightness or weakness) persisted in 32% of the original cohort, but this had reduced to 3% by 2 years, although there were neither controls nor complete follow-up. Muller *et al.* (1958) traced 238 cases of primary aseptic meningitis after between 2 and 12 years. No differences were found between cases and controls on measures of behavioral disturbance or mental health; instead, persistent morbidity was predicted by previous psychological disturbance.

A less favorable prognosis for the survivors of encephalitis is shown by a controlled 5-year follow-up of St. Louis encephalitis (Lawton *et al.*, 1970), a serious insect-borne arbovirus. Neurasthenic and affective symptoms were the most frequently observed sequelae, in particular exhaustion and fatigue, occurring in 35% of cases but only 9% of controls. Similarly, although the parkinsonian sequelae of encephalitis lethargica are well known, von Economo (1931) also described prolonged psychasthenic states with a "striking tendency to fatigue," identical to modern chronic fatigue syndromes. It can be concluded that viral illnesses do convey an increased risk of CFS, but so far this is related to their capacity to cause CNS damage, rather than persistent infection. Although there is a wealth of scientific studies concerning the mechanisms for persistent viral infection (Southern and Oldstone, 1986), such mechanisms have yet to be demonstrated in CFS, although recent speculation on viral persistence in the central nervous system and affective disorder raises exciting possibilities (Webb and Parsons, 1990).

Psychological Vulnerability and Past Psychiatric Illness

Prospective studies remain the best method of assessing the role of psychological vulnerability in the etiology of CFS. For obvious reasons such studies are rare. Nevertheless, a few exist. Six hundred people in employment were psychologically tested prior to the 1957 epidemic of Asian flu (Imboden *et al.*, 1961). All subjects were exposed to the epidemic. Serological surveillance established that those identified as psychologically vulnerable did not have an increased risk of infection, but having done so were ill for a longer period of time. The most common symptom in the "vulnerable group" was tiredness or weakness. Psychological vulnerability was a risk factor for duration of illness and fatigue, although the period of follow-up was short. The findings were replicated twice: first in a prospective study of the effects of immunization (Canter *et al.*, 1972), and later in an extraordinary study (Canter, 1972) in which volunteers were given tularemia. Not only did the "vulnerable" group report more symptoms, but the actual duration of fever was longer, which raises questions about the interaction between host and pathogen yet to be answered.

The less satisfactory alternative is to use the presence of past psychiatric history as a retrospective marker of psychological vulnerability. This is a reasonable strategy, as underascertainment is more likely than overascertainment, but it must be emphasized that it is still open to selection bias. It appears that between 40 and 60% of CFS patients seen in hospital practice have experienced previous episodes of psychiatric disorder before the commencement of their CFS (Taerk *et al.*, 1987; Katon *et al.*, 1988; Wessely and Powell, 1988; Kruesi *et al.*, 1989), with only one study giving discrepant results (Hickie *et al.*, 1990). This is particularly intriguing since two studies (Kruesi *et al.*, 1989; Katon *et al.*, 1988) looked at patients chosen on the basis of abnormal serology. This may be a result of selection bias and chance, or may again reflect a complex host–virus interaction that remains largely unexplored (Straus, 1988).

Multifactorial Models

It is becoming clear that neither an exclusively organic nor psychiatric model will explain the clinical picture of CFS. There are several conditions in which models have been developed that incorporate both organic and psychological factors, for example the outcome of minor head injury (Lishman, 1987) and chronic pain (Fordyce, 1976). Furthermore, such models also allow for different factors to have differing relevance over time. We have argued for a similar model in CFS (Wessely *et al.*, 1989; Wessely, 1990a), emphasizing the role of postmorbid variables, such as attributions, coping styles, inappropriate treatment, and the like. We have also argued that cognitive and behavioral explanations analogous to those advanced in chronic pain are relevant to CFS, and have described cycles of depression, misattribution, inactivity, and further fatigue as contributing to the persistence of CFS (Wessely *et al.*, 1989; Butler *et al.*, 1991). Only further work will tell how accurate such models are.

Some support comes from the preliminary findings of the studies of White (1989) previously mentioned. In a large cohort of patients followed up after developing primary EBV, the predictors of CFS differed with time. At 2 months, fatigue was associated with a decrease in IgG capsular antigen response, and also a decrease in IgM to viral capsular antigen. However, this was not the case at 6 months. Instead, fatigue at 6 months was predicted by psychiatric illness before the infective episode. The preliminary conclusion is that immune factors are associated with immediate fatigue, but past psychiatric history predisposes to fatigue states of longer duration. Such findings are also consistent with a model in which short- and long-term prognosis are influenced by very different factors. Further analysis of this important multidisciplinary study is awaited with interest.

At this stage it is impossible to quote reliable figures on the prognosis of CFS. Although all studies to date emphasize the poor prognosis, all are prevalent studies based on hospital samples, and thus will overestimate duration. Nevertheless, the general experience is conveyed by Behan and Behan (1988): "Most of the cases seen do not improve, give up their work and become permanent invalids." There is evidence of diagnostic stability over time (Macy and Allen, 1933–1934; Wheeler *et al.*, 1950), although, given the protean nature of fatigue, a small number will continue to develop more clear-cut neurological diagnoses during follow-up (Wessely and Thomas, 1990). A poor prognosis is also noted in primary care, and over 50% remain symptomatic at 1 year (Kroenke *et al.*, 1988; Nelson *et al.*, 1987). Finally, some have used evidence of poor outcome as proof of the neurological origin of CFS (Ramsay, 1986; Hyde and Bergmann, 1988). In fact, persistent morbidity does not serve to discriminate between psychiatric and neurological causes of fatigue.

However, all such conclusions remain tentative. Case definition is variable, follow-up rarely systematic, and samples unrepresentative. Those whose CFS is associated with affective disorder (a substantial number, if not the majority) may have a particularly poor prognosis, since not only is affective disorder of sufficient severity to lead to hospital associated with poor outcome (Lee and Murray, 1988), but persistence of somatic symptoms, especially fatigue, after 1 year of treatment for depression has been associated with persistence of affective disorder for 4 or more years (Cadoret *et al.*, 1980). Conversely, both the absence of somatic symptoms in general, and the absence of fatigue in particular, were associated with better outcome in a study of new psychiatric outpatients (Huxley and Goldberg, 1985). A fuller account of the prognosis of CFS is contained elsewhere (Wessely, 1990a).

THE EVIDENCE FOR "EPIDEMIC" FATIGUE

Although there remain often intense disagreements concerning the nature of sporadic CFS, such disputes seem almost like consensus in the light of the controversy surrounding epidemic forms of CFS. In both Britain and the United States, the appearance of epidemic variants of CFS has led to bitter argument. In Britain, controversy continues to surround the mysterious illness that swept through the staff of the Royal Free Hospital in 1955 (Medical Staff of the Royal Free Hospital, 1957), which is seen by some as mass hysteria (Mausner and Gezon, 1967; McEvedy and Beard, 1970), and by others as evidence of a new organic illness named myalgic encephalomyelitis (Ramsay, 1986). Fortunately, such arguments need not concern us here, because the features of the illness do not correspond with modern definitions of CFS. Fatigue was not a prominent part of the picture: all agree the illness was contagious, while the symptoms were neurological or quasi-neurological depending upon one's interpretation. Most regrettably, the name "myalgic encephalomyelitis" has been attached to this epidemic phenomenon in addition to becoming the leading English synonym for CFS. This serves only to confuse the picture yet further (Byrne, 1988; Wessely and Thomas, 1990).

Different arguments surround a specific outbreak of CFS in the United States, the so-called "Lake Tahoe" epidemic. Reports (Peterson *et al.* 1986) of an outbreak of a fatiguing illness in this area of Nevada led to a rash of popular and scientific articles on a new mystery disease (Barnes, 1986), with intense speculation about a possible link to a new virus. Unlike the Royal Free outbreak, and related episodes, in which there was no doubt about the observed increase in morbidity (instead the controversy was whether the contagion was of emotional distress or infectious agent), at Lake Tahoe it is by no means certain that an epidemic occurred at all. Here the argument is not only the nature of the morbidity, but whether or not it represents an increase over normal rates.

The major problem lies in accurate knowledge of base rates, since time–space clustering can only be interpreted in the light of the distribution of CFS in the whole population. Such information is lacking. Nevertheless, various features suggest that no true increase in morbidity occurred. Cases were only being diagnosed in one practice, and other doctors in the area were not seeing anything unusual (Boly, 1987). In the "epidemic" a number of patients "with fatigue who would not otherwise have traveled to Incline Village for medical care had referred themselves specifically for EBV testing in 1985, thus creating an increase in cases in the area" (Holmes *et al.*, 1987). Part of the explanation may thus be a combination of altered medical perception, increased case finding, and a floating denominator. No transmissible agent has been identified, and the current consensus is against an infectious etiology (Schooley, 1988).

Both altered medical perception and a floating numerator have been noted before in less publicized outbreaks. In an earlier outbreak of "ME," May *et al.* (1980) demonstrated that an "epidemic" was the result of altered medical perception of the normal levels of illness found in an enclosed community, so that the increased case rate reflected an altered threshold rather than new morbidity. Both mechanisms explain another brief epidemic of an "infectious" disease, in which cases resulted from an unreliable laboratory test leading to overdiagnosis. Increased public awareness then led to the expected epidemic of "cases" (Mausner and Gezon, 1967). The role of the media in increasing public awareness of a "new" disease cannot be underestimated, nor can the role of doctors in creating new illnesses (Eisenberg, 1988).

WHY VIRUSES?

If the evidence implicating viruses in the etiology of CFS is less than conclusive, why have such labels as chronic EBV or postviral fatigue achieved such ready acceptance and widespread impact? The idea that viruses may substantially contribute to fatigue states has a long history (Arndi, 1892; Kraepelin, 1902; Savill, 1906). Indeed, faulty research first led to an intense, albeit unsuccessful, search for a fatigue vaccine in the years preceding the outbreak of World War I (Rabinbach, 1982).

The reasons lie in the intuitive appeal of viruses. In the community the commonest reason advanced to explain vague, unexplained symptoms is "a virus" (Pill and Stott, 1981). Such attributions are also on the increase, at the expense of earlier explanatory systems involving personal responsibility. Viruses are by definition external agents: "They originate outside the individual" (Helman, 1978). Helman goes on to write that "The germ has its own volition and cannot be directly controlled by the host. The victim of a germ infection is therefore blameless" (with the possible exception of sexually transmitted diseases).

This is an important concept in understanding CFS. Believing your illness is caused by a virus has many advantages. It lessens guilt and avoids blame. Patients who attribute somatically based symptoms to external causes may be less disturbed by them (Watts, 1982). CFS patients with affective disorder show less guilt but more self-esteem than matched depressed controls (Powell *et al.*, 1990). Finally, all those with clinical experience of CFS patients will recognize that many are firmly convinced of the physical, external origin of their symptoms and resistant to explanations involving psychological mechanisms.

Unfortunately, such attributions also have less desirable consequences. If you believe your symptoms are due to a virus, then it is impossible to exert any control over them, and recovery is left in "the lap of the gods." There is now evidence showing that in a number of diseases external attributions, and external locus of control, are associated with prolonged illness and impaired rehabilitation (Watts, 1982; Partridge and Johnson, 1989). Imboden *et al.* (1959) found that patients who attributed symptoms to "chronic brucellosis," a now-discredited diagnosis, were distinguished by a conviction of organic disease, a reluctance to discuss emotional issues and a preoccupation with somatic symptoms. One of the many factors contributing to the observed poor prognosis of CFS may be the nature of the disease attribution itself (Wessely, 1990a). Levi-Straus concluded that for a sick person to recover from any mysterious illness, it was necessary to have an explicit system of belief and explanation, whose accuracy was irrelevant. What cannot be accepted "are the incoherent and arbitrary pains, which are an alien element in her system." Recovery occurs once such symptoms are integrated within a meaningful system. However, "no such thing happens to our sick when the causes of their diseases have been explained to them in terms of secretions, germs or viruses" (Levi-Straus, 1963).

CONCLUSIONS

The balance between agent and host is important in any infectious disease. Logic suggests that in the condition of post-infectious fatigue, it is the host that may be as, if not more, important than the virus. In this context, one can do little better than repeat Pasteur's aphorism that "la germe c'est ne rien: c'est la terre qui est toute" (Laudenslager, 1987). There is a variety of evidence in favor of his intuition.

The viruses that are claimed to be responsible for fatigue are common. Exposure to EBV is nearly universal. Clinical infection with viruses such as influenza occurs in normal people several times a year, while subclinical infection is even commoner: it is worth repeating the assertion that the ratio of subclinical to clinical severe enterovirus infection is of the order of 1000:1 (Pallansch, 1988). CFS is not associated with a single specific pathogen, but has been reported after a number of infections, not all of them viral (Salit, 1985; Behan and Behan, 1988; Wessely and Powell, 1989). The alleged agents are not normally serious pathogens and although it is true that usually innocuous viruses may rarely cause severe illnesses, in such cases evidence of physical morbidity is easy to find, unlike in cases of chronic fatigue. Finally, many people have an identical clinical fatigue syndrome without apparent clinical exposure.

So far no evidence has been presented of clinical (as opposed to merely laboratory) reactivation or disease progression, despite the fact that many patients have an illness that may persist for decades. Lack of progression allied to the lack of development of frank neurological involvement disproves the occasional analogy with a slow virus infection (Sutton, 1978). On the contrary, George Beard (1880), the first person to describe CFS under the label of neurasthenia, asserted that it was actually associated with increased longevity!

Thus, conclusive evidence of a direct link between viruses and chronic fatigue remains elusive. It is unnecessary to insist on all of Koch's postulates being fulfilled before one accepts that such a link exists (Rivers, 1937), but one must insist on a more basic epidemiological principle: that the cause (viruses) must precede the effect (fatigue). The evidence of psychological vulnerability to CFS, and the role of psychiatric disorder as a possible confounder of the links between immune abnormalities and CFS, suggests that even this is not certain.

Finally, CFS itself appears to be a heterogeneous condition, and most, but not all, cases of CFS seen in general hospitals satisfy criteria for psychiatric illness. In patients with CFS, clinical status is associated more with psychological well-being than any laboratory measure.

WHAT SHOULD BE PRESENTED AT THE NEXT ICVO CONFERENCE?

Probably the greatest current problem in the field of CFS is the paucity of reliable epidemiological data. Currently both prevalence and case–control studies are being initiated in primary care in Scotland, England, and the United States. Only a primary care, if not community based, study can overcome the problems of bias that effectively prevent further progress. The most sophisticated molecular virology will be of little use until previous methodological and epidemiological flaws are overcome.

The second major area for research lies in the role of effect modifiers. It is this author's belief that models involving a single agent and single disease will possess little explanatory power in anything other than a highly selected minority. Work is needed on factors that link agent and host, such as genetic, immunological, and psychosocial premorbid vulnerability, and postmorbid variables including cognitive, behavioral, and social factors. Such work should also concentrate on the change from acute to chronic illness, and from adaptive to maladaptive behaviors. Such an approach implies a dynamic, rather than a static, model of CFS.

ACKNOWLEDGMENT The author is supported by a Wellcome Training Fellowship in Epidemiology.

REFERENCES

Anonymous, 1986, Local woman wants to form support group for those who have this fatiguing disease, *Daily News Miner*, Fairbanks, Alaska, May 23, 1986.

Archer, M., 1987, The post-viral syndrome: A review, *J. R. Coll. Gen. Pract.* **37**:212–214.

Archard, L., Bowles, N., Behan, P., Bell, E., and Doyle, D., 1988, Postviral fatigue syndrome: Persistence of enterovirus in muscle and elevated creatine kinase, *J. R. Soc. Med.* **81**:326–329.

Arndt, R., 1892, Neurasthenia, in: *Dictionary of Psychological Medicine*, Volume II (D. Tuke, ed.), Churchill, London, pp. 840–850.

Baracos, V., Rodemann, H., Dinarello, C., and Goldberg, A., 1983, Stimulation of muscle protein degradation and prostaglandin E_2 release by leukocytic pyrogen (interleukin-1): A mechanism for the increased degradation of muscle proteins during fever, *N. Engl. J. Med.* **308**:553–558.

Barnes, D., 1986, Mystery disease at Lake Tahoe challenges virologists and clinicians, *Science* **234**:541–542.

Barsky, A., Goodson, J., Lane, R., and Cleary, P., 1988, The amplification of somatic symptoms, *Psychosom. Med.* **50**:515–519.

Beard, G., 1880, *A Practical Treatise on Nervous Exhaustion (Neurasthenia)*, William Wood, New York.

Behan, P., and Behan, W., 1988, *The postviral fatigue syndrome*, *CRC Crit. Rev. Neurobiol.* **42**: 157–178.

Behan, P., Behan, W., and Bell, E., 1985, The postviral fatigue syndrome—An analysis of the findings in 50 cases, *J. Infect.* **10**:211–222.

Bell, D., and Bell, K., 1988, Chronic fatigue syndrome, *Ann. Intern. Med.* **109**:167.

Bell, E., Assaad, F., and Esteves, K., 1988a, Neurologic disorders, in: *Coxsackie Viruses: A General Update* (M. Benedelli and H. Friedman, eds.), Plenum Press, New York, pp. 319–337.

Bell, E., McCartney, R., and Riding, M., 1988b, Coxsackie B viruses and myalgic encephalomyelitis, *J. R. Soc. Med.* **81**:329–331.

Boly, W., 1987, Raggedy Ann Town, *Hippokrates* **July/August**:31–40.

Borysiewicz, L., 1989, Quoted in Wright, D., Postviral syndrome, *Ciba Found. Bull.* **22:**10.
Bowles, N., Richardson, P., Olsen, E., and Archard, L., 1986, Detection of coxsackie B virus-specific RNA sequences in myocardial biopsy samples from patients with myocarditis and dilated cardiomyopathy, *Lancet* **1:**1120–1123.
Buchwald, D., Sullivan, J., and Komaroff, A., 1987, Frequency of "chronic active Epstein–Barr Virus infection" in a general medical practice, *J. Am. Med. Assoc.* **257:**2303–2307.
Butler, S., Chalder, T., Ron, M., and Wessely, S., 1991, Cognitive–behaviour therapy in the chronic fatigue syndrome, *J. Neurol. Neurosurg. Psychiatry*, **54:**153–158.
Byrne, E., 1988, Idiopathic chronic fatigue and myalgia syndrome (myalgic encephalomyelitis). Some thoughts on nomenclature and aetiology, *Med. J. Aust.* **148:**80–82.
Cadoret, R., Widmer, R., and North, C., 1980, Depression in family practice: Long term prognosis and somatic complaints, *J. Fam. Pract.* **10:**625–629.
Calder, B., Warnock, P., McCartney, R., and Bell, E., 1987, Coxsackie B viruses and the post-viral syndrome: A prospective study in general practice, *J. R. Coll. Gen. Pract.* **37:**11–14.
Canter, A., 1972, Changes in mood during incubation of acute febrile disease and effects of pre-exposure psychological status, *Psychosom. Med.* **34:**424–430.
Canter, A., Cluff, L., and Imboden, J., 1972, Hypersensitive reactions to immunisation inoculations and antecedent psychological vulnerability, *J. Psychosom. Res.* **16:**99–101.
Chen, M., 1986, The epidemiology of self-perceived fatigue among adults, *Prev. Med.* **15:**74–81.
Clare, A., and Blacker, R., 1986, Some problems affecting the diagnosis and classification of depressive disorders in primary care, in: *Mental Illness in Primary Care Settings* (M. Shepherd, G. Wilkinson, and P. Williams, eds.), Tavistock, London, pp. 7–26.
Compston, N., 1978, An outbreak of encephalomyelitis in the Royal Free Hospital Group, London, in 1955, *Postgrad. Med. J.* **54:**722–724.
Cox, B., Blaxter, M., Buckle, A., Fenner, N., Golding, J., Huppert, F., Nickson, J., Roth, M., Stark, J., Wadsworth, M., and Whichelon, M., 1987, *The Health and Lifestyle Survey*, Health Promotion Research Trust, London.
Dana, C., 1904, The partial passing of neurasthenia, *Boston Med. Surg.* **60:**339–344.
David, A., Wessely, S., and Pelosi, A., 1988, Post-viral fatigue: Time for a new approach, *Br. Med. J.* **296:**696–699.
Dawson, J., 1987, Royal Free Disease: Perplexity continues, *Br. Med. J.* **294:**327–328.
Dawson, J., 1989, Brainstorming the postviral fatigue syndrome, *Br. Med. J.* **297:**1151.
DeLisi, L., Nurnberger, J., Goldin, L., Simmons-Alling, S., and Gershon, E., 1986, Epstein–Barr virus and depression, *Arch. Gen. Psychiatry* **43:**815–816.
Dew, M., Dunn, L., Bromet, E., and Schulberg, H., 1988, Factors affecting help-seeking during depression in a community sample, *J. Affect. Disord.* **14:**223–234.
Dinarello, C., 1984, Interleukin-1, *Rev. Infect. Dis.* **6:**51–95.
Dowden, C., and Johnson, W., 1929, Exhaustion states, *J. Am. Med. Assoc.* **93:**1702–1706.
Dunnell, K., and Cartwright, A., 1972, *Medicine Takers, Prescribers and Hoarders*, Routledge & Kegan Paul, London.
Eisenberg, L., 1988, The social construction of mental illness, *Psychol. Med.* **18:**1–9.
Evans, W., Meredith, C., Cannon, J., Dinarella, C., Fontrera, W., Hughes, V., Jones, B., and Knuttsen, H., 1986, Metabolic changes following eccentric exercise in trained and untrained men, *J. Appl. Physiol.* **61:**1864–1868.
Fegan, K., Behan, P., and Bell, E., 1983, Myalgic encephalomyelitis—Report of an epidemic, *J. R. Coll. Gen. Pract.* **33:**335–337.
Fordyce, W., 1976: *Behavioural Methods for Treating Chronic Pain and Illness*, Mosby, St. Louis.
Ganguli, R., and Rabin, B., 1989, Increased serum interleukin 2 receptor concentration in schizophrenic and brain-damaged subjects, *Arch. Gen. Psychiatry* **46:**292.
Goldberg, D., and Huxley, P., 1980, *Mental Illness in the Community*, Tavistock, London.

Hall, W., and MacPhee, D., 1985, Do Vietnam veterans suffer from toxic neurasthenia? *Aust. N. Z. J. Psychiatry* **19**:19–29.

Halpin, D., and Wessely, S., 1989, VP-1 antigen in chronic postviral fatigue syndrome, *Lancet* **1**:1028–1029.

Havard, C., 1985, Lassitude, *Br. Med. J.* **290**:1161–1162.

Hellinger, W., Smith, T., Van Scoy, R., Spitzer P., Forgacs, P., and Edson, R., 1988, Chronic fatigue syndrome and the diagnostic utility of Epstein–Barr virus early antigen, *J. Am. Med. Assoc.* **260**:971–973.

Helman, C., 1978, Feed a cold and starve a fever, *Culture Med. Psychiatry* **7**:107–137.

Henle, W., Henle, G., Andersson, J., Ernberg, I., Klein, G., Horwitz, C., Marklund, G., Rymo, I., Wellinder, C., and Straus, S., 1987, Antibody responses to Epstein–Barr virus-determined nuclear antigen (EBNA) -1 and EBNA-2 in acute and chronic Epstein–Barr virus infection, *Proc. Nat. Acad. Sci. USA* **84**:570–574.

Hickie, I., Lloyd, A., Wakefield, D., and Parker, G., 1990, The psychiatric status of patients with chronic fatigue syndrome, *Br. J. Psychiatry* **156**:534–540.

Holmes, G., Kaplan, J., Stewart, J., Hunt, B., Pinsky, P., and Schonberger, S., 1987, A cluster of patients with a chronic mononucleosis-like syndrome. Is Epstein–Barr virus the cause? *J. Am. Med. Assoc.* **257**:2297–2303.

Holmes, G., Kaplan, J., Gantz, N., Komaroff, A., Schonbergen, L., Straus, S., Jones, J., Dubois, R., Cunningham-Rundles, C., Pahwa, S., Tusaro, G., Zegano, L., Purtilo, D., Brown, N., Schooley, R., and Brus, I., 1988, Chronic fatigue syndrome: A working case definition, *Ann. Intern. Med.* **108**:387–389.

Horwitz, C., Henle, W., Henle, G., Rudnick, H., and Latts, E., 1985, Long-term serological follow-up of patients for Epstein–Barr virus after recovery from infectious mononucleosis, *J. Infect. Dis.* **151**:1150–1153.

Hotchin, N., Read, R., Smith, D., and Crawford, D., 1989, Active Epstein–Barr infection in post-viral fatigue syndrome, *J. Infect.* **18**:143–150.

Huxley, P., and Goldberg, D., 1985, Social versus clinical prediction in minor psychiatric disorders, *Psychol. Med.* **5**:96–100.

Hyde, B., and Bergmann, S., 1988, Akureyi disease (myalgic encephalomyelitis), forty years later, *Lancet* **2**:1191–1192.

Imboden, J., 1972, Psychosocial determinants of recovery, *Adv. Psychosom. Med.* **8**:142–155.

Imboden, J., Canter, A., and Cluff, L., 1959, Brucellosis. III. Psychologic aspects of delayed convalescence, *Arch. Intern. Med.* **103**:406–414.

Imboden, J., Canter, A., and Cluff, L., 1961, Convalescence from influenza: A study of the psychological and clinical determinants, *Arch. Intern. Med.* **108**:115–121.

Jenkins, R., Smeeton, N., and Shepherd, M., 1988, Classification of mental disorder in primary care, *Psycholog. Med. Monogr.* **12**.

Johnson, R., 1982, *Virus Infections of the Central Nervous System*, Raven Press, New York, p. 192.

Jones, J., and Miller, B., 1987, The postviral asthenia syndrome, in: *Viruses, Immunity and Mental Health* (E. Kurstak, Z. Lipowski, and P. Morozov, eds.), Plenum Medical, New York, pp. 441–451.

Jones, J., Williams, M., Schooley, R., Robinson, C., and Glaser, R., 1988, Antibodies to Epstein–Barr virus specific DNase and DNA polymerase in the chronic fatigue syndrome, *Arch. Intern. Med.* **148**:1957–1960.

Katon, W., Riggs, R., Gold, D., and Corey, L., 1988, Chronic fatigue syndrome: A collaborative virologic, immunologic and psychiatric study, Presented at the American Psychiatric Association, Montreal, Canada.

Kibler, R., Lucas, D., Hicks, M., Poulos, B., and Jones, J., 1985, Immune function in chronic active Epstein–Barr virus infection, *J. Clin. Immunol.* **5**:46–54.

Kiecolt-Glaser, J., Speicher C., Holliday, J., and Glaser, R., 1984, Stress and the transformation of lymphocytes by Epstein–Barr virus, *J. Behav. Med.* **7**:1–12.

King, D., and Cooper, S., 1989, Viruses, immunity and mental disorder, *Br. J. Psychiatry* **154**:1–7.

Komaroff, A., Straus, S., Gantz, N., and Jones, J., 1989, The chronic fatigue syndrome, *Ann. Intern. Med.* **110**:407–408.

Kraepelin, E., 1902, *Clinical Psychiatry* (trans. R. Defendorf), Macmillan & Co., London.

Kroenke, K., Wood, D., Mangelsdorff, D., Meier, N., and Powell, J., 1988, Chronic fatigue in primary care: Prevalence, patient characteristics and outcome, *J. Am. Med. Assoc.* **260**:929–934.

Kruesi, M., Dale, J., and Strauss, S., 1989, Psychiatric diagnoses in patients who have chronic fatigue syndrome, *J. Clin. Psychiatry* **50**:53–56.

Laudenslager, M., 1987, Psychosocial stress and disease, in: *Viruses, Immunity and Mental Health* (E. Kurstak, Z. Lipowski, and P. Morozov, eds.), Plenum Medical, New York, pp. 391–402.

Lawton, A., Rich, T., Mclendon, S., Gates, E., and Bond, J., 1970, Follow-up studies of St. Louis encephalitis in Florida: Reevaluation of the emotional and health status of the survivors five years after acute illness, *South. Med. J.* **63**:66–71.

Lee, A., and Murray, R., 1988, The long-term outcome of Maudsley depressives, *Br. J. Psychiatry* **153**:741–751.

Lepow, M., Coyne, N., Thompson, L., Carver, D., and Robbins, F., 1962, A clinical, epidemiological and laboratory investigation of aseptic meningitis during the four year period 1955–58, II, *N. Engl. J. Med.* **266**:1188–1193.

Levi-Straus, C., 1963, *Structural Anthropology*, Basic Books, New York, pp. 186–205.

Lishman, A., 1987, *Organic Psychiatry*, Blackwell, Oxford.

Lloyd, A., Wakefield, D., Boughton, C., and Dwyer, J., 1988a, What is myalgic encephalomyelitis? *Lancet* **1**:1286–1287.

Lloyd, A., Hales, J., and Gandevia, S., 1988b, Muscle strength, endurance and recovery in the post-infection fatigue syndrome, *J. Neurol. Neurosurg. Psychiatry* **51**:1316–1322.

Lloyd, A., Hanni, A., and Wakefield, D., 1988c, Interferon and myalgic encephalomyelitis, *Lancet* **1**:471.

Lynch, S., and Seth, R., 1989, Postviral fatigue syndrome and the VP-1 antigen, *Lancet* **2**:1160–1161.

MacDonald, L., Mann, A., and Thomas, H., 1987, Interferons and mediators of psychiatric morbidity: An investigation in a trial of recombinant alpha interferon in hepatitis B carriers, *Lancet* **2**:1175–1178.

McEvedy, C., and Beard, A., 1970, Royal Free epidemic of 1955: A reconsideration, *Br. Med. J.* **1**:7–11.

Macy, J., and Allen, E., 1933–1934, Justification of the diagnosis of chronic nervous exhaustion, *Ann. Intern. Med.* **7**:861–867.

Manu, P., Matthews, D., and Lane, T., 1988a, The mental health of patients with a chief complaint of chronic fatigue: A prospective evaluation and follow-up, *Arch. Intern. Med.* **148**:2213–2217.

Manu, P., Lane, T., and Matthews, D., 1988b, The frequency of the chronic fatigue syndrome in patients with symptoms of persistent fatigue, *Ann. Intern. Med.* **109**:554–556.

Mausner, J., and Gezon, H., 1967, Report on a phantom epidemic of gonorrhoea, *Am. J. Epidemiol.* **85**:320–331.

May, J., and Kline, P., 1988, Problems in using an adjective checklist to measure fatigue, *J. Person. Individ. Diff.* **9**:831–832.

May, P., Donnan, S., Ashton, J., Ogilvie, M., and Rolles, C., 1980, Personality and medical perception in benign myalgic encephalomyelitis, *Lancet* **2**:1122–1124.

Medical Staff of the Royal Free Hospital, 1957, An outbreak of encephalomyelitis in the Royal Free Hospital Group, London, in 1955, *Br. Med. J.* **2**:895–904.

Meijer, A., Zakay-Rones, Z., and Morag, A., 1988, Post-influenzal psychiatric disorder in adolescents, *Acta Psychiatr. Scand.* **76**:176–181.

Merlin, T., 1986, Chronic mononucleosis: Pitfalls in the laboratory diagnosis, *Hum. Pathol.* **17**:2–8.

Miller, H., 1987, Quoted in Dixon, B., Scientifically speaking, *Br. Med. J.* **294:**317.

Monk, T., 1989, A visual analogue scale technique to measure global vigor and affect, *Psychiatry Res.* **27:**89–99.

Montgomery, G., 1983, Uncommon tiredness among college undergraduates, *J. Consult. Clin. Psychol.* **51:**517–525.

Morag, A., Tobi, M., Ravid, A., Revel, M., and Schaffner, A., 1982, Increased (2′5′)-oligo-A-synthetase activity in patients with prolonged illness associated with serological evidence of persistent Epstein Barr virus infection, *Lancet* **1:**744.

Morrison, J., 1980, Fatigue as a presenting complaint in family practice, *J. Fam. Pract.* **10:**795–801.

Morte, S., Castilla, A., Civeira, M., Serrano, M., and Prieto J., 1988, Gamma-interferon and chronic fatigue syndrome, *Lancet* **2:**623–624.

Muir, P., Nicholson, F., Tilzey, A., Signy, M., English, T., and Banatvala, J., 1989, Chronic relapsing pericarditis and dilated cardiomyopathy: Serological evidence of persistent enterovirus infection, *Lancet* **1:**804–807.

Muller, R., Nylander, I., Larsson, L., Widen, L., and Frankenhauser, M., 1958, Sequelae of primary aseptic meningoencephalitis: A clinical sociomedical, electroencephalographic and psychological study, *Acta Psychiatr. Scand. Suppl.* **126:**1–115.

Murdoch, J., 1988, The myalgic encephalomyelitis syndrome, *Fam. Pract.* **5:**302–306.

Nelson, E., Kirk, J., McHugo, G., Douglass, R., Ohler, J., Wasson, J., and Zubkoff M., 1987, Chief complaint fatigue: A longitudinal study from the patient's perspective, *Fam. Pract. Res. J.* **6:** 175–188.

Pallansch, M., 1988, Epidemiology of group B coxsackieviruses, in: *Coxsackie Viruses: A General Update* (M. Benedelli and H. Friedman, eds.), Plenum Press, New York, pp. 399–415.

Parish, J., 1978, Early outbreaks of "epidemic neuromyasthenia," *Postgrad. Med. J.* **54:**711–717.

Partridge, C., and Johnson, M., 1989, Perceived control of recovery from disability: Measurement and prediction, *Br. J. Clin. Psychol.* **28:**53–59.

Peterson, D., Cheney, P., Ford, M., Hunt, B., and Reynolds, G., 1986, Chronic fatigue possibly related to Epstein–Barr virus—Nevada, *Morbidity Mortality Weekly Reports* May 30.

Pill, R., and Stott N., 1981, Concepts of illness cause and responsibility, *Soc. Sci. Med.* **16:**43–52.

Powell, R., Dolan, R., and Wessely, S., 1990, Attributions and self esteem in depression and the chronic fatigue syndrome. *J. Psychosomatic Res.*, in press.

Rabinbach, A., 1982, The body without fatigue: A nineteenth century utopia, in: *Political Symbolism in Modern Europe: Essays in Honour of George Mosse* (S. Drescher, D. Sabean, and A. Sharlin, eds.), Transaction Books, London, pp. 42–62.

Ramsay, M., 1986, *Postviral Fatigue Syndrome: The Saga of Royal Free Disease*, Gower Medical, London.

Rivers, T., 1937, Viruses and Koch's postulates, *J. Bacteriol.* **33:**1–12.

Rothman, K., 1986, *Modern Epidemiology*, Little, Brown, Boston.

Rubin, L., Kurman, C., and Fritz, M., 1985, Soluble interleukin 2 receptors are released from activated human lymphoid cells in vitro, *J. Immunol.* **135:**3172–3177.

Salit, I., 1985, Sporadic post-infectious neuromyasthenia, *Can. Med. Assoc. J.* **133:**659–663.

Savage, G., 1875, Overwork as a cause of insanity, *Lancet* **July 24:**127.

Savill, T., 1906. *Clinical Lectures on Neurasthenia*, Henry J. Glaisher, London.

Schooley, R., 1988, Chronic fatigue syndrome: A manifestation of Epstein–Barr virus infection? in: *Current Clinical Topics in Infectious Diseases*, Volume 9 (J. Remington and M. Swartz, eds.), McGraw–Hill, New York, pp. 126–146.

Seligmann, J., Abramson, P., Shapiro, D., Gosnell, M., and Hager, M., 1986, Malaise of the '80s: The puzzling and debilitating Epstein–Barr virus, *Newsweek* **October 27:**105–106.

Shepherd, M., Cooper, B., Brown, A., and Kalton, G., 1981, *Psyciatric Illness in General Practice*, 2nd ed., Oxford University Press, London, pp. 113–115.

Shweder, R., 1988, Suffering in style: A review of Arthur Kleiman, social origins of distress and disease, *Culture Med. Psychiatry* **12**:479–497.

Sinclair, A., 1988, ME misery and the new stress syndrome, *South China Morning Post*, December 1.

Smith, A., Tyrrell, D., Coyle, K., and Higgins, P., 1988, Effects of interferon alpha on performance in man: A preliminary report, *Psychopharmacology* **96**:414–416.

Smith, D., 1989, *Understanding M.E.*, Robinson, London.

Southern, P., and Oldstone, M., 1986, Medical consequences of persistent viral infection, *N. Engl. J. Med.* **314**:359–367.

Stokes, M., Cooper, R., and Edwards, R., 1988, Normal strength and fatigability in patients with effort syndrome, *Br. Med. J.* **297**:1014–1018.

Straus, S., 1988, The chronic mononucleosis syndrome, *J. Infect. Dis.* **157**:405–412.

Straus, S., Tosato, G., Armstrong, G., *et al.*, 1985, Persisting illness and fatigue in adults with evidence of Epstein–Barr virus infection, *Ann. Intern. Med.* **102**:7–16.

Straus, S., Dale, J., Tobi, M., Lawley, T., Preble, O., Blaese, M., Hallahan, C., and Henle, W., 1988, Acyclovir treatment of the chronic fatigue syndrome: Lack of efficacy in a placebo-controlled trial, *N. Engl. J. Med.* **319**:1692–1698.

Sutton, R., 1978, Ill defined neurological diseases of possible viral origin, *Postgrad. Med. J.* **54**: 747–751.

Swartz, M., 1988, The chronic fatigue syndrome—One entity or many? *N. Engl. J. Med.* **319**:1726–1728.

Taerk, G., and Abbey, S., 1989, Depression in neuromyasthenia (myalgic encephalomyelitis), Abstracts of the spring quarterly meeting of the Royal College of Psychiatrists, Leeds, April 4.

Taerk, G., Toner, B., Salit, I., Garfinkel, P., and Ozersky, S., 1987, Depression in patients with neuromyasthenia (benign myalgic encephalomyelitis), *Int. J. Psychiatry Med.* **17**:49–56.

Taylor, J., 1907, Management of exhaustion states in men, *Int. Clin.* **17**:36–50.

Tobi, M., Morag, A., Ravid, A., Chowers, I., Feldman-Weiss, V., Michaeli, Y., Ben-Chetrit, E., Shalit, M., and Knobler, H., 1982, Prolonged atypical illness associated with serological evidence of persistent Epstein–Barr infection, *Lancet* **1**:61–64.

Tobler, I., Borberly, A., Schwyzer, M., and Fontana, A., 1984, Interleukin-1 derived from astrocytes enhances slow wave activity in sleep EEG of the rat, *Eur. J. Pharmacol.* **104**:191–192.

von Economo, C., 1931. *Encephalitis Lethargica: Its Sequelae and Treatment*, Oxford University Press, London, pp. 109–110.

Watts, F., 1982, Attributional aspects of medicine, in: *Attributions and Psychological Change* (C. Antaki and C. Brewin, eds.), Academic Press, New York, pp. 35–155.

Webb, H., and Parsons, L., 1990, Esoteric virus infections, *Current Opinion in Neurology and Neurosurgery* **3**:223–228.

Wells, F., 1908, A neglected measure of fatigue, *Am. J. Psychol.* **19**:345–358.

Wessely, S., 1990a, The natural history of chronic fatigue and myalgia syndromes, in: *Psychological Disorders Frequently Seen in General Medical Settings* (N. Sartorius, ed.), World Health Organisation, Hans Huber, Bern, pp. 82–97.

Wessely, S., 1990b, "Old Wine in New Bottles": Neurasthenia and "M.E.", *Psychol. Med.* **20**:35–53.

Wessely, S., and Powell, R., 1989, Fatigue syndromes: A comparison of chronic "postviral" fatigue with neuromuscular and affective disorders, *J. Neurol. Neurosurg. Psychiatry* **52**:940–948.

Wessely, S., and Thomas, P. K., 1990, The chronic fatigue syndrome ("myalgic encephalomyelitis" or "postviral fatigue"), in: *Recent Advances in Neurology*, Volume 6 (C. Kennard, ed.), Churchill Livingstone, Edinburgh, pp. 85–132.

Wessely, S., David, A., Butler, S., and Chalder, T., 1989, The management of the chronic "post-viral" fatigue syndrome, *J. R. Coll. Gen. Pract.* **39**:26–29.

Wheeler, E., White, P., Reed, E., and Cohen, M., 1950, Neurocirculatory asthenia (anxiety neurosis, effort syndrome, neurasthenia), *J. Am. Med. Assoc.* **142**:878–889.

White, P., 1989, Psychiatric illness following glandular fever, Abstract presented at the spring quarterly meeting of the Royal College of Psychiatry, Leeds, April 4.

Wilson, P., Kusumakar, V., McCartney, R., and Bell, E., 1989, Features of coxsackie B virus (CBV) infection in children with prolonged physical and psychological morbidity, *J. Psychosom. Res.* **33**:29–36.

Wright, D., 1989, Postviral syndrome, *CIBA Found. Bull.* **22**:10.

Yousef, G., Bell, E., Mann, G., Murgesan, V., Smith, D., McCartney, R., and Mowbray, J., 1988, Chronic enterovirus infection in patients with postviral fatigue syndrome, *Lancet* **1**:146–150.

Chapter **22**

The Suppression of Recurrent Herpes Simplex Virus Infections with Lithium Carbonate

Jay D. Amsterdam and Greg Maislin

INTRODUCTION

There has been considerable interest in the possibility that some psychiatric disorders may be caused by viral infections (Kurstak *et al.*, 1987), and that some psychotropic drugs may possess antiviral activity (Chang, 1975; Wunderlich *et al.*, 1980; Bohn *et al.*, 1983; Patou *et al.*, 1986). In particular, several lines of evidence indicate that lithium salts may possess antiviral activity, especially toward herpes simplex virus (HSV). For example, several clinical reports have suggested that lithium may suppress the reactivation of latent HSV and reduce the number of recurrent infections (Lieb, 1979; Skinner, 1983; Gilis, 1983), while several *in vitro* studies have demonstrated that lithium can inhibit the replication of HSV by interfering with DNA synthesis (Skinner *et al.*, 1980; Hartley, 1983; Bach and Specter, 1988; Buchan *et al.*, 1988). In view of these interesting reports, we

Jay D. Amsterdam • *Depression Research Unit, Department of Psychiatry, University of Pennsylvania School of Medicine, Philadelphia, Pennsylvania 19104, and The Wistar Institute, Philadelphia, Pennsylvania 19104.* Greg Maislin • *Depression Research Unit, Department of Psychiatry, University of Pennsylvania School of Medicine, Philadelphia, Pennsylvania 19104.*

performed a series of clinical studies to examine the putative anti-herpesvirus activity of lithium carbonate in humans.

STUDY ONE: A RETROSPECTIVE EXAMINATION OF THE ANTI-HERPESVIRUS ACTIVITY OF LITHIUM CARBONATE AND OTHER ANTIDEPRESSANT DRUGS IN AFFECTIVE DISORDER PATIENTS

Methods

Subjects

We examined a total of 236 affective disorder patients: 177 taking long-term lithium carbonate and 59 taking other antidepressant medications on a chronic basis. The mean (± S.D.) age of the lithium patients with 46 ± 13 years and the mean duration of lithium therapy was 101 ± 67 months. The mean age of the patients taking other antidepressants was 48 ± 15 years and the mean duration of medication use was 55 ± 54 months. All subjects fulfilled Research Diagnostic Criteria (Spitzer *et al.*, 1978) for either past or present major depressive disorder, primary endogenous or bipolar subtype. None of the patients were psychotic or demented, and all had taken medication for a minimum of 12 months. Evaluations were performed in a consecutive, naturalistic fashion with some patients in the midst of an affective episode and others in remission. All of the subjects were in good physical health, and none had a recent history of significant neurologic, immunologic, or infectious disease.

Procedure

Each subject was administered a structured interview to assess the presence (and past history) of infectious diseases, with specific attention given to estimating the frequency of recurrence of herpesvirus infections. Responses were recorded on a standardized report form for pooled data analyses.

Statistical Procedures

Subjects with labial herpes infections at any time before or during drug treatment constituted the primary study group. We calculated the proportion of subjects with any reduction in the number of herpes episodes per year, as well as the mean within-subject change in the lithium and nonlithium groups. A chi-square statistic was used to test for differences in the proportions, and odds ratios (with 95% confidence interval) were used to measure the magnitude of group differences.

Pooled T test (or t tests for unequal variances) and the Wilcoxon rank sum test were used to examine group differences for the mean change in yearly herpes infection rates. The within-group treatment effects over time were examined using the paired t test and Wilcoxon sign rank test.

Because we used retrospective data, we constructed a model comparing lithium versus nonlithium differences adjusted for several potentially confounding variables including: age, concomitant medication, concurrent medical illness; a history of rubeola (measles), rubella (German measles), myxovirus (mumps), herpes zoster (chickenpox), Epstein–Barr virus (mononucleosis), and hepatitis infection; allergies to food, pollen, and drugs; and the average number of common colds per year prior to treatment. The test was constructed using a logistic regression model with any reduction in herpes infections as the dependent variable and the listed factors as the independent variables. This analysis was repeated for the mean change in herpes infection rates using multiple linear regression.

Finally, we separated out those patients who reported never having experienced labial herpes infection prior to treatment to determine if there was a difference in the proportion of patients with a first-time occurrence during treatment.

Results

Ninety subjects reported the presence of recurrent labial herpes infections: 63 (36%) in the lithium group and 27 (46%) taking other antidepressants ($\chi^2 = 1.94$; $p = 0.16$). These findings are similar to prior estimates of labial herpes infections in the general population (Ship *et al.*, 1977). The mean pretreatment frequency of labial herpes infections (1.6 ± 2.6 episodes/year) significantly diminished during lithium therapy (0.8 ± 1.8 episodes/year) ($p < .001$), while there was no significant change in the frequency of herpes infections during treatment with other antidepressants ($p = 0.6$) (Table 1). However, the statistical significance of this

Table 1. Analysis of the Mean Frequency of Herpes Infections per Year

	Pretreatment	During treatment		Difference	
Lithium	1.61 ± 2.04	0.80 ± 2.56		0.82 ± 1.81	$p < 0.001$[a]
Other antidepressants	2.58 ± 3.09	2.10 ± 4.86		0.48 ± 3.92	$p = 0.53$[b]
	$T = 1.50$	$T = 1.30$	$T = 0.42$		
	$df = 36.2$	$df = 32.3$	$df = 30.9$		
	$p = 0.14$	$p = 0.20$	$p = 0.68$[c]		

[a]Wilcoxon Sign Rank Test $p < 0.0001$.
[b]Wilcoxon Sign Rank Test $p < 0.08$
[c]Wilcoxon Rank Sum Test $p = 0.36$; estimated difference after adjustment for factors in "*a*" using multiple linear regression was 1.04 (2.41) ($T = 1.60$, $df = 64$, $p = 0.12$).

observation could not be completely established because the difference between treatment groups did not achieve significance (Table 1). Overall, however, 45 of 63 (71%) lithium subjects reported a decline in the number of herpes infections, while 18 subjects (29%) reported no change or an increased number of infections. In contrast, 14 of 27 (52%) nonlithium patients had fewer herpes infections during treatment while 13 (48%) reported no change or an increased number of infections. Thus, slightly more lithium patients reported a reduction of Herpes infections compared to those taking other antidepressants ($\chi^2 = 3.21$; $p = 0.07$).

The odds ratio of a reduction in herpes infections between the two treatment groups was 2.3 (0.9–5.9) ($p = 0.07$), indicating that evidence of a difference (before adjustment for confounding variables) was modest. Although complete data were not available for 10 subjects, the remaining patients had an unadjusted odds ratio of 3.5 (1.2–10.0) and an adjusted ratio of 3.6 (1.1–12.6) suggesting that the group comparisons were probably unaffected by the potentially confounding variables. Therefore, these clinical factors did not substantially contribute to the finding of a marginal difference in herpes infection rates between the lithium and nonlithium subjects.

Finally, more nonlithium subjects reported a primary labial herpes infection during treatment (11%) compared to patients on lithium (3%), although this difference failed to achieve statistical significance ($p < 0.09$).

STUDY TWO: A PROSPECTIVE, RANDOMIZED, TRIPLE-BLIND, PLACEBO-CONTROLLED TRIAL OF LITHIUM CARBONATE IN PREVENTING RECURRENT GENITAL HERPES INFECTIONS

Background

In general, HSV type 2 is more likely to be reactivated than HSV type 1, and when it is present in the genital area, it can recur eight to ten times more frequently than genital herpes type 1 infections (Reeves *et al.*, 1981). Moreover, at least 80% of women with genital herpesvirus infections will experience a recurrence within 1 year, with the average frequency being four episodes per year (Corey and Spear, 1986).

Although acyclovir has been shown to be effective in suppressing recurrent genital herpes infections (Reichman *et al.*, 1984; Straus *et al.*, 1984; Kinghorn, 1988; Mertz *et al.*, 1988; Mostov *et al.*, 1988), many patients fail to respond or are intolerant to the drug, and questions remain concerning its long-term safety in women of child-bearing potential (Sacks, 1987). Consequently, alternative treatments for preventing recurrent genital herpes infections would be of interest.

Several case reports have suggested that lithium may reduce the number of labial herpes infections (Lieb, 1979; Gilis, 1983), and this speculation was confirmed in study one (Amsterdam *et al.*, 1989) (*vide supra*). In addition, Skinner (1983) reported on a clinical trial comparing the topical application of lithium succinate ointment to placebo during repeated outbreaks of genital herpes infections, and observed a statistically significant reduction in the duration and severity of infections.

The observation that chronic lithium therapy may reduce the frequency of recurrent labial herpes infections, together with the *in vitro* demonstration that lithium (at a concentration of 7.5 mM) could reduce herpesvirus DNA replication without disturbing host cell replication (Skinner *et al.*, 1980; Buchan *et al.*, 1988), led us to initiate the following prospective, triple-blind, placebo-controlled study examining the prophylactic efficacy of daily lithium therapy in suppressing recurrent genital herpesvirus infections.

Methods

Subjects

Ten women with a mean (± S.D.) age of 37 ± 12 years (range: 18 to 63 years) were selected based upon the presence of a minimum of six infections in the year prior to treatment. Their mean duration of illness was 4.1 ± 3.5 years. In the year preceding treatment, they had an average of 0.9 ± 0.2 episode per month, and an average episode duration of 8.4 ± 4.0 days. Nine of the subjects had prior treatment for recurrent genital herpes infections: five had taken 2-deoxyglucose and nine had taken acyclovir. None of the subjects responded to the 2-deoxyglucose and only two reported a partial response to acyclovir. The remaining patients were either intolerant to acyclovir or failed to respond to the drug. Half of the patients had received more than one prior treatment and 70% had failed to respond to any prior treatment.

Procedure

Genital herpes infections were diagnosed and confirmed prior to treatment, and all prior antiviral medication was discontinued before entering the study.

Patients were randomly assigned to receive either lithium carbonate or identical placebo, and the study was conducted under triple-blind conditions (for the patients, gynecologist, and psychopharmacologist). Each subject received 12 consecutive months of lithium therapy, as well as 6 months of placebo either prior to, or after lithium therapy.

The frequency, severity, and duration of each herpes infection were recorded using a structured, self-rated daily calendar, as well as by gynecologic examinations and viral cultures (when feasible). Symptom severity ratings ranged from (+1) very mild (e.g., prodromal symptoms without obvious lesion) to (+5) very severe (e.g., extreme pain, dysuria, generalized malaise), and episode duration was recorded from the onset of prodromal symptoms to complete cessation of the episode.

Statistical Procedures

The analyses examined the number of herpes episodes per month, the total duration of all episodes per month, the average duration of each episode, the maximum symptom severity experienced during the month, and the "severity index" (the ratio of total illness duration to the maximum severity) per month.

We estimated the monthly change of each parameter using least squares by computing linear regressions as a function of months on lithium. The statistical significance of the average change was then assessed using the Wilcoxon signed rank test because these tests did not assume that the estimated slope coefficients were normally distributed. The magnitude of the change over time was estimated by medians, and the variability of the change was estimated by the minimum and maximum values. Analyses were also performed on the mean and standard deviation values using the one-sample t test.

The randomized clinical trial component of the study compared the 6 months of placebo for group one, to the first and second 6-month epochs of lithium treatment using pooled t tests [unless the variables were significantly different ($p < 0.05$ for the F test) in which case the t test for unequal variances was used).

Finally, within-patient changes were assessed over time, by comparing the averages for the first and second 6-month epochs of lithium to each other and to the pre- and post-treatment placebo periods using paired t tests.

Results

Efficacy

The mean ($\pm$ S.D.) daily lithium dosage was 587 $\pm$ 49 mg (range: 150 mg to 900 mg daily) and the average plasma lithium concentration was 0.51 mEq/liter (range: 0.38 $\pm$ 0.20 mEq/liter to 0.59 $\pm$ 0.27 mEq/liter) for all subjects.

We observed a significant reduction in the total duration of all episodes per month ($p < 0.01$), the average duration of each herpes infection ($p < 0.01$), the maximum symptom severity ($p < 0.01$), and the clinical "severity index" score ($p < 0.004$) (Table 2). The onset of lithium prophylaxis was gradual and the duration of each episode declined by about 0.5 day per month during lithium therapy.

Table 3 displays results from the randomized clinical trial component of the study. There was no significant difference in any of the treatment measurements when the first 6 months of lithium was compared to placebo. However, there was a significant reduction in the number of herpes episodes per month ($p < 0.04$), the

Table 2. Change per Month over 1 Year of Treatment with Lithium Carbonate ($N = 10$)[a]

	Mean (median)	S.D. (Minimum)	S.D. (Maximum)	Signed-rank p value (t test)
Number of episodes	−0.03	0.05		0.09
	(−0.03)	(−0.13)	(0.03)	(0.09)
Total duration all episodes per month	−0.51	0.58		<0.02
	(−0.47)	(−1.97)	(0.06)	(<0.01)
Average duration each episode	−0.43	0.43		0.01
	(−0.44)	(−1.45)	(0.09)	(<0.01)
Maximum severity all episodes per	−0.14	(−0.30)	0.12	<0.01
month	(−0.15)		(0.05)	(<0.01)
Severity index	−1.92	1.30		<0.002
	(−1.78)	(−3.52)	(0.08)	(<0.004)

[a]Change per month estimated using least squares by linear regression.

Table 3. Randomized Clinical Trial Results ($N = 5$)[a,b]

	Placebo	Lithium therapy: First 6 months	Lithium therapy: Second 6 months
Number of episodes	1.33	0.80	0.45
	(0.68)	(0.38)	(0.20)
Placebo vs. 1st		$T = -1.54$, $df = 8$ $p = 0.16$	
Placebo vs. 2nd		$T = -3.00$, $df = 4.8$ $p < 0.04$	
Total duration all episodes	8.13	7.23	2.36
per month	(4.52)	(3.90)	(1.36)
Placebo vs. 1st		$T = -0.34$, $df = 8$ $p = 0.78$	
Placebo vs. 2nd		$T = -2.85$, $df = 8$ $p < 0.04$	
Average duration each	6.04	9.23	4.72
episode	(2.27)	(2.25)	(1.57)
Placebo vs. 1st		$T = 1.15$, $df = 8$ $p = 0.06$	
Placebo vs. 2nd		$T = -2.85$, $df = 8$ $p = 0.31$	
Maximum severity of all	2.67	1.68	0.65
episodes per month	(1.18)	(0.60)	(0.33)
Placebo vs. 1st		$T = -1.66$, $df = 8$ $p = 0.13$	
Placebo vs. 2nd		$T = -4.00$, $df = 4.7$ $p < 0.02$	
Severity index	16.80	15.23	3.36
	(10.27)	(6.83)	(2.57)
Placebo vs. 1st		$T = -0.28$, $df = 8$ $p = 0.78$	
Placebo vs. 2nd		$T = -3.00$, $df = 4.5$ $p < 0.04$	

[a]Values are means (S.D.).
[b]Pooled t test or t test for unequal variance.

total duration of all episodes per month ($p < 0.04$), the maximum symptom severity per month ($p < 0.02$), and the clinical "severity index" score ($p < 0.04$) during the second 6 months of lithium therapy.

Finally, within-subject analyses demonstrated statistically significant reductions for each patient when the first and second 6-month epochs of lithium treatment were compared (Tables 4 and 5).

Overall, side effects during lithium therapy were mild and remarkably well tolerated, and no one had to discontinue treatment because of an adverse event.

Report of Cases

Case One

A thirty-one-year-old woman with a 12-year history of genital herpes infections recurring at monthly intervals with a duration of 10–12 days, and a 5-year history of recurrent herpes infections of the pharynx, face, and hands occurring either simultaneously with the genital infections or at separate times. She had failed to respond to prior suppressive therapy with oral acyclovir and 2-deoxyglucose. In the present study she had no response to placebo therapy, but by the fourth month of lithium at 900 mg daily (mean lithium level of 0.59 mEq/liter), she ceased having extragenital infections, and during the subsequent 8 months had only three very mild genital herpes outbreaks lasting an average of 6 days. Interestingly, this subject had previously received lithium for 3 years for affective illness and reported a similar response at that time.

Table 4. Analysis of 6-Month Averaged Data[a]

	A Pretreatment placebo (N = 5)	B First 6 months lithium treatment (N = 10)	C Second 6 months lithium treatment (N = 10)	D Posttreatment placebo (N = 4)
Number of episodes	1.33 (0.68)	0.78 (0.38)	0.58 (0.45)	1.50 (1.58)
Total duration	8.13 (4.52)	6.47 (3.70)	3.36 (3.40)	3.21 (1.50)
Average duration	6.04 (2.27)	8.20 (2.20)	4.69 (2.12)	4.40 (2.90)
Maximum severity	2.67 (1.18)	1.86 (0.76)	1.04 (1.07)	1.29 (0.48)
Severity index	16.80 (10.27)	15.21 (7.40)	6.17 (7.80)	4.93 (3.29)

[a]Values are means (S.D.).

Table 5. Within-Patient Analysis of 6-Month Averaged Data[a,b]

	A minus B (N = 5)	A minus C (N = 5)	B minus C (N = 10)	C minus D (N = 4)
Number of episodes	0.60 (0.43)	0.66 (0.35)	0.21 (0.37)	−1.08 (1.55)
	<0.04	<0.02	0.11	0.26
Total duration	2.58 (3.25)	3.91 (3.75)	3.10 (3.38)	−0.96 (2.68)
	0.15	0.08	<0.02	0.53
Average duration	−1.09 (1.54)	1.39 (2.88)	3.51 (2.61)	0.32 (3.30)
	0.19	0.34	<0.003	0.86
Maximum severity	0.71 (0.70)	1.31 (0.86)	0.82 (0.91)	−0.67 (0.68)
	0.09	<0.03	<0.02	0.14
Severity index	1.94 (7.26)	8.15 (11.54)	9.04 (7.31)	−1.23 (5.51)
	0.58	0.19	<0.004	0.69

[a]Values are means (S.D.).
[b]Paired t test.

Case Two

A forty-seven-year-old woman with a 3.5-year history of genital herpes infections recurring 11 times in the year preceding the study. The average duration of each episode was 5 days. She was treated with a lithium dose of 300 mg daily (mean plasma lithium level of 0.38 mEq/liter). By the fourth month of therapy the herpes outbreaks had ceased and during the subsequent 8 months she experienced only one mild episode lasting 3 days.

DISCUSSION

The present observations of a significant reduction in the number, duration, and severity of recurrent herpes infections during chronic lithium therapy complement prior clinical reports suggesting an antiviral activity for lithium (Lieb, 1979; Gilis, 1983; Skinner, 1983). Similarly, a number of *in vitro* studies have demonstrated that lithium affects the replication of herpesvirus DNA and viral protein synthesis. For example, Skinner *et al.* (1980) added lithium chloride to herpes-infected baby hamster kidney cells and observed a substantial reduction in virus replication at a lithium concentration of 5 mM, with complete inhibition of viral replication at 30 mM. Lithium also reduced viral DNA replication at 7.5 mM (a concentration which permitted host cell replication), and completely inhibited viral DNA replication at 30 mM.

Other mechanisms for the antiviral action of lithium have been postulated and include: the replacement of magnesium ion as an enzyme cofactor in viral protein synthesis (Bach and Specter, 1988), inhibition of viral DNA polymerase (Skinner *et al.*, 1980), alterations in lymphocyte and macrophage function (Friedenberg and Marx, 1980), a reduction of T-suppressor lymphocyte activity (Shenkman *et al.*, 1987), altered prostaglandin E_1 and free fatty acid synthesis (Horrobin, 1980; Horrobin *et al.*, 1988), and altered host cell membrane dynamics which would reduce the likelihood of virus penetration into the cell (Gosztonyi and Ludwig, 1984; Shaskan *et al.*, 1988). Furthermore, the antiviral activity of lithium appears to be limited to the lithium ion *per se*, affecting primarily DNA, but not RNA viruses (Skinner *et al.*, 1980; Buchan *et al.*, 1988).

The observation that lithium can reduce the recurrence rate of labial herpes infections, together with the *in vitro* finding that herpesvirus DNA replication is reduced at 7.5 mM lithium (Skinner *et al.*, 1980) suggested to us the possibility that chronic lithium administration might suppress the recurrence of genital herpes infections at clinically acceptable plasma lithium concentrations.

The reactivation of latent herpesvirus has often been attributed to psychological and physiological stress (Landmann *et al.*, 1984; Glaszer *et al.*, 1985; Schleifer *et al.*, 1985) and one could speculate that it is the beneficial effect of lithium on mood stability that might enhance the overall immune competence of an individual and diminish the likelihood of recurrent viral infections (Fernandez and Fox, 1980; Sengar *et al.*, 1982; Drob *et al.*, 1986). This possibility might be particularly important in patients with chronic psychiatric illness. Although we did not directly measure immune competence in either study, there was no indication that any subject was immunocompromised. Furthermore, while both patient groups from study one reported fewer viral infections during antidepressant treatment, the lithium patients reported fewer herpes infections ($p < 0.07$), suggesting the possibility of a more specific anti-herpesvirus action for lithium. Furthermore, in study two all of the subjects were psychiatrically healthy at the time of treatment, and many of the subjects were maintained at a plasma lithium level that was less than that required for controlling mood disorders.

In conclusion, the present results indicate that long-term lithium administration can substantially reduce the frequency of labial herpes infections ($p < 0.001$), and marginally diminish the recurrence rate of herpes infections when compared to other antidepressant medications ($p = 0.07$). More importantly, the findings from our prospective study show that lithium therapy at low doses can significantly reduce the duration of recurrent genital herpes infections ($p < 0.01$), reduce the maximum severity of each episode ($p < 0.01$), and diminish the clinical "severity index" score ($p < 0.004$). These data suggest that long-term lithium prophylaxis may be an effective treatment for preventing recurrent genital herpesvirus infections.

ACKNOWLEDGMENTS This work was supported, in part, by B. S. R. grant S07-RR-65415-28 awarded by the Biomedical Research Support Grant Program, Division of Research Resources at the N. I. H.; and The Jack Warsaw Fund for Research in Biological Psychiatry, Hospital of the University of Pennsylvania, Philadelphia. The authors extend their appreciation to William Dyson, M.D., Janusz Rybakowski, M.D., and Larry Potter, A.B., for providing clinical material and technical assistance with these studies.

REFERENCES

Amsterdam, J. D., Maislin, G., and Rybakowski, J., 1989, Possible anti-viral action of lithium carbonate in herpes simplex virus infections, *Biol. Psychiatry* **27**:477–453.

Bach, R. O., and Specter, S., 1988, Antiviral activity of the lithium ion with adjuvant agents, in: *Lithium: Inorganic Pharmacology and Psychiatric Use* (N. J. Birch, ed.), IRL Press, Oxford, pp. 91–92.

Bohn, W., Rutter, G., Hohenberg, H., and Mannweller, K., 1983, Inhibition of measles virus budding by phenothiazines, *Virology* **130**:44–55.

Buchan, A., Randall, S., Hartley, C. E., Skinner, G. R. B., and Fuller, A., 1988, Effect of lithium salts on the replication of viruses and non-viral microorganisms, in: *Lithium: Inorganic Pharmacology and Psychiatric Use* (N. J. Birch, ed.), IRL Press, Oxford, pp. 83–92.

Chang, T.-W., 1975, Suppression of herpetic recurrence by chlorpromazine, *N. Engl. J. Med.* **293**:153–154.

Corey, L., and Spear, P. G., 1986, Infections with herpes simplex viruses, *N. Engl. J. Med.* **314**:686–691.

Drob, S., Bernard, H., Lifshutz, H., and Nierenberg, A., 1986, Brief group psychotherapy for herpes patients: A preliminary study, *Behav. Ther.* **17**:229–238.

Fernandez, L. A., and Fox, R. A., 1980, Perturbation of the human immune system by lithium, *Clin. Exp. Immunol.* **41**:527–532.

Friedenberg, W. R., and Marx, J. J., 1980, The effect of lithium carbonate on lymphocyte, granulocyte, and platelet function, *Cancer* **45**:91–97.

Gilis, A., 1983, Lithium in herpes simplex, *Lancet* **2**:1209–1210.

Glaser, R., Kiecolt-Glaser, J. K., Speicher, C. E., and Holliday, J. E., 1985, Stress, loneliness, and changes in herpesvirus latency. *J. Behav. Med.* **8**:249–260.

Gosztonyi, G., and Ludwig, H., 1984, Neurotransmitter receptors and viral neurotropism, *Neuropsychiatr. Clin.* **3**:107–114.

Hartley, C. E., 1983, The effect of lithium on herpes simplex virus replication, *Med. Lab. Sci.* **40**:406.

Horrobin, D. F., 1980, Lithium in the control of herpesvirus infections, in: *Lithium: Current Applications in Science, Medicine, and Technology* (R. O. Bach, ed.), Wiley, New York, pp. 397–406.

Horrobin, D. F., Jenkins, D. K., Mitchell, J., and Manku, M. S., 1988, Lithium effects on essential fatty acid and prostaglandin metabolism, in: *Lithium: Inorganic Pharmacology and Psychiatric Use* (N. J. Birch, ed.), IRL Press, Oxford, pp. 173–176).

Kinghorn, G. R., 1988, Long-term suppression with oral acyclovir of recurrent herpes simplex virus infections in otherwise healthy patients. A European multicenter study, *Am. J. Med.* **85**(Suppl. 2A):26–29.

Kurstak, E., Lipowski, Z. J., and Morozov, P. V. (eds.), 1987, *Viruses, Immunity, and Mental Disorders*, Plenum Medical, New York.

Landmann, R. M. A., Muller, F. B., Perini, C. H., Wesp, M., Erne, P., and Buhler, F. R., 1984, Change in immunoregulatory cells induced by psychological and physical stresses: relationship to plasma catecholamines, *Clin. Exp. Immunol.* **58**:127–135.

Lieb, J., 1979, Remission of recurrent herpes infection during therapy with lithium, *N. Engl. J. Med.* **301**:942.

Mertz, G. J., Jones, C. C., Mills, J., Fife, K. H., Lemon, S. M., Stapleton, J. T., Hill, E. L., and Davis, G., 1988, Long-term acyclovir suppression of frequently recurring genital herpes simplex virus infection. A multicenter double-blind trial, *J. Am. Med. Assoc.* **260**:201–206.

Mostov, S. R., Mayfield, J. L., Marr, J. J., and Drucker, J. L., 1988, Suppression of recurrent genital herpes by single daily dosages of acyclovir, *Am. J. Med.* **85**(Suppl. 2A):30–33.

Patou, G., Crow, T. J., and Taylor, G. R., 1986, The effects of psychotropic drugs on synthesis of DNA and the infectivity of herpes simplex virus, *Biol. Psychiatry* **21**:1221–1225.

Reeves, W. C., Corey, L., Adams, H. G., Vontver, L. A., and Holmes, K. K., 1981, Risk of recurrence after first episode of genital herpes: relation to HSV type and antibody response, *N. Engl. J. Med.* **305**:315–319.

Reichman, R. C., Badger, G. J., Mertz, G. J., Corey, L., Richman, D. D., Connor, J. D., Redfield, D., Savoia, M. C., Oxman, M. N., Bryson, Y., Tyrrell, D. L., Portnoy, J., Creigh-Kirk, T., Keeney, R. E., Ashikaga, T., and Dolin, R., 1984, Treatment of recurrent genital herpes simplex infections with oral acyclovir: A controlled trial, *J. Am. Med. Assoc.* **251**:2103–2107.

Sacks, S. L., 1987, The role of oral acyclovir in the management of genital herpes, *Can. Med. Assoc.* **136**:701–707.

Schleifer, S. J., Keller, S. E., Siris, S. G., and Davis, K. L., 1985, Depression and immunity. Lymphocyte function in ambulatory depressed patients, hospitalized schizophrenic patients, and patients hospitalized for herniorrhaphy, *Arch. Gen. Psychiatry* **42**:129–133.

Sengar, D. P. S., Waters, B. G. H., Dunne, J. V., and Bouer, I. M., 1982, Lymphocyte subpopulations and mitogenic responses of lymphocytes in manic-depressive disorders, *Biol. Psychiatry* **17**:1017–1022.

Shaskan, E. G., Oreland, L., and Wadell, G., 1985, Dopamine receptors and monoamine oxidase as virion receptors, *Perspect. Biol. Med.* **27**:239–250.

Shenkman, L., Borkowsky, W., Holzman, R. S., and Shopsin, B., 1987, Enhancement of lymphocyte and macrophage function in vitro by lithium chloride, *Clin. Immunol. Immunopathol.* **10**:187–192.

Ship, I. I., Miller, M. F., and Ram, C., 1977, A retrospective study of recurrent herpes labialis (RHL) in a professional population, 1958–1971, *Oral Surg.* **44**:723–730.

Skinner, G. R. B., 1983, Lithium ointment for genital herpes, *Lancet* **2**:288.

Skinner, G. R. B., Hartley, C., Buchan, A., Harper, L., and Gallimore, P., 1980, The effects of lithium chloride on the replication of herpes simplex virus, *Med. Microbiol. Immunol.* **168**:139–148.

Spitzer, R. L., Endicott, J., and Robins, E., 1978, Research Diagnostic Criteria: Rationale and reliability, *Arch. Gen. Psychiatry* **35**:773–782.

Straus, S. E., Takiff, H. E., Seidlin, M., Bachrach, S., Lininger, L., DiGiovanna, J. J., Wester, K. A., Smith, H. A., Lehrman, S. N., Greagh-Kirk, T., and Alling, D. W., 1984, Suppression of frequently recurring genital herpes. A placebo controlled double-blind trial of oral acyclovir, *N. Engl. J. Med.* **310**:1545–1550.

Wunderlich, V., Fey, F., and Sydow, V. S., 1980, Antiviral effect of haloperidol on Rauscher murine leukemia virus, *Arch. Geschwulstforsch.* **50**:758–762.

Chapter **23**

Suppressive Effect of Alcohol on Normal Lymphocyte Proliferative Response to HIV Antigens

Madhavan P. N. Nair, Stanley A. Schwartz, Ziad A. Kronfol, Raveendran Pottathil, Edgar P. Heimer, and John F. Greden

INTRODUCTION

Previous studies have shown that chronic alcohol intake is associated with abnormalities of humoral and cellular immune functions (Mutchnick and Lee, 1988; McKeever *et al.*, 1988). Infection by the human immunodeficiency virus (HIV) causes profound dysfunction of cellular and humoral immune responses (Rosenberg and Fauci, 1989). Recent studies suggest that several cofactors such as other coincident infections, malnutrition, use of recreational drugs such as marijuana, cocaine, alcohol, and the like may exist in the natural history of HIV infection and development of AIDS. The present investigation is based on the

Madhavan P. N. Nair • *Departments of Pediatrics, Epidemiology, and Psychiatry, the Alcohol Research Center, and Midwest AIDS Biobehavioral Research Center, University of Michigan, Ann Arbor, Michigan 48109.* Stanley A. Schwartz • *Departments of Pediatrics and Epidemiology, the Alcohol Research Center, and Midwest AIDS Biobehavioral Research Center, University of Michigan, Ann Arbor, Michigan 48109.* Ziad A. Kronfol and John F. Greden • *Department of Psychiatry, the Alcohol Research Center, and Midwest AIDS Biobehavioral Research Center, University of Michigan, Ann Arbor, Michigan 48109.* Raveendran Pottathil and Edgar P. Heimer • *Hoffman–LaRoche, Inc., Nutley, New Jersey 07110.*

hypothesis that alcohol may reduce the host's immune response to HIV infection and increase the progression of the disease to clinical AIDS. We examined the effect of alcohol on natural killer (NK) cell activities and lymphocyte proliferative response (LPR) of lymphocytes from normal donors to peptides derived from the HIV.

MATERIALS AND METHODS

Peripheral blood lymphocytes were separated from healthy (HIV^-) nonalcoholic individuals aged 20–40 years old and used for NK and LPR. NK activity was determined in a direct ^{51}Cr release assay as described previously (Nair *et al.*, 1986) whereas LPR was determined using a [^3H]-thymidine assay as described elsewhere (Nair *et al.*, 1988).

RESULTS

In view of the finding that alcoholics are highly susceptible to various infections and because of a possible association between AIDS and alcohol abuse (Stimmel, 1987; Seigel, 1986), we examined the effect of alcohol on NK activity of purified NK cells. As shown in Table 1, isolated large granular lymphocytes precultured for 72 hr with 0.3% ethanol (EtOH) demonstrated significant suppression ($p < 0.5$) of NK activity.

Our previous studies demonstrated that both recombinant and synthetic HIV peptides can stimulate lymphocyte proliferative responses and can suppress polyclonal immunoglobulin production by normal lymphocytes (Nair *et al.*, 1988). In

Table 1. Effect of Alcohol on NK Activity of Large Granular Lymphocytes (LGL)[a]

Treatment of lymphocytes	% cytotoxicity	
—	27.7 ± 4.0	
EtOH 0.1%	28.7 ± 5.7	(N.S.)
0.2%	20.3 ± 3.4	(N.S.).
0.3%	16.4 ± 3.3	($p < 0.05$)

[a]Lymphocytes were precultured with different concentrations of EtOH for 72 hr, washed, and tested for their NK activity against K562 target cells at 2.5:1 E:T cell ratio. LGL were prepared on a discontinuous density gradient of Percoll as described (Nair *et al.*, 1986). The least dense fraction of lympyhocytes banding at the 37.5% Percoll interface consistently showed the highest NK activity and was used as LGL. Recovery of the cell was ~ 85% of the input and the yield was 7 to 10% at the 37.5% Percoll interface. Seventy-five to eighty percent of the cells were positive as demonstrated by HNK-I monoclonal antibody positivity. Values are mean ± S.D. of three experiments performed in triplicate.

view of the hypothesis that alcohol may be a cofactor in reducing the immune response to HIV infection, potentially enhancing progression to clinical AIDS (Seigel, 1986; MacGregar, 1987; Stall, 1987), we examined the effect of alcohol on proliferative responses of peripheral blood lymphocytes (PBL) to HIV-specific peptides. Data presented in Table 2 demonstrate that normal PBL stimulated separately with 5 ng/ml of env-gag and env 80-DHFR peptide showed a peak response between 72 and 96 hr of incubation as determined by [^{3}H]-thymidine incorporation.

In a dose-dependent lymphocyte proliferative response study, env-gag, a recombinant HIV fusion peptide, produced significant proliferation at 5, 10, and 50 ng/ml, the peak response being at 5–10 ng/ml (Table 3). Lymphocytes precultured with eng-gag plus alcohol at 0.2 and 0.3% concentration showed a significant suppression of LPR.

PBL precultured with 5, 10, and 50 ng/ml of env 80-DHFR, another HIV recombinant peptide which corresponds to the superconserved region of gp41, also showed proliferative responses which were significantly inhibited by alcohol at a concentration of 0.3% (Table 4).

CONCLUDING REMARKS

NK cell activity is considered to be a primary host defense mechanism against tumors and viral infections. Earlier studies showed that patients with AIDS demon-

Table 2. Kinetics of Peripheral Blood Lymphocyte (PBL) Proliferative Response to Env-gag and Env 80-DHFR Peptide[a]

Lymphocyte treatment	Period of incubation (hr) 24	48	72	96
Media[b]	1,254 ± 435[c]	2,361 ± 510	2,456 ± 1,392	1,956 ± 821
Env-gag[d]	4,367 ± 572	10,376 ± 1,123	19,132 ± 2,894	13,461 ± 2,017
	($p < 0.01$)[e]	($p < 0.002$)	($p < 0.005$)	($p < 0.005$)
Env 80-DHFR[f]	5,632 ± 912	14,832 ± 3,310	23,635 ± 3,941	11,367 ± 2,891
	($p < 0.01$)	($p < 0.025$)	($p < 0.005$)	($p < 0.025$)

[a]PBL ($2 - 10^5$) were cultured separately with or without 5 ng/ml of either env-gag or env 80-DHFR for 24 to 96 hr and proliferation was measured by [^{3}H]thymidine incorporation.
[b]Lymphocytes precultured in media alone.
[c]Values represent mean cpm ± S.D. of three separate experiments performed in triplicate.
[d]PBL precultured with env-gag peptide, a fusion product that contains 80 amino acids from gp41 and 190 amino acids from P24 of HIV.
[e]The statistical significance in mean values was determined by single-tailed Student's t test when lymphocytes cultured in media alone were compared with env-gag or env 80-DHFR peptide-treated cultures.
[f]PBL precultured with env 80-DHFR peptide, a synthetic oligonucleotide-based recombinant envelope gene product which corresponds to the superconserved region of gp41.

Table 3. Effect of Alcohol on HIV Peptide, Env-Gag-Induced Lymphocyte Proliferative Response[a]

	Env-gag concentrations (ng/ml)			
	0	5	10	50
Control[b]	2,105 ± 1,485[c]	18,311 ± 1,210 ($p < 0.001$)[d]	19,311 ± 1,833 ($p < 0.002$)	13,671 ± 1,303 ($p < 0.01$)
EtOH 0.1%[e]	2,136 ± 1,811 (N.S.)[f]	19,731 ± 1,014 (N.S.)	18,343 ± 1,819 (N.S.)	13,867 ± 1,319 (N.S.)
0.2%[g]	1,936 ± 1,120 (N.S.)	12,364 ± 1,180 ($p < 0.025$)	13,210 ± 1,940 ($p < 0.05$)	9,860 ± 956 ($p < 0.05$)
0.3%[h]	2,078 ± 830 (N.S.)	11,321 ± 1,735 ($p < 0.025$)	10,320 ± 1,763 ($p < 0.025$)	8,397 ± 689 ($p < 0.025$)

[a]PBL (2×10^5) were cultured with different concentrations of the recombinant HIV peptide, env-gag, ± alcohol for 72 hr. Proliferation was measured by [^{3}H]thymidine incorporation.
[b]PBL cultured in absence of EtOH.
[c]Values represent mean cpm ± S.D. of three separate experiments performed in triplicate.
[d]The statistical significance in mean values was determined by single-tailed Student's *t* test when either control lymphocytes were compared with env-gag-treated cultures or lymphocytes precultured with env-gag were compared with lymphocytes precultured with env-gag ± alcohol.
[e]PBL cultured in media containing 0.1% alcohol.
[f]Not statistically significant.
[g]PBL cultured in media containing 0.2% alcohol.
[h]PBL cultured in media containing 0.3% alcohol.

Table 4. Effect of Alcohol on HIV Peptide, Env 80-DHFR-Induced Lymphocyte Proliferative Responses[a]

	Env 80-DHFR concentrations (ng/ml)			
	0	5	10	50
Control[b]	1,836 ± 679[c]	19,367 ± 3,411 ($p < 0.01$)[d]	11,391 ± 1,167 ($p < 0.002$)	8,679 ± 910 ($p < 0.002$)
EtOH 0.1%[e]	2,210 ± 1,132 (N.S.)[f]	20,134 ± 2,413 (N.S.)	12,331 ± 1,371 (N.S.)	8,716 ± 1,339 (N.S.)
0.2%[g]	2,019 ± 892 (N.S.)	17,632 ± 3,748 (N.S.)	9,038 ± 870 (N.S.)	6,321 ± 765 (N.S.)
0.3%[h]	1,733 ± 567 (N.S.)	11,016 ± 873 ($p < 0.05$)	8,144 ± 630 ($p < 0.05$)	5,636 ± 525 ($p < 0.025$)

[a]PBL (2×10^5) were cultured with different concentrations of the recombinant HIV peptide, env 80-DHFR, ± alcohol for 72 hr. Proliferation was measured by [^{3}H]thymidine incorporation.
[b]PBL cultured in absence of EtOH.
[c]Values represent mean cpm ± S.D. of three separate experiments performed in triplicate.
[d]The statistical significance in mean values was determined by single-tailed student's *t* test when either control lymphocytes were compared with env 80-DHFR-treated cultures or lymphocytes precultured with env 80-DHFR were compared with lymphocytes precultured with env 80-DHFR + alcohol.
[e]PBL cultured in media containing 0.1% alcohol.
[f]Not statistically significant.
[g]PBL cultured in media containing 0.2% alcohol.
[h]PBL cultured in media containing 0.3% alcohol.

strate decreased NK cell activity. Because of the inhibitory effect of alcohol on various immunologic functions of normal lymphocytes as well as the observed depressed immune status of both alcoholic and AIDS patients, alcohol should be considered as a potential cofactor in the natural history of HIV infection and disease progression. Our studies have demonstrated that alcohol can suppress NK cell activity of normal lymphocytes. Further, we have shown that alcohol at intoxicating levels (0.2 to 0.3%) can suppress LPR to recombinant HIV peptides. The mechanisms by which normal lymphocytes undergo proliferative response to HIV peptides and the suppressive effect of alcohol on NK and LPR to HIV peptides are not clearly understood. Our studies, however, present preliminary evidence that alcohol can suppress the host's immune response to HIV peptides, suggesting that alcohol may act as a cofactor in the natural history of HIV infection and progression to clinical AIDS.

ACKNOWLEDGMENTS We express our appreciation to Denise DuPrie for expert secretarial assistance. This work was supported in part by National Institutes of Health grants MH42988, 1 P50 AA07378, 1 P50 MH43654, and 2 RO1 CA35922.

REFERENCES

MacGregar, R. R., 1987, Alcohol and drugs as cofactors for AIDS, *Adv. Alcohol Substance Abuse* **7**(2):47–71.

McKeever, Y., Mahony, C. O., Whelan, C. A., Weir, D. G., and Feighery, C., 1988, Helper and suppressor T lymphocyte function in severe alcoholic liver disease, *Clin. Exp. Immunol.* **60:** 39–48.

Mutchnick, M. G., and Lee, H., 1988, Impaired lymphocytes proliferative response to mitogen in alcoholic patients. Absence of a relationship to liver disease activity, *Alcoholism Clin. Exp. Res.* **12:**155–158.

Nair, M. P. N., Cilik, J. M., and Schwartz, S. A., 1986, Histamine-induced suppressor factor inhibition of NK cells. Reversal with interferon and interleukin 2, *J. Immunol.* **136:**2456–2462.

Nair, M. P. N., Pottathil, R, Heimer, E. P., and Schwartz, S. A., 1988, Immunoregulatory activities of human immunodeficiency virus (HIV) proteins. Effect of HIV recombinant and synthetic peptides on immunoglobulin synthesis and proliferative responses by normal lymphocytes, *Proc. Natl. Acad. Sci. USA* **85:**6498–6502.

Rosenberg, Z. R., and Fauci, A. S., 1989, Immunopathogenic mechanisms of HIV infection, *Clin. Immunol. Immunopathol.* **50:**5149–5156.

Seigel, L., 1986, AIDS relationship to alcohol and other drugs, *J. Substance Abuse Treatment* **3:** 271–274.

Stall, R., 1987, The prevention of HIV infection associated with drug and alcohol use during sexual activity, *Adv. Alcohol Substance Abuse* **7**(2):73–89.

Stimmel, B., 1987, AIDS, alcohol and heroin; a particularly deadly combination, *Adv. Alcohol Substance Abuse* **6**(3):1–5.

Part **V**

Animal Models in Virus Neuropathology

Chapter 24

Herpes Simplex Virus Type 1 Transcription during Latent Infections of Mouse and Man

Implications for Dementia

Anne M. Deatly, Ashley T. Haase, and Melvyn J. Ball

INTRODUCTION

Latent herpesvirus infections are generally described to have three stages: establishment, maintenance, and reactivation. Since 1929 when Goodpasture postulated that latent herpesvirus infections are established in the nervous system, we have known the sites where latent infections are established but the events by which latent infections are established, maintained, and reactivated remain a mystery. To completely understand the latency phenomena of herpesviruses, we must understand not only the role of the virus during the latent infection, but also the contribution of the infected cell or tissue to this process.

In this report, we describe the present understanding of the role of the virus

Anne M. Deatly • *Department of Microbiology, Mount Sinai School of Medicine, New York, New York 10029.* Ashley T. Haase • *Department of Microbiology, University of Minnesota, Minneapolis, Minnesota 55455.* Melvyn J. Ball • *Departments of Pathology, Clinical Neurological Sciences, and Psychiatry, University of Western Ontario, London, Ontario N6A 5C1, Canada.*

during the maintenance and reactivation stages of herpesvirus latency in the peripheral and central nervous systems. In addition, we present some studies attempting to understand the role of the infected cell during the maintenance and reactivation stages of herpesvirus latency. Finally, we present some ideas about the role of herpesvirus latency in dementia disease states, specifically Alzheimer's disease.

THE ROLE OF THE VIRUS DURING THE MAINTENANCE STAGE

The mouse eye model system (Knotts *et al.*, 1974) has been used to study the maintenance stage of herpesvirus latency because of the lack of spontaneous reactivation (Hill, 1985). Mice are inoculated with herpes simplex virus type 1 (HSV-1) (10^6–10^7 pfu per eye) following corneal scarification (Fraser *et al.*, 1986). The virus replicates at the site of inoculation and travels along the ophthalmic nerve to the trigeminal ganglion in the peripheral nervous system (Fraser *et al.*, 1986; Deatly *et al.*, 1988). The virus then enters the CNS in the pontine region of the brain stem where the trigeminal nerve root is located (Fraser *et al.*, 1986; Deatly *et al.*, 1988). Latent HSV-1 infections are established not only in the trigeminal system of the CNS but also in other areas such as the raphe nucleus, the pontine reticular formation, cerebellum, hippocampus, and entorhinal cortex (Stroop *et al.*, 1984; Deatly *et al.*, 1988).

The latent viral DNA exists in a episomal structure (Mellerick and Fraser, 1988) in which the ends of the linear virion genome are joined (Rock and Fraser, 1983, 1985). Since there is no detectable viral replication during latency, it has been assumed that the viral DNA is maintained in a silent state waiting for a stimulus to activate DNA replication, resulting in a recurrent herpesvirus lytic infection.

Transcription during a lytic or acute herpesvirus infection is temporally regulated (Honess and Roizman, 1974). The virion protein Vmw65 or αTIF (transcription-inducing factor) gene product initiates the transcriptional cascade by inducing the synthesis of the five immediate early transcripts (Batterson and Roizman, 1983). The immediate early gene products then transactivate the synthesis of early transcripts. These early gene products are involved in viral DNA replication which precedes late viral transcription. To determine the role of the virus during herpesvirus latency, we investigated whether there was transcription of any or all of the latent viral genome. Trigeminal ganglia were removed from mice at 5 days postinoculation (acute infections) or 1 month or later (latent infections), and the transcriptional programs during acute and latent infections were investigated by *in situ* hybridization. Using a total genomic probe, it was determined that transcription of the HSV-1 genome was occurring during latency (Stroop *et al.*, 1984). To determine if the latent transcripts were limited to a certain gene class or region of the genome, sections of trigeminal ganglia were hybridized with probes encoding different gene classes and different regions of the genome. Results from these experiments indicated that the repeat region of the genome which brackets the long unique sequence encoded the only latent transcripts (Deatly *et al.*, 1987, 1988). Further experimentation using small subfragment probes from this region demonstrated that the major latent transcriptional region either coincides with or overlaps one of the major immediate early regulatory genes, the infected cell polypeptide O (ICPO) gene. Some minor latent transcripts also mapped to regions both upstream and downstream from this one (Deatly *et al.*, 1987, 1988, unpublished data). Using single-stranded probes from the ICP0 region, Stevens and colleagues determined that the abundant latent RNA(s) are synthesized from the strand complementary to that of ICP0 RNA (Stevens *et al.*, 1987).

The latent RNA(s) is produced abundantly and continuously during herpesvirus latency as evident by comparing the trigeminal ganglia from animals infected for different lengths of time (Deatly *et al.*, 1987; Puga and Notkins, 1987). Wagner *et al.* (1988) have estimated between 10^4 and 10^6 copies of this RNA in latently infected neurons. In addition, this RNA is found predominantly in the nucleus of latently infected cells (Deatly *et al.*, 1987; Stevens *et al.*, 1987) and the majority is not polyadenylated (Spivack and Fraser, 1987; Wagner *et al.*, 1988).

From these studies, it became clear that the latent viral genome is not silent, and that the transcriptional program during the maintenance stage of herpesvirus latency is limited to one region of the genome. The latent RNA(s) is also produced in lytic infections but only in very low abundance (Spivack and Fraser, 1987, 1988). Therefore, the restricted latent transcriptional program is different from the temporal cascade observed during a normal lytic infection, indicating that the controls regulating the two different programs must be different. Stevens *et al.* (1987) have suggested that the major latent transcript functions through an antisense mechanism, hybridizing to the ICP0 mRNA and therefore blocking the lytic cascade of gene expression.

It appears that the production of a specific latent RNA(s) (or potentially a latent protein) is necessary for the maintenance of herpesvirus latency. However, Stevens and colleagues have demonstrated that latent herpesvirus infections are established when the latency-associated transcript promoter has been deleted (Javier *et al.*, 1988). In addition, Steiner *et al.* (1989) have performed experiments infecting mice with 1704 (HSV-1 variant) virus, a virus lacking the latency-associated transcript region. Latent infections are established (in the absence of the latency-associated RNAs) because explanted trigeminal ganglia reactivate from 1704-infected mice. However, reactivation times are greater compared to the time to reactivate from wild-type-infected mice. These results indicate that these latency-associated transcripts may not be active in establishing or maintaining latency but rather may aid in the reactivating process. At present, we still do not understand the role of the latent transcript(s) in establishing, maintaining, or even reactivating a latent herpesvirus infection.

THE ROLE OF THE INFECTED CELL DURING THE MAINTENANCE AND REACTIVATION STAGES

The contribution of the infected cell to herpesvirus latency was examined by studying differences in reactivation between latent infections established in PNS and CNS tissues. Explant cocultivation assays were used to monitor virus reactivation from PNS and CNS tissues of latently infected mice. Trigeminal ganglia (PNS tissue) and brain stem (CNS tissue) were explanted and separately placed onto monolayers of permissive CV-1 cells. The supernatant from these cultures was then removed after an appropriate incubation time and assayed for infectious virus. At 7 days postexplant, 100% (40/40) of the PNS tissues yielded reactivated virus, but at up to 15 days postexplant, none (0/6) of the CNS tissues yielded reactivated virus (Deatly *et al.*, 1988).

For reactivation to occur, regulation of virus gene expression would have to be altered from the tightly controlled restricted transcription observed during the maintenance stage of latency to that of the temporally regulated cascade expression of the different gene classes. To determine whether the difference in reactivation of virus from these two different tissues was due to differences in the viral infection or to differences in the infected cell types, we compared the transcriptional program of latent infections established in the PNS and CNS by *in situ* hybridization. We performed a similar study of transcription during latency with mouse brain stem tissues as we had with the trigeminal ganglia to ascertain whether a difference in the latent transcriptional program could account for the difference in reactivation efficiencies. These experiments demonstrated that HSV-1 RNA present in latently infected CNS cells mapped to the same region of the genome as observed in the PNS cells (Deatly *et al.*, 1988). These results did not reveal any difference in the latent transcriptional programs of the PNS and CNS; however, different latent RNAs from the same region could be produced in these different tissues to affect reactivation. This possibility remains to be investigated.

These results lead us to hypothesize that the difference in reactivation efficiencies between the PNS and CNS tissues is at the level of the infected cells rather than differences in transcription during the latent infection. The reduced number of lower density of latently infected cells in the CNS relative to the PNS may reduce the possibility for reactivation to occur. Another possibility is that different cellular factors in the CNS and PNS might play a role in reactivation differences. It is also possible that the two tissues differ in their ability to survive in explant culture. Consistent with this is the finding that neurons of the CNS do not have the same ability as neurons of the PNS to repair nerve processes (Grafstein, 1975; Benfey and Aguayo, 1982). The required metabolic change in the host cell for the reactivation to occur may be related to the ability of the host cell to repair itself (Hill, 1985). Clearly further work is needed to understand the very complex viral–host interaction during herpesvirus latency.

THE POTENTIAL ROLE OF HERPESVIRUSES IN NERVOUS SYSTEM DISORDERS

Latent herpesvirus infections are believed not to have any adverse effects on the host cells. However, latent herpesviruses can be reactivated following appropriate stimuli (Hill, 1983), and this reactivated virus growing lytically could have negative effects on the host cell. Reactivation of virus in the CNS could lead to destruction of specific neuronal cells (Townsend and Baringer, 1978; Price, 1985) which could interfere with intracellular communication within these tissues. We speculate that if reactivation of HSV-1 occurred from neurons of the trigeminal ganglia (the most common site of latent infection), the virus could then travel to the CNS. The CNS is a highly complex organ in which the cellular structure and morphology are important for efficient intracellular communication. Because these cells do not divide, any invasion (either by a virus or the immune system) could easily disrupt or interfere with normal cellular functions or even destroy the cells (ter Meulen *et al.*, 1984). Cumulative effects of these reactivation events in specific areas could play a role in slowly progressing CNS diseases (Ball, 1982). Others have speculated that herpesvirus infections may play a role in human CNS diseases of unknown etiologies, including multiple sclerosis (Koprowski and Warren, 1978; Martin, 1981; Vahlne *et al.*, 1985; Martin *et al.*, 1988), Bell's palsy (Adour *et al.*, 1975; Brodie, 1979; Vahlne *et al.*, 1981), psychiatric disorders (Sequiera *et al.*, 1979), trigeminal neuralgia (Finelli, 1975), and temporal lobe epilepsy (Oxbury *et al.*, 1972). HSV-1 has been isolated from the CSF of patients with meningitis and encephalitis (Tenser, 1984). In fact, HSV is the most common cause of viral encephalitis. At present, it is not known whether this CNS disease is caused by a primary herpesvirus infection or a reactivated latent infection.

THE POTENTIAL ROLE OF HERPESVIRUS LATENCY IN DEMENTING DISEASES

In organic dementias such as Alzheimer's disease, the degeneration and the dropout of the neuronal cells in the areas of the hippocampus, basal ganglia, and neocortex affect intracellular communication within the CNS which impairs memory processes, resulting in the dementia state. We speculate that recurrent herpesvirus reactivation events may play a role in the degeneration of specific areas of the CNS and may cause a dementia state like Alzheimer's disease.

Latent herpesvirus infections are (1) common infections which correlate with the high incidence of Alzheimer's disease cases, (2) found in the same areas of the CNS as those of the characteristic neurofibrillary changes of Alzheimer's disease (Deatly *et al.*, 1988; Stroop *et al.*, 1984), (3) predominantly found in neuronal cells (Deatly *et al.*, 1988) which are the cells in Alzheimer's disease which degenerate into neuritic plaques and tangles, and (4) the lymphocytic infiltrate present in areas around latently infected cells may indicate viral activity in these tissues. Also, McGeer *et al.* (1987) reported immunohistological data showing reactive microglia near Alzheimer's disease plaques, perhaps resulting from an immune reaction to a viral infection.

In support of the hypothesis that HSV may be associated with Alzheimer's disease, herpesvirus DNA has been detected by hybridization analysis in the CNS of normal patients (Fraser *et al.* 1981; Efstathiou *et al.*, 1986) and two patients with chronic psychiatric disorders and neuropathological changes characteristic of Alzheimer's disease dementia (Sequiera *et al.*, 1979). Others have had less success in detecting HSV-1 DNA in CNS tissue from Alzheimer's disease patients using solution hybridization (Middleton *et al.*, 1980), Southern blot analysis (Pogo *et al.*, 1987), dot blot hybridization techniques (Taylor *et al.*, 1984) and *in situ* hybridization (Elizan and Casals, 1987). Immunocytochemical analysis to detect antigens in Alzheimer's disease tissues has detected occasional HSV-1-infected cells (Mann *et al.*, 1981; Esiri, 1982).

We have taken advantage of the latency associated HSV-1 transcript(s) which are synthesized continuously and abundantly during latent HSV infections (Deatly *et al.*, 1987, 1988; Stevens *et al.*, 1987; Puga and Notkins, 1987) to use as a marker for latent herpesvirus infections in disease tissue. We have employed *in situ* hybridization using a probe from the region that encodes the latent HSV-1 RNAs, and hybridized 21 sets of trigeminal ganglia from Alzheimer's disease patients and 19 sets from non-Alzheimer's disease control patients. Eighty-one percent of the Alzheimer's disease patients had detectable latent HSV-1 infections in their trigeminal ganglia compared to 47% of the control patients (Deatly *et al.*, 1990). Statistical analysis of the data demonstrated that the difference was significant ($p < 0.05$). The frequency of HSV-1 latent infections in our control population (47%) is in line with other *in situ* hybridization data using control or normal human trigeminal ganglia (Gordon *et al.*, 1987; Croen *et al.*, 1987; Steiner *et al.*, 1988; Stevens *et al.*, 1988) as well as the estimates derived from sensitive explant assays, where theoretically a single latently infected cell could be detected with the amplification of viral replication accompanying reactivation. In several large and carefully conducted surveys, HSV was recovered from 40% to 62.5% of human trigeminal ganglia (Lonsdale *et al.*, 1980; Lewis *et al.*, 1982). These results are lower than the incidence of neutralizing antibody to HSV in the American adult population, which varies from 30 to 95% depending on age, geographic location, and socioeconomic status (Nahmias and Roizman, 1973; Koprowski, 1978; Whitley, 1985). The high incidence (90%) of neutralizing antibody in adults 60 years or older (Johnson, 1982; Stuart-Harris, 1983), which exceeds the recovery of virus and detection of latency transcripts, may be accounted for by latent infection of other sites or possibly an antibody cross-reaction with HSV-2.

Our evidence for a larger pool of latently infected neurons in the trigeminal ganglia of the Alzheimer's disease population in this study, and previously reported lower incidences of dementia in populations from Japan (Wang, 1977; Warren *et al.*, 1978) and Czechoslovakia (Libikova *et al.*, 1975) where ganglionic virus recovery and CSF herpes antibody are also lower, strengthen the suspicion that HSV might play a role in the pathogenesis of Alzheimer's disease.

In an attempt to show an association of latent herpesviruses with Alzheimer's disease pathology, we have analyzed the hippocampus of three Alzheimer's disease patients who had HSV-1 latently infected neurons in their trigeminal ganglia. We hybridized every 15th–20th tissue section (40–100 total sections) from these hippocampi with a probe to detect the abundant HSV-1 latent RNA(s) but were unable to find any hippocampal pyramidal neurons expressing HSV-1 RNA(s) (Deatly *et al.*, 1990). Moreover, we have also investigated the possibility of detecting HSV-1 latently infected cells in the brain stems of these patients with the rationale that the virus could initiate its damaging effects in an area along the pathway from the PNS to CNS at some distance from the sites of neuropathologic damage. Again, we were unable to detect any neuronal cells expressing latent HSV-1 RNA in the pons or medulla from two Alzheimer's disease patients (Deatly *et al.*, 1990).

The results of these experiments demonstrate that latent HSV-1 RNA is not present in the hippocampus or brain stem of three end-stage Alzheimer's disease tissues. However, we cannot rule out the possibility that a herpesvirus is involved in an earlier stage of dementia in Alzheimer's disease.

Acknowledgments We acknowledge Dr. Nigel W. Fraser in whose laboratory the mouse studies were performed. We thank Dr. Richard Peluso for critical reading of the manuscript; Dr. Peter Fewster for the statistical analysis; the members of the Dementia Study group, University of Western Ontario for their cooperation; and Drs. C. Anderson, D. Banerjee, J. Frei, B. Garcia, C. Guiraudon, D. G. Perkins, and A. C. Wallace for pathological assistance. This work was supported by grants from the NIH to A.T.H. (NS21580) and to M.J.B. (AG03047) and by funds from the Atkinson Charitable Foundation of Toronto to M.J.B. A.M.D. was supported by NIH Training Grant T32 CA09138-13.

REFERENCES

Adour, K. K., Bell, D. N., and Hilsinger, R. L., 1975, Herpes simplex virus in idiopathic facial paralysis (Bell palsy). *J. Am. Med. Assoc.* **233:**527–530.

Ball, M. J., 1982, Limbic predilection in Alzheimer dementia: Is reactivated herpesvirus involved? *Can. J. Neurol. Sci.* **9:**303–306.

Batterson, W., and Roizman, B., 1983, Characterization of the herpes simplex virion-associated factor responsible for induction of α genes, *J. Virol.* **46:**371–377.

Benfey, M., and Aguayo, A. J., 1982, Extensive elongation of axons from rat brain into peripheral nerve grafts, *Nature* **296:**150–152.

Brodie, S. W., 1979, Virology studies and Bell's palsy, *J. Laryngol. Otol.* **93:**563–568.

Croen, K. D., Ostrove, J. M., Dragovic, L. J., Smialek, J. E., and Straus, S. E., 1987, Latent herpes simplex virus in human trigeminal ganglia. Detection of an immediate early gene "anti-sense" transcript by *in situ* hybridization, *N. Engl. J. Med.* **317:**1427–1432.

Deatly, A. M., Spivack, J. G., Lavi, E., and Fraser, N. W., 1987, RNA from an immediate early region of the HSV-1 genome is present in the trigeminal ganglia of latently infected mice, *Proc. Natl. Acad. Sci. USA* **84:**3204–3208.

Deatly, A. M., Spivack, J. G., Lavi, E., O'Boyle, D. R., II, and Fraser, N. W., 1988, Latent herpes simplex virus type 1 transcripts in peripheral and central nervous system tissues of mice map to similar regions of the viral genome, *J. Virol.* **62:**749–756.

Deatly, A. M., Haase, A. T., Fewster, P. H., Lewis, E., and Ball, M. J., 1990, Human herpes virus infections and Alzheimer's disease, *Neuropathol. Appl. Neurobiol.* **16:**213–223.

Efstathiou, S., Minson, A. C., Field, H. J., Anderson, J. R., and Wildy, P., 1986, Detection of herpes simplex virus-specific DNA sequences in latently infected mice and in humans, *J. Virol.* **57:** 446–455.

Elizan, T. S., and Casals, J., 1987, The viral hypothesis in Parkinson's disease and in Alzheimer's disease, in: *Viruses, Immunity and Mental Disorders* (E. Kurstak, Z. J. Lipowski, and P. Morozov, eds.), Plenum Medical, New York, pp. 47–59.

Esiri, M. M., 1982, Herpes simplex encephalitis: An immunohistological study of the distribution of viral antigen within the brain, *J. Neurol. Sci.* **54:**209–226.

Finelli, P. F., 1975, Herpes simplex virus and the human nervous system: Current concepts and review, *Milit. Med.* **140:**765–771.

Fraser, N. W., Lawrence, W. C., Wroblewska, Z., Gilden, D. H., and Koprowski, H., 1981, Herpes simplex virus type 1 DNA in human brain tissue, *Proc. Natl. Acad. Sci. USA* **78:**6461–6465.

Fraser, N. W., Deatly, A. M., Mellerick, D. M., Muggeridge, M. I., and Spivack, J. G., 1986, Molecular biology of latent HSV-1, in: *Human Herpesvirus Infections* (C. Lopez and B. Roizman, eds.), Raven Press, New York, pp. 39–54.

Goodpasture, E. W., 1929, Herpetic infection, with special reference to involvement of the nervous system, *Medicine* **7:**223–233.

Gordon, Y. J., Johnson, B., Romanowski, E., and Araullo-Cruz, T., 1988, RNA complementary to herpes simplex virus type 1 ICP0 gene demonstrated in neurons of human trigeminal ganglia, *J. Virol.* **62:**1832–1835.

Grafstein, B., 1975, The nerve cell body response to axotomy, *Exp. Neurol.* **48:**32–51.

Hill, T. J., 1983, Herpesviruses in the central nervous system, in: *Viruses and Demyelinating Diseases* (C. Mims, ed.), Academic Press, New York, pp. 29–45.

Hill, T. J., 1985, Herpes simplex virus latency, in: *The Herpesviruses*, Volume 4 (B. Roizman, ed.), Plenum Press, New York, p. 175–240.

Honess, R. W., and Roizman, B., 1974, Regulation of herpesvirus macromolecular synthesis. I. Cascade regulation of the synthesis of three groups of viral proteins, *J. Virol.* **14:**8–19.

Javier, R. T., Stevens, J. G., Dissette, V. B., and Wagner, E. K., 1988, A herpes simplex virus transcript abundant in latently infected neurons is dispensable for establishment of the latent state, *Virology* **166:**254–257.

Johnson, R. T., 1982, Herpesvirus infections, in: *Viral Infections of the Nervous System* (R. T. Johnson, ed.), Raven Press, New York, pp. 129–157.

Knotts, F. B., Cook, M. L., and Stevens, J. G., 1974, Pathogenesis of herpetic encephalitis in mice after ophthalmic inoculation, *J. Infect. Dis.* **130:**16–27.

Koprowski, H., 1978, Possible role of herpes virus in the chronic CNS diseases, in: *ICN-UCLA Symposia on Molecular and Cellular Biology*, Volume 11 (J. G. Stevens, G. J. Todaro, and C. F. Fox, eds.), Academic Press, New York, pp. 691–699.

Koprowski, H., and Warren, K. G., 1978, Can a defective herpes simplex virus cause multiple sclerosis? *Perspect. Biol. Med.* **22**:10–18.

Lewis, M. E., Warren, K. G., Jeffrey, V. M., and Shnitka, T. K., 1982, Factors affecting recovery of latent herpes simplex virus from human trigeminal ganglia, *Can. J. Microbiol.* **28**:123–129.

Libikova, H., Pogady, J., Wiedermann, V., and Breier, S., 1975, Search for herpetic antibodies in the cerebrospinal fluid in senile dementia and mental retardation, *Acta Virol.* **19**:493–495.

Lonsdale, D. M., Brown, S. M., Lang, J., Subak-Sharpe, J., Koprowski, H., and Warren, K. G., 1980, Variations in herpes simplex virus isolated from human ganglia and a study of clonal variation in HSV-1, *Ann. N.Y. Acad. Sci.* **354**:291–308.

Mann, D. M. A., Yates, D. O., Davies, J. S., and Hawkes, J., 1981, Viruses, parkinsonism and Alzheimer's disease, *J. Neurol. Neurosurg. Psychiatry* **4**:651.

Martin, J., 1981, Herpes simplex virus 1 and 2 and multiple sclerosis, *Lancet* **2**:777–781.

McGeer, P. L., Itagaki, S., Tago, H., and McGeer, E. G., 1987, Reactive microglia in patients with senile dementia of the Alzheimer type are positive for the histocompatibility glycoprotein HLA-DR, *Neurosci. Lett.* **79**:195–200.

Martin, J. R., Holt, R. K., and Webster, H., 1988, Herpes simplex-related antigen in human demyelinative disease and encephalitis, *Acta Neuropathol.* **76**:325–337.

Mellerick, D. M., and Fraser, N. W., 1988, Physical state of the latent herpes simplex virus genome in a mouse model system. Evidence suggesting an episomal state, *Virology* **158**:265–275.

Middleton, P. J., Petric, M., Kozak, M., Rewcastle, N. B., Crapper, M., and McLachlan, D. R., 1980, Herpes simplex viral genome and senile and presenile dementias of Alzheimer and Pick, *Lancet* **1**:1038.

Nahmias, A. J., and Roizman, B., 1973, Infection with herpes-simplex viruses 1 and 2, *N. Eng. J. Med.* **289**:781–789.

Oxbury, J. M., Matthews, W. B., and MacCallum, F. O., 1972, Herpes simplex and temporal lobe epilepsy, *Br. Med. J.* **3**:288.

Pogo, B. G. T., Casals, J., and Elizan, T. S., 1987, A study of viral genomes and antigens in brains of patients with Alzheimer's disease, *Brain* **110**:907–915.

Price, R. W., 1985, Herpes simplex virus latency: Adaptation to the peripheral nervous system. II, *Cancer Invest.* **3**:389–403.

Puga, A., and Notkins, A. L., 1987, Continued expression of a poly (A+) transcript of herpes simplex virus type 1 in trigeminal ganglia of latently infected mice, *J. Virol.* **61**:1700–1703.

Rock, D. L., and Fraser, N. W., 1983, Detection of HSV-1 genome in the central nervous system of latently infected mice, *Nature* **302**:523–525.

Rock, D. L., and Fraser, N. W., 1985, Latent herpes simplex virus type 1 DNA contains two copies of the virion DNA joint region, *J. Virol.* **55**:849–852.

Sequiera, L. W., Jennings, L. C., Carasco, L. H., Lord, M., Curry, A., and Sutton, R. N. P., 1979, Detection of herpes simplex viral genome in brain tissue, *Lancet* **2**:608–612.

Spivack, J. G., and Fraser, N. W., 1987, Detection of herpes simplex virus type 1 transcription during latent infections in mice, *J. Virol.* **61**:3841–3847.

Spivack, J. G., and Fraser, N. W., 1988, Expression of a herpes simplex virus type 1 latency-associated transcript in the trigeminal ganglia of mice during acute infection and reactivation of latent infection, *J. Virol.* **62**:1479–1485.

Steiner, I., Spivack, J. G., O'Boyle, D. R., II, Lavi, E., and Fraser, N. W., 1988, Latent herpes simplex virus type 1 transcription in human trigeminal ganglia, *J. Virol.* **62**:3493–3496.

Steiner, I., Spivack, J. G., Lirette, R. P., Brown, S. M., MacLean, A. R., Subak-Sharpe, J. H., and Fraser, N. W., 1989, Herpes simplex virus type 1 latency-associated transcripts are evidently not essential for latent infections, *EMBO J.* **8**:505–511.

Stevens, J. G., Wagner, E. K., Devi-Rao, G. B., Cook, M. L., and Feldman, L. T., 1987, RNA complementary to a herpesvirus α gene mRNA is prominent in latently infected neurons, *Science* **235**:1056–1059.

Stevens, J. G., Harr, L., Porter, D. D., Cook, M. L., and Wagner, E. K., 1988, Prominence of the herpes simplex virus latency-associated transcript in trigeminal ganglia from seropositive humans, *J. Infect. Dis.* **158**:117–123.

Stroop, W. G., Rock, D. L., and Fraser, N. W., 1984, Localization of herpes simplex virus in the trigeminal and olfactory systems in the mouse central nervous system during acute and latent infections by *in situ* hybridization, *Lab. Invest.* **51**:27–38.

Stuart-Harris, Sir C., 1983, The epidemiology and clinical presentation of herpes virus infections, *J. Antimicrob. Chemother.* **12**(Suppl. B), 1–8.

Taylor, G. R., Crow, T. J., Markakis, D. A., Lofthouse, R., Neeley, S., and Carter, G. I., 1984, Herpes simplex virus and Alzheimer's disease: A search for virus DNA by spot hybridisation, *J. Neurol. Neurosurg. Psychiatry* **47**:1061–1065.

Tenser, R. B., 1984, Herpes simplex and herpes zoster nervous system involvement, *Neurol. Clin.* **2**:215–240.

ter Meulen, V., Carter, M. J., Wege, H., and Watanabe, R., 1984, Mechanisms and consequences of virus persistence in the human nervous system, *Ann. N.Y. Acad. Sci.* **436**:86–97.

Townsend, J. J., and Baringer, J. R., 1978, Central nervous system susceptibility to herpes simplex virus infection, *J. Neuropathol. Exp. Neurol.* **37**:255–262.

Vahlne, A., Edstrom, S., Arstila, P., Beran, M., Enjell, H., Nylen, O., and Lycke, E., 1981, Bell's palsy and herpes simplex, *Arch. Otolaryngol.* **107**:79–81.

Vahlne, A., Edstrom, S., Hanner, P., Anderson, O., Svennerholm, B., and Lycke, E., 1985, Possible association of herpes simplex virus infection with demyelinating disease, *Scand. J. Infect. Dis. Suppl.* **47**:16–21.

Wagner, E. K., Devi-Rao, G. B., Feldman, L. T., Dobson, A. T., Zhang, Y.-F., Flanagans, W. F., and Stevens, J. G., 1988, Physical characterization of the herpes simplex virus latency-associated transcript in neurons, *J. Virol.* **62**:1194–1202.

Wang, H. S., 1977, Dementia of old age, in: *Aging and Dementia* (W. L. S. Smith and M. Kinsbourne, eds.), Spectrum Publications, New York, pp. 1–24.

Warren, K. G., Wroblewska, Z., Okabe, H., Brown, S. M., Gilden, D. H., Koprowski, H., Rorke, L. B., Subak-Sharpe, J., and Yonezawa, T., 1978, Virology and histopathology of the trigeminal ganglia of Americans and Japanese, *Can. J. Neurol. Sci.* **5**:425–430.

Whitley, R. J., 1985, Epidemiology of herpes simplex viruses, in: *The Herpesviruses*, Volume 3 (B. Roizman, ed.), Plenum Press, New York, pp. 1–44.

Chapter **25**

Effects of Stress on a Murine Neurotropic Retrovirus Infection

W. P. Paré, D. S. Robbins, J. L. Martin, and P. M. Hoffman

INTRODUCTION

Psychological and environmental factors have long been recognized as affecting health and disease (Monjan and Collector, 1977; Riley, 1981; Sklar and Anisman, 1980; Weiner, 1977; Wolf and Goodell, 1968). The immune system is also quite responsive to environmental perturbations. Many investigators have documented changes in the immune system resulting from stressful stimulation (Ader, 1981; Cooper, 1984; Monjan, 1981; Riley, 1981; Rogers *et al.*, 1979). Susceptibility to infectious diseases is also influenced by exposure to environmental stressors (Amkraut *et al.*, 1971; Friedman *et al.*, 1969; Locke and Hornig-Rohan, 1983; Rasmussen *et al.*, 1957; Yamada *et al.*, 1964). Given that variations in the immune response and susceptibility to infectious disease have been related to stress exposure, it is reasonable to consider the possibility that stress may be involved in the pathogenesis and clinical expression of the acquired immunodeficiency syndrome (AIDS) (Britton, 1986; Locke *et al.*, 1984; Risenberg, 1986; Stein, 1985). The

W. P. Paré • *Veterans Administration Medical Center, Perry Point, Maryland 21902.* D. S. Robbins, J. L. Martin, and P. M. Hoffman • *Veterans Administration Medical Center, Baltimore, Maryland 21218.*

discovery that a human retrovirus (HIV) infection can cause AIDS in man has focused attention on animal retrovirus infections as models of AIDS. The fact that murine retroviruses (MuLV) can cause immunodeficiency (Mosier *et al.*, 1985) and neurodegeneration (Hoffman *et al.*, 1981) makes them useful as models for human retrovirus infections. The question of how stress may be related to the development and clinical manifestations of AIDS can be formed with basic investigations using these animal models.

The neurotropic MuLV model chosen for this study utilizes a biologically cloned ectopic MuLV (Cas-Br-M MuLV) isolated from wild mice (Hartley and Rowe, 1976). Inoculation of newborn inbred NFS/N mice results in a well-defined syndrome of progressive tremor, hind limb weakness, and paralysis (Hoffman *et al.*, 1981). The disease onset and progression rate are virus-dose and host age dependent. Maturation of host T-cell immunity, particularly the MuLV-specific cytotoxic T-cell response, appears to play a major role in age-dependent susceptibility and resistance to neurodegeneration (Hoffman *et al.*, 1984; Robbins *et al.*, 1989).

Virus replication occurs earliest in splenic megakaryocytes and lymphoid cells and dissemination to brain capillary endothelial cells can be detected by 3 weeks postinfection (Hoffman *et al.*, unpublished). Viral proteins can be identified in glial and endothelial cells but not in neurons (Hoffman *et al.*, 1988). Spongiform vacuolation, gliosis, and neuronal vacuolation and dropout begin at 4 weeks postinfection and become progressively more severe over time. The gray matter–white matter junction of the spinal cord, brain stem, and cerebellum are the most affected areas (Hoffman *et al.*, unpublished).

Prior to the development of neurological symptoms such as tremors and weakness, abnormal behavior such as aggressiveness and hyperactivity had been observed in infected mice. These observations reinforced our suspicions that environmental and psychological variables might influence the expression of symptoms in infected mice and that these mice might be sensitive to stress effects. Consequently, we wanted to test the hypothesis that psychological stress during the latent period following MuLV infection would adversely affect disease outcome by accelerating immune dysfunction, neurological symptom expression, and behavioral abnormalities. However, we are aware that stress is a very complex process with subtle effects. This research program, of necessity, had to first address very basic variables, such as the impact of housing and handling. Therefore, the first study evaluated the effects of housing condition on the clinical and neuropathological expression of Cas-Br-M MuLV infection.

EXPERIMENT 1

At 4 days of age, Cas-Br-M MuLV (1×10^5 pfu/mouse) was inoculated i.p. into Swiss mice ($n = 45$). At 23 days of age, mice were assigned to either group housing ($n = 35$) which included 5 mice per cage, or isolated housing ($n = 10$) with only one mouse per cage. Housing was provided by standard Plexiglas cages measuring 12 × 16 × 28 cm. All mice had continuous access to food and water and light conditions were artificially maintained between 0600 and 1800 hr. Twenty days later and every week thereafter, all mice were evaluated for clinical symptoms of disease. These symptoms included two levels of splay foot, two levels of tremor, spasticity, and paralysis. For scoring purposes, these symptoms were arranged in order of symptom severity with early signs of splay foot receiving a score of 1 at the low end of the scale, and paralysis receiving a score of 6 at the high end of the scale. The symptom severity rating scale is summarized in Table 1. After 10 weeks all mice were sacrificed and assayed for pathology and virus levels.

All mice had histopathological evidence of MuLV-induced neurodegeneration including gliosis, vacuolation, and neuronal dropout. The symptom severity scores were analyzed for possible differences between groups, but this analysis failed to reveal any significant differences. These data are illustrated in Fig. 1.

Possible explanations for these negative results are that: (1) outbred Swiss mice do not express a spectrum of neurological symptoms broad enough to detect subtle differences due to stress or that (2) the housing treatment did not have a significant influence on the expression of the disease and a more intense stressor is required in order to demonstrate any possible stress effects. We elected to investigate the second possibility. Consequently, we exposed mice to grid shock, which we assumed was more stressful than group housing. Shock was presented using either an acute or a chronic schedule.

EXPERIMENT 2

The second study used 21 male Swiss mice. Animals were inoculated when 4 days old, as in Experiment 1. At weaning, mice were housed either 3 or 4 per cage. At 26 days of age, mice were randomly assigned to either the acute stress, chronic stress, or a no-stress control treatment ($n = 7$). Stress consisted of placing mice individually in small plastic boxes (measuring 17 × 17 × 20 cm) with grid floors

Table 1. Symptom Severity Rating Scale

Symptom	Score
Splay	1
Splay tremor	2
	3
	4
Spasticity	5
Paralysis	6

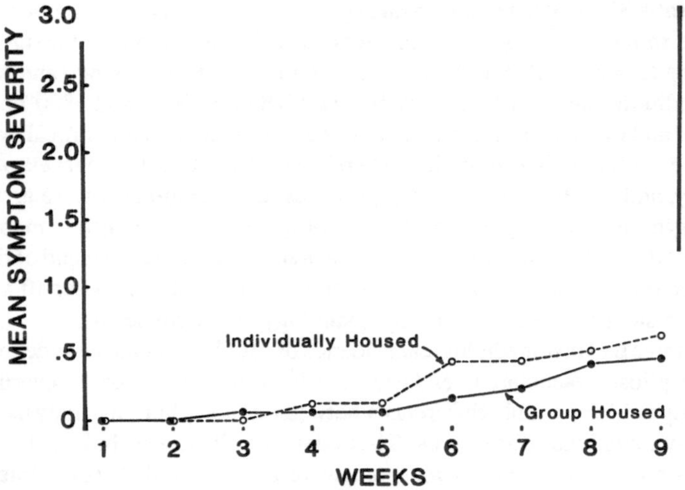

Figure 1. Mean symptom severity scores for group-housed and individually housed mice.

and subjecting the animal to 60 6-sec shocks (0.15 mA) with an average interval between shocks of 1 min. Mice in the acute stress treatment condition were exposed to the stress schedule only once on day 28. Mice in the chronic stress schedule were exposed to the stress schedule on 5 consecutive days each week for 10 weeks. The no-stress control mice remained in home cages and were not exposed to grid shock. All mice were examined for clinical symptoms on day 80 and weekly for the next 3 weeks. When the mice were 104 days old, all animals were sacrificed in order to determine virus levels and to conduct pathological examinations.

These examinations revealed that all mice, 100 days after the inoculation, had nervous system pathology. However, the symptom severity scores yielded different results. These data are illustrated in Fig. 2 and show that disease severity was greater for no-stress control mice. Analysis of these data, using a Kruskal–Wallis design, revealed that symptom severity was significantly less for chronic stress mice as compared to acute and control mice for the first examination day ($H = 6.91$, $df = 2, p < 0.05$), the second examination day ($H = 9.71$, $df = 2, p < 0.01$), and the third examination day ($H = 12.38, df = 2, p < 0.01$). Mice exposed to the acute stress treatment had significantly lower symptom severity scores as compared to controls for the second examination day ($H = 4.58, df = 2, p < 0.05$) and the third examination day ($H = 6.21$, $df = 2$, $p < 0.05$). Thus, it would appear that stress had an attenuating effect on the clinical manifestations of the disease and this effect was more robust for chronic stress as compared to acute stress.

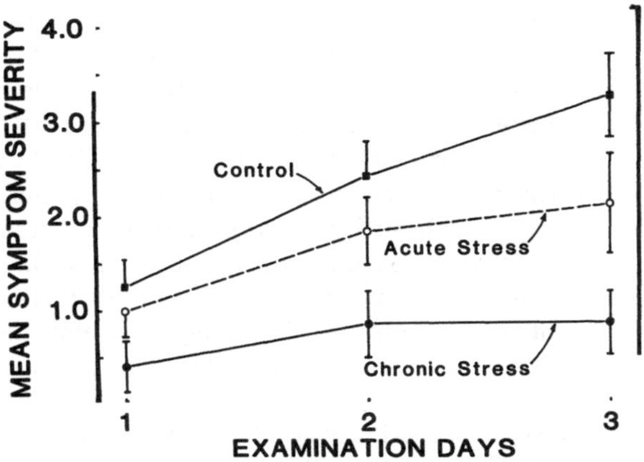

Figure 2. Mean (± S.E.) symptom severity scores for mice exposed to chronic shock stress, acute shock stress, or a no-stress control condition.

DISCUSSION

These data provided only partial confirmation of our initial hypothesis. The first study produced very low symptom severity scores, and in the second study, all mice showed evidence of the disease on the basis of the pathological exam, but group differences emerged when the clinical symptom severity scores were compared by treatment group. Regarding the latter discrepancy, one possible explanation is the fact that the pathological exams were conducted only at the end of the experiment and this strategy favored positive pathological results. Obviously, an experimental design that sacrifices subgroups of mice at different time periods throughout the study would address this problem. Another concern which would address the results from both experiments, is the fact that Swiss mice do not readily manifest all the neurologic symptoms associated with Cas-Br-M MuLV infection (Hoffman *et al.*, 1981; Hoffman and Morse, 1985). NFS/N mice more consistently demonstrate the full spectrum of neurologic symptoms associated with Cas-Br-M MuLV infection (Hoffman and Morse, 1985) and this strain should be used in subsequent studies.

Besides these procedural issues, there are other issues which should be considered before research on this topic is pursued. Our basic hypothesis must be reexamined. On the basis of the published literature we assumed that stress would produce differences in the clinical expression of target tissue injury associated with MuLV infection. We also assumed that group housing would be stressful and consequently would produce an effect. However, it is possible that housing can certainly produce an effect, but the effects may not be attributable to housing *per se*. For example, Rabin *et al.* (1987) were successful in producing an altered immune reactivity in group- versus single-housed mice. However, they argued that the effect was not stress-mediated since blood corticosterone levels were not significantly different between groups, leading them to conclude that "the psychologic and genetic variables associated with this effect remained to be determined" (Rabin *et al.*, 1987). These reports emphasize the fact that any stress–behavioral effect must involve very complicated mediating mechanisms. The problem is further complicated if the temporal relationship between the inoculation event and the stress event is manipulated. Justice (1985) reviewed this literature and concluded that different outcomes are obtained depending on whether the animal was first inoculated, or first exposed to a stressor. Thus, the temporal sequence of events is critical.

The results of our second experiment also force a reexamination of our initial hypothesis. If we disregard momentarily that the symptom severity data and the pathology data were collected at different times, we note that stress had an effect only with one dependent variable, the symptom severity data, and none with the pathology data. This suggests that stress effects may be studied far more critically if we adopt dependent variables which are capable of discriminating between experimental treatments. Crnic and Pizer (1988) have demonstrated that behavioral response categories such as hyperactivity, and passive avoidance learning are sufficiently sensitive to detect subtle effects such as occur following herpes simplex type 1 infection. This suggests that subsequent research on the effects of stress on the MuLV model should use behavioral parameters which may be more sensitive than our symptom severity scale. With this in mind, we have initiated developmental studies wherein the behavior of Cas-Br-M MuLV-infected mice is monitored for changes in daily motor activity, open-field behavior, and chronic avoidance learning. We hope these studies will provide some information regarding the effect of Cas-Br-M MuLV infection on motor, affective, and cognitive processes.

REFERENCES

Ader, R. (ed.), 1981, *Psychoneuroimmunology*, Academic Press, New York.

Amkraut, A. A., Soloman, G. F., and Kraemer, H. C., 1971, Stress, early experience and adjuvant-induced arthritis in the rat, *Psychosom. Med.* **33**:203–214.

Britton, S., 1986, Psychosocial aspects of HTLV-III infections, *Scand. J. Soc. Med.* **14**:211–212.

Cooper, E. L. (ed.), 1984, *Stress, Immunity, and Aging*, Dekker, New York.

Crnic, L. S., and Pizer, L. I., 1988, Behavioral effects of neonatal herpes simplex type I infection of mice, *Neurotoxicol. Teratol.* **10**:381–386.

Friedman, S. B., Glasgow, L. A., and Ader, R., 1969, Psychosocial factors modifying host resistance to experimental infections, *Ann. N.Y. Acad. Sci.* **164**:381–393.

Hartley, J. W., and Rowe, W. P., 1976, Naturally occurring murine leukemia viruses in wild mice: Characterization of a new "amphotropic" class, *J. Virol.* **19**:19–25.

Hoffman, P. M., and Morse, H. C., III, 1985, Host genetic determinants of neurologic disease in murine retrovirus infection, *J. Virol.* **53**:40–43.

Hoffman, P. M., Ruscetti, S. K., and Morse, H. C., III, 1981, Pathogenesis of paralysis and lymphoma associated with a wild mouse retrovirus infection. Part I. Age-and-dose-related effects in susceptible laboratory mice, *J. Neuroimmunol.* **1**:275–285.

Hoffman, P. M., Robbins, D. S., and Morse, H. C., III, 1984, Role of immunity in age-related resistance to paralysis after murine retrovirus infection, *J. Virol.* **52**:734.

Hoffman, P. M., Pitts, D. M., Bilello, J A., and Cimino, E. F., 1988, Retrovirus induced motor neuron degeneration, *Rev. Neurol.* **144**:676–679.

Justice, A., 1985, Review of the effects of stress on cancer in laboratory animals. Importance of time of stress application and type of tumor, *Psychol. Bull.* **98**:108–138.

Locke, S. E., and Hornig-Rohan, M., 1983, *Mind and immunity: Behavioral Immunology*, Institute for the Advancement of Health, New York.

Locke, S. E., Krans, L., Leurman, J., Hurat, M. W., Heisel, J. S., and Williams, L. M., 1984, Life change stress, psychiatric symptoms, and natural killer cell activity, *Psychosom. Med.* **46**: 441–453.

Monjan, A. A., 1981, Stress and immunologic competence: Studies in animals, in: *Psychoneuroimmunology* (R. Ader, ed.), Academic Press, New York, pp. 185–228.

Monjan, A A., and Collector, M. I., 1977, Stress-induced modulation of the immune response, *Science* **196**:307–308.

Mosier, E. E., Yetter, R. A., and Morse, H. C., III, 1985, Retroviral induction of acute lymphoproliferative disease and profound immunosuppression in adult C57 BL/6 mice, *J. Exp. Med.* **161**: 766–784.

Rabin, B. S., Lyte, M., and Harriel, E., 1987, The influence of mouse strain and housing on the immune response, *J. Neuroimmunol.* **17**:11–16.

Rasmussen, A. F., Jr., Marsh, J. T., and Brill, N. Q., 1957, Increased susceptibility to herpes simplex in mice subjected to avoidance-learning stress or restraint, *Proc. Soc. Exp. Biol. Med.* **96**:183–189.

Riley, V., 1981, Psychoneuroendocrine influences on immunocompetence and neoplasia, *Science* **212**:1100–1109.

Risenberg, D. E., 1986, Can mind affect body defenses against disease? Nascent specialty offers a host of tantalizing clues, *J. Am. Med. Assoc.* **256**:313–317.

Robbins, D. S., Bilello, J. A., and Hoffman, P. M., 1989, Pathogenesis and treatment of neurotropic murine leukemia virus infections, in: *HTLV-I and the Nervous System* (G. C. Roman, J. C. Vernant, and M. Deane eds.), Liss, New York, pp. 575–587.

Rogers, M. P., Dubey, D., and Reich, P., 1979, The influence of the psyche and the brain on immunity and disease susceptibility: A critical review, *Psychosom. Med.* **41**:147–164.

Sklar, L. S., and Anisman, H., 1980, Social stress influences tumor growth, *Psychosom. Med.* **42**: 347–365.

Stein, M., 1985, Depression and immunity, *Arch. Gen. Psychiatry* **42**:129–233.

Weiner, H., 1977, *Psychobiology and Human Disease*, Elsevier/North-Holland, Amsterdam.

Wolf, S., and Goodell, H., 1968, *Harold G. Wolfs Stress and Disease*, Thomas, Springfield, Ill.

Yamada, A., Jensen, M. M., and Rasmussen, A. F., Jr., 1964, Stress and susceptibility to viral infections. III. Antibody response and viral retention during avoidance learning stress, *Proc. Soc. Exp. Biol. Med.* **116**:677–680.

Chapter 26

The Effect of Cold or Isolation Stress on Neuroinvasiveness and Neurovirulence of an Avirulent Variant of West Nile Virus (WN-25)

D. Ben-Nathan, S. Lustig, and G. Feuerstein

INTRODUCTION

Stress has been defined by Selye (1950, 1957) as a nonspecific response to internal and external stimuli that induces hormonal changes which lead to depression of the immune system. Since stress alters the chemical balance of the body, it probably influences the development of diseases through its effect on the immune system. In order to understand the influence of physical or nonphysical stress on the susceptibility of mice to viral infections, we used avirulent West Nile virus.

D. Ben-Nathan and S. Lustig • *Department of Virology, Israel Institute for Biological Research, Ness-Ziona, Israel.* G. Feuerstein • *Department of Neurology, USUHS, Bethesda, Maryland 20814.*

West Nile virus (WNV) is a member of the flavivirus genus, of the family Flaviviridae. As a flavivirus it contains a nonsegmented single-stranded 42 S RNA and three virion polypeptides, one of which is a glycoprotein (Forterfield *et al.*, 1978). WNV is widely distributed throughout Asia, Africa, and parts of Europe (Monath, 1986). It is a neurotropic arbovirus (Weiner *et al.*, 1970) and is capable of endemic spread (Hayes *et al.*, 1982; Goldblum *et al.*, 1954). Wild birds are the primary host but high antibody levels in a variety of animals including man indicate a broad infection spectrum; in man the morbidity rate is low and severe cases of encephalitis occur only occasionally, but subclinical infection is common (Chamberlain, 1980). In parts of Africa, up to 70% of the human population may possess antibodies (Chamberlain, 1980). A variant of WNV, designated WN-25, has been isolated from a WNV-persistent infection in mosquito cell cultures (Halevy *et al.*, 1986). WN-25 showed no differences from WNV in serology tests (HI, NT, and RIA), buoyant density, surface charge, and RNA fingerprints. Both strains grew equally well in BHK and Vero cell cultures.

The ratios of plaque-forming units to HA, antigenic mass (RIA), and LD50 by intracerebral (i.c.) route in suckling and adult mice were similar for both strains. The lethality of both strains in suckling mice by the i.p. route was similar. In adult mice, WNV was as lethal by i.p. as by i.c. inoculation, whereas WN-25 was completely nonlethal when injected i.p. No infectious virus could be found in the brains of the WN-25-injected mice although all became immune (Halevy *et al.*, 1986).

Environmental or physical stress is known to affect the immune system. For example, starvation (Ben-Nathan *et al.*, 1977) cortisol injection (Parillo and Fauci, 1979), cold or isolation stress (Ben-Nathan and Feuerstein, 1988a, 1990) can cause involution of lymphoid organs such as thymus, spleen, and lymph nodes through activation of the pituitary–adrenocortical axis (Friedman and Glasgow, 1966). Further, interferon production is suppressed in stress situations (Jensen, 1973), and T-helper lymphocyte levels are reduced under various types of stress (Kiecolt-Glaser *et al.*, 1984; Sapse, 1984). In fact, stress paradigms such as avoidance behavior have already been shown to exacerbate several infectious agents, including herpes simplex virus (Rasmussen *et al.*, 1957), Coxsackie B_1 virus (Johnson *et al.*, 1963), and vesicular stomatitis virus (Jensen and Rasmussen, 1963).

The following studies explored the interaction of physical (cold) and social (isolation) stress situations on the course of WNV encephalitis, including brain and spleen virus level, mortality, and lymphoid organ development.

WNV and WN-25 have been chosen as a model for studying the interaction of stress on viral infections since they provide a reproducible and predictable model in mice, and allow one to address neurovirulence and neuroinvasiveness, two phenomena which have been little studied in the past.

MATERIALS AND METHODS

Viruses

WNV

The original strain of virus was isolated from a human case of WNV infection (Goldblum *et al.*, 1954). The virus stock was prepared and assayed in Vero cells in our laboratory. The virus stock used for the experiments contained 3×10^8 plaque-forming units (PFU)/ml. The intracerebral titer (LD_{50}) was 1.3×10^7/ml and 6.9×10^6 mouse i.p. LD_{50}/ml.

WN-25

Aedes aegypti cultures (kindly provided by Dr. Peleg) were infected with an input of about one PFU per cell of WNV from mouse brain suspension. The infected culture was subcultured once or twice a week and the virus progeny harvested. At passage 25 the virus was plaque purified on Vero cells (three times), regrown in $C_{6/36}$ (*Aedes albopictus* cell line) and later on Vero cells (Halevy *et al.*, 1986).

Mice

Charles River outbred ICR mice (CD1) were obtained at the age of 21 days (10–12 g. body wt) and kept in our vivarium until the age of 27 to 42 days. In all studies, mice of the same age and batch were used.

Virus Inoculation

Each mouse was inoculated with 0.2 ml (i.p.) of WNV containing 20–200 PFU or with WN-25 200,000 PFU/mouse. The virus dilutions were performed using inactivated rabbit serum (10%) in 0.09% saline containing penicillin (1000 U/ml). Groups of 6–18 mice were used and the results calculated according to the method of Reed and Muench (1938).

Stress

Cold Stress

Mice were placed for 5 min/day in cold water (1 ± 0.5°C). The mice could stand in the water, which was 3 cm deep. WNV was inoculated and the mice immediately exposed to the cold stress. Stress continued every day until day 8 to 10 postinoculation. For mortality rate, mice were observed until the end of the experiment (21 days) and for brain virus level, mice were sacrificed 7 or 8 days after inoculation.

Isolation

Mice were housed in individual cages soon after inoculation until the end of the experiment or sacrificed for brain virus level. Control mice were housed six per cage. All mice received the same dose of WNV or "WN-25."

Tissue Cultures

Vero Cells

The Vero cell line was derived from kidneys of a normal African green monkey. The cells are grown in Dulbecco's modified Eagle medium (DMEM) containing 10% fetal calf serum (FCS).

BHK Cells

A baby hamster kidney (BHK) cell line is grown in Eagle's F-12 medium supplemented with 10% tryptose broth and 10% calf serum.

Isolation of WNV from the Spleen and Brain of Infected Mice

Each brain or spleen was rinsed in cold PBS and sonicated; the virus suspension was centrifuged at 3000 rpm for 10 min. The supernatant was aliquoted into plastic tubes and stored at −70°C for further processes. In experiments where brains were pooled, six brains from each group were assayed to determine brain virus level. The virus level in the blood, brain, or spleen was determined by titration of virus in Vero cells or in BHK cell line.

Organ Weights

Mice were individually weighed on day 7 postinoculation. The mice were sacrificed and the thymus and spleen immediately removed and weighed aseptically. The spleens and brains of each group were individually rinsed in cold PBS (1 ml per spleen and 2 ml per brain) containing 2% FCS and penicillin (1000 U/ml).

Titration of Virus in Tissue Cultures

For demonstration of WNV plaques in Vero cells the original plaque technique of Dulbecco and Vogt (1956) was used. A dilution of virus is added to Vero cell monolayers in petri dishes and incubated at 37°C for 1 hr to permit viral adsorption. The monolayer is overlaid with MEM×2 and tragacanth (gum tragacanth grade III G-1128, Sigma) containing 2% FCS and 2.4% $NaHCO_3$. The cultures were incubated (37°C, 5% CO_2) for 72 hr. Plaques are counted after staining the monolayer with neutral red (0.05%). The same procedure was followed for BHK cells. All plaques were counted by a blinded investigator.

In Vivo Assay

Virus lethality was determined by i.p. injection of the virus (0.2 ml). The titer of the virus was calculated according to the mortality recorded within 14 days (Reed and Muench, 1938).

Data Analysis

All data in text and figures are mean values ± S.E.M. for the indicated number of mice. Data were analyzed by ANOVA followed by the Student–Newman–Keul test for *a posteriori* multiple comparisons or by the Kruskal–Wallis test followed by the Mann–Whitney U test, where appropriate. The Fisher exact probability test was used for survival analysis. Data were considered significant for $p < 0.05$.

RESULTS

The Effect of Cold or Isolation Stress on Mortality of Mice Inoculated with Avirulent WNV

The purpose of these experiments was to determine the effect of stress on the mortality of mice after inoculation with avirulent WNV (WN-25). Each mouse was inoculated i.p. with 200,000 PFU. The results of these experiments are presented in Table 1. The results show that exposure of inoculated mice to both kinds of stress markedly increased the mortality as compared to control mice. In mice which were exposed to cold or isolation stress, the mortality rate was 58 and 54%, respectively, as compared to 0% in control mice ($p < 0.05$). Death of mice started on day 7 to day 12.

Table 1. Effect of Cold or Isolation Stress on Mortality Rate of Mice Inoculated with Avirulent WNV

	Experiment 1		Experiment 2		Experiment 3		Total	
Treatment group	D/T[a]	%	D/T	%	D/T	%	D/T	%
Control	0/8	0	0/10	0	0/10	0	0/28	0
Isolation	4/8	50	6/12	50	5/8	62.5	15/28	53.6*
Cold Do+Vdo[b]	5/8	62.5	6/10	60	4/8	50	15/26	58*

[a]D/T, dead/total.
[b]Five minutes a day at 1 ± 0.5°C; Do = start of cold stress; Vdo = inoculation on Do.
*$p < 0.05$ compared to control.

Effect of Cold or Isolation Stress on Brain WN-25 Virus Level 8 Days after Inoculation and Exposure

These experiments were performed to determine brain virus level in control and stressed mice. Moreover, we tested if there was a correlation between the level of virus in the brain and the mortality rate. As shown in Table 2, virus titers in the brain of stressed mice which were inoculated i.p. (200,000 PFU) were similar to those found in mice which received i.c. injections of only 200 PFU. The brain virus level of control mice showed a titer of 1.5 ($\log_{10}$PFU) whereas the virus titers in the brain of isolation- or cold-stressed mice were 7.4 and 8.9 ($\log_{10}$PFU), respectively. In mice inoculated i.c., the mortality rate was 100% as compared to 0% in control (i.p. inoculated) mice. The brain virus levels in surviving mice from the groups which were inoculated i.p. and exposed to stress were similar to the levels found in the control group (i.c.).

Character of WM-25 after Isolation from the Brain of Stressed Mice

After i.c. injection of WN-25 into mice, the virus which was isolated from the brain of infected mice does not change its virulence. Therefore, we wanted to know the virulence of WN-25 isolated from stressed mouse brain after i.p. injection. This question was studied by experiments aimed at testing if the virus increased its replication rate or changed its virulence in stressed mice. Our data show (Table 3) that virus isolated from the brain of stressed mice was very virulent even after i.p. injection. Table 3 summarizes the virus titers in brains of control and stressed mice. These titers were determined by PFU in tissue cultures and by *in vivo* assay in which mice were inoculated i.c. or i.p. and the LD_{50} measured. Both WNV and WN-25 levels were higher in brains of stressed mice as compared to control (nonstressed) mice. The brain virus levels in stressed mice (WN-25 inoculated i.p.) were sevenfold higher as compared to controls. In the *in vivo* assay, the level

Table 2. Effect of Isolation or Cold Stress on Mortality and Brain "WN-25" Virus Level on Day 8 after Inoculation and Exposure

Treatment group	N	% dead	Log no. PFU/brain
Control (i.p.)[a]	20	0	1.54 ± 0.95
Control (i.c.)[b]	20	100	8.40 ± 0.14*
Isolation (i.p.)	20	55*	7.43 ± 0.70*
Cold (i.p.)	20	60*	8.97 ± 0.23*

[a]Each mouse was inoculated i.p. with 200,000 PFU.
[b]Each mouse was inoculated i.c. with 200 PFU.
*$p < 0.05$ compared to control.

Table 3. Titration of WNV and "WN-25" Isolated from Mouse Brain after Exposure to Cold Stress

Virus strain	Vero cells (PFU/ml)	LD_{50}/ml	
		Mouse i.c.	Mouse i.p.
WNV[a]	5×10^8	1.3×10^7	6.98×10^6
WNV + cold[b]	1.75×10^9	ND	5.62×10^8
WN-25	2.5×10^8	3×10^8	$<10^2$
WN-25 + cold	1.7×10^9	4×10^8	1.33×10^8
WN-25 (i.c.)[a]	7.5×10^8	2.6×10^8	$<10^3$

[a]Wild type.
[b]Five minutes a day at 1 ± 0.5°C for 8 days.
[c]Mice were inoculated i.c. and the brain suspension was tested in mice and tissue culture.

(i.p. LD_{50}) increased by 10^6 indicating extreme virulence. The data clearly show that in stressed mice the avirulent WN-25 strain becomes virulent and reaches higher titer than the original WNV in control mice.

Spleen and Brain Virus Level in Stress and Dexamethasone-Treated Mice

As was shown previously (Ben-Nathan and Feuerstein, 1988a, b), there is a correlation between virus level in the spleen and brain of stressed mice. In these experiments we tested brain and spleen WN-25 virus levels in control and stressed mice. The data in Table 4 show significantly higher virus level in both organs of stressed mice as compared to control mice; in control mice the brain virus titer was 2.2 as compared to 7.5 ($\log_{10}$ PFU) in isolated mice.

In contrast to the brain, no virus was detected in the spleen of control mice whereas the virus titer in the spleen of isolated mice was 3.4 ($\log_{10}$ PFU).

Table 4. Titration of WN-25 Virus Isolated from Brain and Spleen of Mice after Exposure to Isolation Stress or Dexamethasone Injection

Treatment group	Log_{10} PFU/organ		Body weight (g)	Spleen (mg)	Thymus (mg)
	Brain	Spleen			
Control	2.2 ± 0.8	0	18.5 ± 5.4	113.4 ± 5.4	59.7 ± 5.7
Isolation	7.5 ± 0.5*	3.4 ± 0.4	16.6 ± 1.1	47.8 ± 5.5*	19.2 ± 3.8*
Dexamethasone[b]	7.4 ± 0.6*	0	15.3 ± 1.2	38.3 ± 5.9*	11.6 ± 2.2*

[a]Day 8 after inoculation. $N = 8$ in each group.
[b]Two injections of 1 mg/kg, 3 hr before virus inoculation and 2 days after inoculation.
*$p < 0.05$.

The effect of stress could be mediated by immunosuppression. Therefore, we tested the immunosuppressive drug dexamethasone (D-1756, Sigma) for its effect on mortality and virus titers.

Table 5 demonstrates mortality, brain and spleen virus levels in control and dexamethasone-treated mice. Mice inoculated with WN-25 and dexamethasone (1 mg/kg) had a mortality of 67% as compared to 0% in control mice. The virus level in the brain of the dexamethasone-treated group was similar to the level in the stressed mice. The results show that dexamethasone significantly reduced lymphoid organ weight (spleen and thymus) as observed previously in cold- or isolation-stressed mice (Ben-Nathan and Feuerstein, 1988b).

Dexamethasone mimicked the effect of stress on mortality rate and brain virus level. Nevertheless, no virus was found in the spleen of mice injected with dexamethasone or in control mice, whereas in stressed mice, virus was detected in the spleen (3.4 log_{10} PFU).

DISCUSSION

In the present study we used a WNV variant (WN-25) which lost its neuroinvasiveness in comparison to WNV. The difference between WNV and WN-25 is

Table 5. Effect of Dexamethasone on Mortality and Brain Virus Level

Treatment group	Dead/total	% dead	Log_{10} PFU/organ	
			Brain	Spleen
Control	0/8	0	2.18 ± 0.8 (8)	0 (8)
Dexamethasone[a]	8/12*	67	6.85 ± 0.5 (8)*	0 (8)

[a]1 mg/kg, 3 hr before virus inoculation and 2 days after virus inoculation.
*$p < 0.05$.

particularly obvious when the virus is injected i.p. into weaning mice. Thus, 10 PFU of WNV is equivalent to 1 LD_{50} of WNV whereas doses of WN-25 up to 2 × 10^5 PFU did not produce mortality.

Our data also show significant differences in mortality rates from WN-25 infection in stressed versus nonstressed mice. Exposure of mice to cold or isolation stress increased mortality from 0% in control mice to 54–58% in the various stress paradigms. The increased mortality in stressed mice was associated with higher levels of WN-25 in the brain. This finding suggests that in stressed mice, WN-25 increased its replication and virulence. These changes were not detected in control mice.

After primary replication in mice, Toga neurotropic viruses can reach the CNS either by secondary replication in the endothelial cells of brain capillaries or by infected lymphocytes which may pass through the capillary wall (Monath, 1983; Wolinsky and Johanson, 1980; Albrect, 1968; Johanson and Mins, 1968). From our studies we found a significantly higher virus titer in the spleen of stressed mice (3.4 $\log_{10}$ PFU) as compared to control mice (0).

To our knowledge, there are no other studies that have considered the effect of individual housing or cold stress on mortality of mice inoculated with avirulent virus. It is known that stress conditions affect the immune system and cause immunosuppression (Sapse, 1984; Johnson *et al.*, 1963; Friedman *et al.*, 1970) through involution of lymphoid organs (Ben-Nathan *et al.*, 1977; Parillo and Fauci, 1979; Ben-Nathan and Feuerstein, 1988a), possibly mediated by increased activity of the pituitary–adrenocortical axis (Parillo and Fauci, 1979; Selye, 1950; Friedman and Glasgow, 1966). It appears that stress situations act by enhancing virus replication in lymphocytes as shown in the spleen of stressed mice. Since lymphocytes can pass through the blood–brain barrier, the larger fraction of infected lymphocytes in stressed mice could contribute to higher virus titers also in the brain. This possibility, however, awaits further clarification by more direct evidence on the mode of immune cell penetration into the CNS.

The immunosuppressive drug dexamethasone exhibited the same effect on mortality and brain virus titers as in stressed mice. Furthermore, after an i.c. injection of WN-25 into mice, the virus which was isolated from the brain of these mice had no virulence by i.p. inoculation as the parent WN-25. Nevertheless, we found that the virus which was isolated from the brain of stressed mice after i.p. inoculation was extremely virulent even by i.p. inoculation of as little as 10 PFU into normal nonstressed mice.

Therefore, we suggest that immunosuppression caused by stress conditions induce a selection process in the WN-25 population and permit the virus to proliferate in the lymphocytes and to invade the brain.

In another system (Akov *et al.*, 1987; Kobiler *et al.*, 1989) we have shown that blood–brain barrier modulation leads to direct invasion of the brain and causes death through encephalitis by WN-25 after i.v. inoculation. Moreover, in the latter case the virus which was found in the brain was similar to the original WN-25.

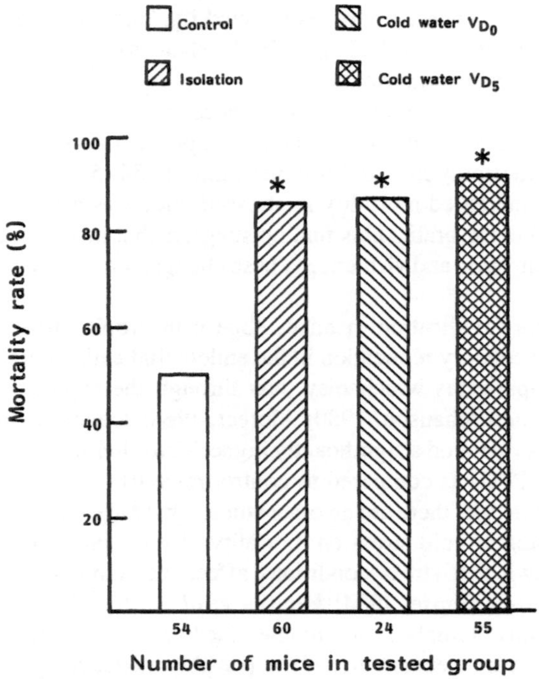

Figure 1. The effect of cold or isolation stress on mortality rate of mice inoculated with WNV.

In previous studies using WNV wild type (Ben-Nathan and Feuerstein, 1988a,b, 1990) we have shown that exposure of mice to cold or isolation stress increased the mortality from 47% in control to 85–100% in stressed groups (Fig. 1). Furthermore, the brain virus levels were 100-fold higher compared to control mice. The results in the present study using avirulent (WN-25) virus show dramatic differences between stressed and control mice (Table 6, Ben-Nathan *et al.*, 1989). The brain virus level in stressed mice increased by 6.0 $\log_{10}$ PFU compared to control mice.

This finding suggests that both physical and nonphysical stress situations enhance WN-25 virus replication followed by change in neuroinvasiveness and neurovirulence. Future studies should investigate the influence of environmental physical and psychological stress on outbreak of viral diseases.

Table 6. The Effect of Cold or Isolation Stress on Mortality, Brain and Spleen WN and WN-25 Virus Levels

Treatment group	WNV				WN-25			
	Mortality		Log_{10} PFU organ[b]		Mortality		Log_{10} PFU/organ	
	D/T[a]	%	Brain	Spleen	D/T	%	Brain	Spleen
Control	17/36	47	5.8 ± 0.5	2.2 ± 0.5	0/28	0	1.5 ± 1	0
Isolation	46/54*	85	8.6 ± 0.6*	3.8 ± 0.1*	15/28*	54	7.4 ± 0.7*	3.4 ± 0.4*
Cold	21/24*	88	8.8 ± 0.7*	3.8 ± 0.2*	15/26*	58	8.9 ± 0.2*	3.7 ± 0.3*

[a]D/T, dead/total mice.
[b]Six mice were used for virus level.
*$p < 0.01$ compared to control.

ACKNOWLEDGMENTS We thank Ms. E. Lupu for her technical assistance.

REFERENCES

Akov, Y., Halevy, M., and Lustig, S., 1987, Neuroinvasiveness of West Nile virus strains and the use of the blood brain barrier (BBB), 7th International Congress of Virology, Edmonton, Canada, p. 74.

Albrect, P., 1968, Pathogenesis of neurotropic arbovirus infections, *Curr. Top. Microbiol. Immunol.* **43**:44–91.

Ben-Nathan, D., and Feuerstein, G., 1988a, Effect of cold or isolation stress on mortality of mice to West Nile virus, Annual Meeting of the Israel Society for Microbiology, Isr. J. Med. Sci. p. 393.

Ben-Nathan, D., and Feuerstein, G., 1988b, Stress enhancement of viral encephalitis, FASEB 72nd Annual Meeting, Las Vegas, p. 935.

Ben-Nathan, D., and Feuerstein, G., 1990, The influence of cold or isolation stress on resistance of mice to West Nile Virus, *Experientia* **46**:285–290.

Ben-Nathan, D., Heller, E. D., and Perek, M., 1977, The effect of starvation on antibody production of chicks, *Poult. Sci.* **56**:1468–1471.

Ben-Nathan D., Lustig, S., and Feuerstein, G., 1989, The influence of cold or isolation stress on neuroinvasiveness and virulence of an attenuated variant of West Nile Virus, *Arch. Virol.* **109**:1–10.

Chamberlain, R. W., 1980, Epidemiology of arthropod-borne togaviruses: The role of arthropods as hosts and vectors and of vertebrate hosts in natural transmission cycles, in: *The Togaviruses: Biology, Structure, Replication* (R. W. Schlesinger, ed.), Academic Press, New York, pp. 175–227.

Dulbecco, R., and Vogt, M., 1956, Plaque formation and isolation of pure lines with poliomyelitis viruses, *J. Exp. Med.* **99**:167–182.

Forterfield, J. S., Casals, J., Chuma Kov, M. P., Gaidamovich, S. Y., Hannouon, C., Holmes, T. H., Horzinek, M. C., Mussay, M., Oker-Bloom, N., Russel, P. K., and Trent, D. W., 1978, Togaviridae, *Intervirology* **9**:129–148.

Friedman, S. B., and Glasgow, L. A., 1966, Psychologic factor and resistance to infectious disease, *Pediatr. Clin. North Am.* **13**:315–335.

Friedman, S. B., Glasgow, L. A., and Adir, R., 1970, Differential susceptibility to viral agent in mice housed alone or in group, *Psychosom. Med.* **32**:285–299.

Goldblum, N., Sterk, V. V., and Paderski, B., 1954, West Nile fever: The clinical features of the disease and the isolation of West Nile virus from the blood of nine human cases, *Am. J. Hyg.* **59**:89–103.

Halevy, M., Lustig, S., and Akov, Y., 1986, Neuroinvasiveness and replication in murine macrophages of two West Nile virus (WNV) strains, Annual Meeting of the Israel Society for Microbiology, *Isr. J. Med. Sci.* **22**:148.

Hayes, C. G., Bagar, S., Ahmed, T., Chowdhry, M. A., and Reisen, W. K., 1982, West Nile virus in Pakistan. I. Sero-epidemiological studies in Pungab province, *Trans. Soc. Trop. Med. Hyg.* **76**:431–435.

Jensen, M. M., 1973, Possible mechanisms of impaired interferon production in stressed mice, *Proc. Soc. Exp. Biol. Med.* **142**:820–823.

Jensen, M. M., and Rasmussen, A. F., 1963, Stress and susceptibility to viral infections. II. Sound stress and susceptibility to vesicular stomatitis virus, *J. Immunol.* **90**:21–23.

Johanson, R. T., and Mins, C. A., 1968, Pathogenesis of viral infection of the nervous system, *N. Engl. J. Med.* **278**:84–92.

Johnson, T., Lavender, J. F., Multin, E., and Rasmussen, A. F., 1963, The influence of avoidance-learning stress on resistance to coxsackie B virus in mice, *J. Immunol.* **91**:569–575.

Kiecolt-Glaser, J. K., Speicher, C., Holliday, J. E., and Glaser, R., 1984, Stress and the transformation of lymphocytes by Epstein–Barr virus, *J. Behav. Med.* **7**:1–11.

Kobiler, D., Lustig, S., Gozes, Y., Ben-Nathan, D., and Akov, Y., 1989, Sodium dodecyl-sulphate induces a breach in the blood brain barrier and enables a West Nile virus variant to penetrate into mouse brain, *Brain Res.* **496**:314–316.

Monath, T. P., 1983, Mode of entry of neurotropic arboviruses into the CNS, *Lab. Invest.* **48**(4):399.

Monath, T. P., 1986, Pathobiology of the Flaviviruses, in: *The Togaviridae and Flaviviridae* (S. Schlesinger and M. J. Schlesinger eds.), Plenum Press, New York, 375–440.

Parillo, J. E., and Fauci, A. S., 1979, Mechanisms of glucocorticoid action on immune processes, *Am. Rev. Pharmacol. Toxicol.* 19:279–301.

Rasmussen, A. F., March, J. T., and Brill, N. Q., 1957, Increased susceptibility to herpes simplex in mice subjected to avoidance-learning stress or restraint, *Proc. Soc. Exp. Biol. Med.* **96**:183–189.

Reed, L. G., and Muench, M., 1938, A simple method of estimating fifty percent endpoints, *Am. J. Hyg.* **27**:493–497.

Sapse, A. T., 1984. Stress cortisol, interferon and stress diseases. I. Cortisol as the cause of stress diseases, *Med. Hypothesis* **13**:31–44.

Selye, H., 1950, *The Physiology and Pathology of Exposure to Stress*, Acta. Inc. Montreal.

Selye, H., 1957, Implications of stress concept, *N.Y. State J. Med.* **1957**:2139–2145.

Weiner, L. P., Cole, G. A., and Nathanson, N., 1970, Experimental encephalitis following peripheral inoculation of West Nile virus in mice of different ages, *J. Hyg.* **68**:435–446.

Wolinsky, J. S., and Johanson, R. T., 1980, Role of viruses in chronic neurological diseases, *Compr. Virol.* **16**:257.

Index